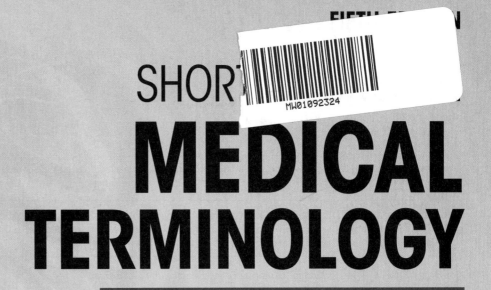

FIFTH EDITION

SHORT
MEDICAL
TERMINOLOGY

Engage, Learn, Apply, Reflect

Judi L. Nath

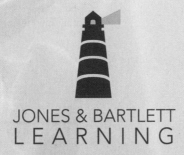

JONES & BARTLETT
LEARNING

World Headquarters
Jones & Bartlett Learning
25 Mall Road
Burlington, MA 01803
978-443-5000
info@jblearning.com
www.jblearning.com

Jones & Bartlett Learning books and products are available through most bookstores and online booksellers. To contact Jones & Bartlett Learning directly, call 800-832-0034, fax 978-443-8000, or visit our website, www.jblearning.com.

Substantial discounts on bulk quantities of Jones & Bartlett Learning publications are available to corporations, professional associations, and other qualified organizations. For details and specific discount information, contact the special sales department at Jones & Bartlett Learning via the above contact information or send an email to specialsales@jblearning.com.

27325-0

Production Credits

Vice President, Product Management: Marisa R. Urbano
Vice President, Content Strategy and Implementation: Christine Emerton
Director, Product Management: Matthew Kane
Product Manager: Bill Lawrensen
Director, Content Management: Donna Gridley
Manager, Content Strategy: Carolyn Pershouse
Content Strategist: Ashley Malone
Content Coordinator: Jessica Covert
Director, Project Management and Content Services: Karen Scott
Manager, Program Management: Kristen Rogers
Project Manager: Angela Montoya
Project Manager: Belinda Thresher
Digital Project Specialist: Carolyn Downer
Marketing Manager: Mark Adamiak
Content Services Manager: Colleen Lamy
Vice President, Manufacturing and Inventory Control: Therese Connell
Product Fulfillment Manager: Wendy Kilborn
Composition: Straive
Project Management: Straive
Cover and Text Design: Briana Yates
Media Development Editor: Faith Brosnan
Rights & Permissions Manager: John Rusk
Rights Specialist: Robin Silverman
Cover: © Magic mine/Shutterstock
Chapter Opener: © Matthew25/Shutterstock.
Printing and Binding: Lakeside Book Company

Library of Congress Cataloging-in-Publication Data
Library of Congress Cataloging-in-Publication Data unavailable at time of printing.

LCCN: 2022045884

6048

Printed in the United States of America
27 26 25 24 23   10 9 8 7 6 5 4 3 2 1

This book is dedicated to students who
challenge themselves. Thank you!

Brief Contents

New to This Edition   xi

Author's Preface   xv

User's Guide   xvii

Reviewers   xix

Acknowledgments   xxi

CHAPTER 1   **Analyzing Medical Terms** 1

CHAPTER 2   **Common Prefixes and Suffixes** 9

CHAPTER 3   **Organization of the Body**.........................27

CHAPTER 4   **The Integumentary System** 39

CHAPTER 5   **The Skeletal System** 59

CHAPTER 6   **The Muscular System** 87

CHAPTER 7   **The Nervous System** 103

CHAPTER 8   **The Special Senses of Sight and Hearing** 127

CHAPTER 9   **The Endocrine System** 151

CHAPTER 10   **The Cardiovascular System**.......................171

CHAPTER 11   **The Lymphatic System and Immunity** 199

CHAPTER 12   **The Respiratory System** 215

CHAPTER 13   **The Digestive System**............................239

CHAPTER 14   **The Urinary System** 261

CHAPTER 15   **The Reproductive System** 279

APPENDIX A   Answers to In-Text Questions 307

APPENDIX B   Glossary of Word Parts with Meanings 337

APPENDIX C   Glossary of Abbreviations 343

APPENDIX D   Error-Prone Abbreviations, Symbols, and Dose Designations 347

APPENDIX E   Top 100 Prescribed Medications 351

Index   **355**

Contents

New to This Edition xi
Author's Preface xv
User's Guide xvii
Reviewers xix
Acknowledgments xxi

CHAPTER 1 Analyzing Medical Terms 1
Introduction 1
Acquiring and Using Language Sense 2
Medical Term Parts 2
Analyzing Terms 3

CHAPTER 2 Common Prefixes and Suffixes 9
Introduction 9
Word Roots Introduced in This Chapter 10
Categories of Prefixes 10
   Prefixes of Time and Speed 10
   Prefixes of Direction 11
   Prefixes of Position 11
   Prefixes of Size and Number 12
   Prefixes of Negation 13
Categories of Suffixes 13
   Suffixes Signifying Medical Conditions 13
   Suffixes Signifying Diagnostic Terms, Tests,
     and Surgical Procedures 14
   Suffixes That Signify Medical Practices
     and Practitioners 15
   Suffixes That Denote Adjectives 15

CHAPTER 3 Organization of the Body 27
Introduction 27
Word Parts Related to Body Organization 28
Levels of Organization 28
   Cells 28
   Tissues 28

   Organs 28
   Systems 28
Navigating the Body 28
   Anatomic Position 30
   Directional Terms 30
   Body Planes 32
Body Cavities and Divisions 32
   Divisions of the Abdominopelvic Cavity 32
   Regions of the Spinal Column 34

CHAPTER 4 The Integumentary System 39
Introduction 39
Word Parts Related to the Integumentary
   System 40
Structure and Function 40
Disorders Related to the Integumentary
   System 42
   Burns 42
   Skin Lesions 42
   Inflammatory Disorders 43
   Skin Cancer 43
   Skin Infections 44
   Other Skin Disorders 44
Diagnostic Tests, Treatments, and Surgical
   Procedures 45
Practice and Practitioners 46

CHAPTER 5 The Skeletal System . . 59
Introduction 59
Word Parts Related to the Skeletal System . . . 59
Structure and Function 61
   The Axial Skeleton 62
   The Appendicular Skeleton 63
   Joints 67
Disorders Related to the Skeletal
   System 67
Diagnostic Tests, Treatments, and Surgical
   Procedures 70
Practice and Practitioners 70

CHAPTER 6 The Muscular System **87**

Introduction 87
Word Parts Related to the Muscular System . . 88
Structure and Function 88
  Skeletal Muscle 88
  Smooth Muscle 88
  Cardiac Muscle 90
Disorders Related to the Muscular System . . . 90
  Chronic Disorders 90
  Cumulative Trauma and
    Sports Injuries 90
  Paralysis and Paresis 91
Diagnostic Tests, Treatments, and Surgical
  Procedures 91
Practice and Practitioners 92

CHAPTER 7 The Nervous System **103**

Introduction 103
Word Parts Related to Nervous System 105
Structure and Function 105
  Central Nervous System (CNS) 106
  Peripheral Nervous System (PNS) 107
Disorders Related to the Nervous System . . . 108
  Trauma 108
  Vascular Insults 109
  Tumors 109
  Systemic Degenerative Diseases 109
  Seizures 110
  Behavioral Disorders 110
  Diagnostic Tests, Treatments, and Surgical
    Procedures 110
Practice and Practitioners 111

CHAPTER 8 The Special Senses of Sight and Hearing **127**

Introduction 127
Word Parts Related to the Eye 128
  Structure and Function of the Eye 128
  Disorders Related to the Eye 131
  Diagnostic Tests, Treatments, and Surgical
    Procedures of the Eye 132
  Practice and Practitioners of the Eye 132
Word Parts Related to the Ear 132
  Structure and Function of the Ear 133
  Disorders Related to the Ear 133
  Diagnostic Tests, Treatments, and Surgical
    Procedures of the Ear 134

Practice and Practitioners of the Ear 135
Abbreviations 135

CHAPTER 9 The Endocrine System **151**

Introduction 151
Word Parts Related to the Endocrine
  System 151
Structure and Function 152
  Pituitary Gland 152
  Thyroid Gland and Parathyroid Gland 155
  Adrenal Glands 155
  Pancreas 156
  Gonads 156
Disorders Related to the Endocrine System . 156
  Disorders of the Pituitary Gland 156
  Disorders of the Thyroid Gland 156
  Disorders of the Adrenal Gland 157
  Disorders of the Pancreas 158
Diagnostic Tests, Treatments, and Surgical
  Procedures 158
Practice and Practitioners 158

CHAPTER 10 The Cardiovascular System **171**

Introduction 171
Word Parts Related to the Cardiovascular
  System 172
Structure and Function 173
  The Heart 173
  The Heartbeat 175
  Blood Vessels 177
  Blood 178
Disorders Related to the Cardiovascular
  System 179
  Coronary Artery Disease 179
  Blood Clots 179
  Myocardial Infarction and Congestive
    Heart Failure 179
  Arrhythmias 179
  Hypertension 180
  Blood Disorders 180
Diagnostic Tests, Treatments, and
  Surgical Procedures 180
Practice and Practitioners 180

CHAPTER 11 The Lymphatic System and Immunity **199**

Introduction 199

Word Parts Related to the Lymphatic
  System and Immunity. 200
Structure and Function 201
Disorders Related to the Lymphatic
  System and Immunity. 202
Diagnostic Tests, Treatments, and
  Surgical Procedures. 203
Practice and Practitioners 203

**CHAPTER 12 The Respiratory
System. 215**

Introduction 215
Word Parts Related to the Respiratory
  System. 216
Structure and Function 216
  The Nose, Nasal Cavity, and Paranasal Sinuses . . 216
  The Pharynx and Tonsils. 218
  The Larynx and Trachea 219
  The Trachea, Bronchi, Bronchioles,
    and Alveoli. 219
  The Lungs 219
  The Diaphragm 220
Disorders Related to the Respiratory
  System. 221
  Infectious Disorders. 221
  Obstructive Lung Diseases. 221
  Expansion Disorders 222
Diagnostic Tests, Treatments, and
  Surgical Procedures. 222
Practice and Practitioners 223

**CHAPTER 13 The Digestive
System. 239**

Introduction 239
Word Parts Related to the Gastrointestinal
  System. 240
Structure and Function 241
  Major Organs of the Digestive Tract. 241
  Accessory Organs 243
Disorders Related to the Digestive System . . 244
  Disorders of the Lower Gastrointestinal Tract . . . 244
  Disorders of the Accessory Organs
    of the Digestive System 245
Diagnostic Tests, Treatments, and Surgical
  Procedures 245
Practice and Practitioners 246

CHAPTER 14 The Urinary System. . .261

Introduction 261
Word Parts Related to the Urinary System . . 262
Structure and Function 263
Disorders Related to the Urinary System . . . 264
Diagnostic Tests, Treatments, and
  Surgical Procedures. 264
Practice and Practitioners 265

**CHAPTER 15 The Reproductive
System. 279**

Introduction 279
Word Parts Related to the Reproductive
  System. 279
Structure and Function 280
  The Male Reproductive System 281
  The Female Reproductive System 283
  Pregnancy 284
  Terms Associated with Pregnancy 285
Disorders Related to the Reproductive
  System. 286
  Sexually Transmitted Diseases 286
  Inflammation. 286
  Female Structural Abnormalities 287
  Tumors 287
  Menstrual Cycle Disorders. 288
  Disorders That Affect Males 288
Diagnostic Tests, Treatments, and Surgical
  Procedures 288
Practice and Practitioners 289

**APPENDIX A Answers to In-Text
Questions 307**

**APPENDIX B Glossary of Word
Parts with Meanings 337**

**APPENDIX C Glossary of
Abbreviations 343**

**APPENDIX D Error-Prone
Abbreviations, Symbols, and
Dose Designations 347**

**APPENDIX E Top 100 Prescribed
Medications 351**

Index 355

New to This Edition

This new edition builds on the foundation established in the previous four editions. The reader will find the writing style of this edition easy to follow, with special focus given to ensuring that each page is user friendly, accessible to all learning levels, and sensitive to diversity, equity, and inclusion issues. As an educator, I wanted to be sure that students found the content manageable, interesting, and understandable.

Approach and Content Organization

This section outlines the global changes that were made throughout the entire textbook as well as the chapter-by-chapter changes. Changes across all chapters are introduced first.

Global Changes

- The narrative has been modernized to make the text user-friendly and approachable.
- To engage readers, each chapter begins with a relevant Case Study. This Case Study wraps up at the end of the chapter and is followed by Case Study Application Questions. This follows the model of **Engage, Learn,** and **Apply**.
- A **Reflection** section finishes each chapter and allows readers to think about what they have learned with directed questions.
- Study Tables may contain terms that are not in the narrative; however, most bold-faced terms in the narrative are found in the Study Tables. The book would be unwieldy with text if the terms in the tables were also in the narrative. The most relevant terms were selected for inclusion in the tables.
- All terminology has been updated so that terms are current and match words used in common practice.
- Appendixes A through E have been updated so the information is the most current and nationally recognized.

Basic Chapter Outline

1. Learning Outcomes
2. Case Study
3. Introduction
4. Word Parts Related to the XXX System
5. Structure and Function
6. Quick Check (at least one per chapter)
7. Disorders Related to the XXX System
8. Diagnostic Tests, Treatments, and Surgical Procedures
9. Practice and Practitioners
10. The XXX System Abbreviation Table
11. Sidebar (at least one per chapter)
12. The XXX System Study Table (alphabetized within subheadings)
    - Structure and Function
    - Disorders
    - Diagnostic Tests, Treatments, and Surgical Procedures
    - Practice and Practitioners
13. Case Study Wrap-Up
14. Case Study Application Questions
15. End-of-Chapter Exercises—not all exercises may be present, but the order of exercises is maintained
    - Exercise X-X Labeling
    - Exercise X-X Word Parts
    - Exercise X-X Word Building
    - Exercise X-X Matching
    - Exercise X-X Multiple Choice
    - Exercise X-X Fill in the Blank
    - Exercise X-X Abbreviations
    - Exercise X-X Spelling
    - Exercise X-X Medical Report
16. Reflection

Chapter-by-Chapter Changes

Chapter 1 Analyzing Medical Terms

- New Case Study: Greta's Losing Her Groove
- Updated section on word root, *ped/o*
- Updated Table 1-1
- Updated Table 1-3

Chapter 2 Common Prefixes and Suffixes
- New Case Study: Bear's Bad Day
- Updated Table 2-2
- Updated Table 2-4
- Updated Table 2-5

Chapter 3 Organization of the Body
- New Case Study: Trayvon's Tibia
- Revised Table 3-3
- Revised Table 3-5
- Revised Study Table, Body Position and Directional Terms
- New Terms: sagittal section, transverse section

Chapter 4 The Integumentary System
- New Case Study: Hot Tub Hives
- Revised section on skin cancer
- Revised section on liquid nitrogen

Chapter 5 The Skeletal System
- New Case Study: Fall in February
- Revised section on axial skeleton
- Revised section on joint movements
- New Terms: osteoblast and osteoclast

Chapter 6 The Muscular System
- New Case Study: My Head Is Heavy
- New Abbreviation: MRI
- Updated section on amyotrophic lateral sclerosis (ALS)
- New Terms: blood tests, lumbar puncture, magnetic resonance imaging, muscle biopsy, myopathy, nerve conduction studies, polymyositis, rheumatologist, spinal tap, and urine tests

Chapter 7 The Nervous System
- New Case Study: Pierce Can No Longer Play
- New Abbreviations: CP and MG
- New Terms: amyotrophic lateral sclerosis, cerebral palsy, electromyography, nerve conduction study, spina bifida, and torticollis

Chapter 8 The Special Senses of Sight and Hearing
- New Case Study: Purple Rain
- Updated section on disorders related to the eye
- Changed sidebar information on abbreviations from AU to AS
- New Terms: floaters, retinal detachment, vitrectomy

Chapter 9 The Endocrine System
- New Case Study: Felicity's Fatigue
- New Abbreviations: HbA1c, HRT, and OXT
- Updated diabetes mellitus section
- New Terms: gestational diabetes, lactotropin, parathormone, polyphagia, prediabetes, urinalysis, and vasopressin

Chapter 10 The Cardiovascular System
- New Case Study: Brian's Blood Bruise
- New Abbreviations: DVT, ECG, PA, PE, and US
- Updated MONA to THROMBINS$_2$
- New Terms: cardiac ablation, cardiothoracic surgeon, coronary sinus, deep vein thrombosis, embolism, murmur, physician assistant, pulmonary embolism, thrombus, and thromboembolism

Chapter 11 The Lymphatic System and Immunity
- New Case Study: Piano Playing Petra
- New Abbreviations: CRP test
- New Terms: C-reactive protein (CRP) test, ibuprofen, rheumatologist

Chapter 12 The Respiratory System
- New Case Study: My Child Tastes Salty
- New Abbreviations: CT
- Revised sections on tonsils and respiratory system disorders
- Added a sidebar on the difference between mucous and mucus
- New Terms: hypercapnia, hypercarbia, and mucolytic

Chapter 13 The Digestive System
- New Case Study: Mario's Malaise
- New Abbreviations: BP, GP, HTN, IBD, LGI, UGI, SOB, UC, WBC
- New Terms: colostomy, gastrostomy, H2-receptor antagonists, icterus, ileostomy, inflammatory bowel disease, malaise, ostomy, stool studies, ulcerative colitis, vermiform appendix

Chapter 14 The Urinary System
- New Case Study: Skin Frost
- New Abbreviations: UACR
- Added a sidebar on the origin of the abbreviation GC for gonorrhea
- New Terms: azotemia, continuous ambulatory peritoneal dialysis, extracorporeal dialysis, glucosuria, pararenal fat, renomegaly, uremic frost, uresis, voiding

Chapter 15 The Reproductive System
- New Case Study: Paige's Problematic Pregnancy
- Deleted words: prostatomegaly, trachelitis
- New Terms: Cowper's gland, ductus deferens, estimated date of confinement, estimated date of delivery, gravid, hysterodynia, labor, leiomyoma, orchidectomy, placenta previa, sexually transmitted infection, spermatic cord, testicle, trachelectomy, prostate gland, spermatocyte, spermatozoa

Appendix E Top 100 Prescribed Medications
- Revised table

Other Resources

Online ancillary materials complement the text and provide additional support for student learning.

Student Resources

- Anatomy and Physiology Review Module
- Audio Glossary
- Flash Cards
- Worksheets
- Learning Objectives

Instructor Resources

- Slides in PowerPoint format and Lesson Plans include useful information to facilitate presentation of material by instructors.

- A Test Bank to test students' knowledge of key chapter content.
- Answer Keys to both in-text questions and Worksheets.
- Sample Syllabus
- Image Bank
- Lecture Outlines

Author's Preface

Welcome to the field of medical terminology. This workbook-textbook is intended to teach the language of medicine in an engaging and meaningful way. It is written to represent the real world so that you can move seamlessly from the classroom to actual practice. The approach is based on research that demonstrates how students learn best. To that end, each chapter begins with an engaging case study, followed by ample opportunity for learning and applying, and concludes with reflection. Learning and application use a three-pronged approach: (1) immersion—the terms are presented in context; (2) chunking—the material is given in manageable units; and (3) practice—exercises allow you to check your knowledge and your ability to apply concepts to new situations. Learning word parts is also an essential component of learning medical terms. If you learn the word parts tables, you will be well on your way to knowing medical terms you have never encountered because you can figure them out by breaking apart the new words into their component word parts. This will be quite useful, because not every word you will encounter in your careers is found in this book; but you will be equipped with the knowledge to understand the meaning of new words. Pay special attention to the analysis sections in the Study Tables, as these provide interesting, foundational information for forming medical terms.

While learning medical terminology, you will also learn some basic anatomy (body structures), physiology (body functions), and pathology (body diseases). Because medical terms describe the human body in health and in disease, attaining an elementary understanding of these topics will help you retain a working memory of medical language.

Learning medical terms can be easy if you approach the subject from a proper perspective. Begin by telling yourself that medical terms do not make up a separate language. Medical terms are simply words that you can add to your vocabulary. As with all words, medical words are meant to convey information.

As you enter a medical profession, you will be communicating with other medical professionals and with patients. Therefore, your job will include choosing words and sentence structures that communicate accurate information and reflect a professional attitude. Both your communication skills and your behavior toward patients are very important. As you are about to discover, learning medical terminology can be easy at times and challenging at others. However, if you use the textbook and its ancillaries to their fullest, you will be well on your way to mastering medical terminology.

Judi L. Nath, PhD, CHES
Lourdes University

User's Guide

A Short Course in Medical Terminology, Fifth Edition was developed to provide an easy, efficient, and effective way to learn medical terminology. This User's Guide introduces the features of the book that help the learning experience.

A **logical organization** guides you through the basics of medical terminology, word parts, and word analysis.

Chapters 1 and 2 introduce the basics of word building and set the foundation for learning terms.

Chapters 3–15 offer an overview of each body system and introduce terms that identify the structure and function of that system along with terms that name system disorders, diagnostic tests, treatments, surgical procedures, practice, and practitioners.

Each chapter opens with a list of **Learning Outcomes**. These are measurable educational aims and objectives that indicate what you should be able to do after completing the chapter.

A chapter-specific **Case Study** follows the Learning Outcomes. Opening Case Studies engage you for learning, which prepares you for the **Case Study Application Questions** that are posed after the **Case Study Wrap-Up**.

An introduction and a tabular presentation of **Word Parts** related to a specific body system are presented next.

Word Parts Exercises offer you an opportunity to quickly review the word parts before moving on to new material.

Structure and Function sections with **full-color illustrations** help you learn basic anatomy and physiology using tight text–art integration.

Quick Checks are exercises that help reinforce your knowledge of term parts before studying disorders related to the body systems.

All body system chapters include an **Abbreviations Table**, which lists common abbreviations and their meanings used in the chapter.

Sidebars appear throughout to highlight interesting facts about medical terms and words in general.

All body system chapters include a **Study Table** summarizing terms for reinforcement of the material in an easy-to-reference format. Some terms in the table are not found in the running narrative, but they are important to include for general reference, or the terms are used in the end-of-chapter case study.

The **Case Study Wrap-Up** picks up where the introductory case study left off. This wrap-up provides additional information, using terminology learned in the chapter. It concludes with the **Case Study Application Questions** that allow you to apply your knowledge.

End-of-Chapter Exercises and a **Medical Report** close out each chapter to maximize learning. Exercises include figure labeling, word building, matching exercises, multiple-choice questions, fill in the blank, short answer, true/false, and spelling. The Medical Report and Case Study Wrap-Up provide real-world application of medical terms and give you an opportunity to interact with the chapter material as you would in a clinical setting.

Each chapter concludes with **Reflection** questions. Taking time to reflect and think about what you have just learned is an important piece for long-term growth and learning.

Reviewers

The author and publisher would like to thank the following individuals who helped to review this textbook:

- Joel A. Bloom, PhD, MSE
  University of Houston—College of Education
- David R. Chicoine, DC, MS
  University of New England
- Perla Gilman, MS, MLS (ASCP)
  Bunker Hill Community College
- Dana Griffin, MBA, MLS (ASCP)
  Madonna University
- Kay Smith, MSN, RN
  Bluegrass Community and Technical College

Acknowledgments

With sincere gratitude, I wish to acknowledge all the hard work done by members of the editorial staff. Writing and publishing a textbook requires more than putting fingers to the keyboard. The printed book represents the work of many dedicated individuals, without whom this project could not be completed. To begin, thanks to Product Manager, Bill Lawrensen, for valuing the fourth edition enough that a fifth edition was necessary. Another round of thanks to content strategist, Ashley R. Malone, who was my day-to-day point person; you were always quick to answer and helpful with your responses. Thank you to copy editor, Sheryl Nelson, whose keen eyes aided manuscript preparation. Special thanks to ancillary writer, Anjali Dogra Gray, PhD Textbooks require solid ancillary packages, and her work is greatly appreciated.

CHAPTER 1

Analyzing Medical Terms

LEARNING OUTCOMES

Upon completion of this chapter, you should be able to:

- Discuss the purpose of medical terminology.
- Recognize the four different word parts of medical terms: prefixes, roots, suffixes, and combining forms.
- Define commonly used prefixes, roots, and suffixes introduced in this chapter.
- Divide medical terms into word parts.
- Understand how word parts are put together to make medical terms.
- Recognize the importance of proper spelling, pronunciation, and use of medical terms.
- Apply knowledge gained to Case Study Questions.

CASE STUDY

Greta's Losing Her Groove

Greta is an active 75-year-old female living in a retirement community. She prides herself on her ability to bicycle or walk 5 miles per day, regardless of the weather or who shows up in her exercise group. Lately, she hasn't felt like herself. Whenever she walks, she has severe pain in her right hip, so she is only able to walk about a half mile. Greta finds bicycling a little easier. She also notices that she's been a little forgetful, but she doesn't know why. Greta was a former teacher, so her forgetfulness is frustrating, but not as frustrating as not being able to keep up with her friends. When she couldn't walk to the end of her driveway without experiencing pain, she decided to make an appointment with her geriatrician, Dr. Nayak.

Introduction

There are many ways and various books to help you learn medical terminology. This book is intended for a short course in medical terminology and focuses on medical terms, their definitions, and brief exercises to help you quickly gauge your understanding. That means this book can be worked through in as little as 8 weeks. The goal is to give you all the basics necessary to be successful in your career, while allowing you to have a little fun learning. Not every word in the medical field is found in this book, but their Latin and Greek word parts are found here. These word parts can be combined to make thousands of medical terms, and understanding the basic word parts is the first step toward understanding complete words. While it is possible to memorize the definitions of individual medical words, understanding just the parts that make up the medical word is easier and faster than learning every word because there are fewer word parts than complete words. In fact, approached the right way, medical terminology may be the easiest subject in your program. Learning it takes a bit of thought and an open mind, but it need not involve sweating or paper ripping out of frustration.

Why is medical terminology important? Can't medical professionals just use simple words like "gut" and "cut"? Unfortunately, these aren't always specific enough. Gut can refer to the stomach, small intestine, large intestine, or many parts of the digestive system. If someone has pain in one of these areas, it is important to easily identify that area and have other medical professionals also recognize that specific area. The term "cut" could mean just an incision, or in other cases, it could mean cutting *off* a body part. For example, "She cut her hand" indicates an incision, but "Cut the hand distal to the wrist" could mean an amputation. Fortunately, medical terminology allows us to specifically identify places in the body and even what type of cut it is with words (**Figure 1.1**).

The foundation of medical terminology is learning the four basic word parts: **prefixes**, **roots**, **suffixes**, and **combining forms**. You'll learn how to distinguish among these word parts to combine them into meaningful medical terms.

First, let's examine some medical term characteristics. Most medical terms are derived from Latin and Greek languages. While this may make them seem "foreign" to native English speakers, 75% of *all English words* are derived from Latin and Greek. When looking up a term in the dictionary, its **etymology**, or word origin, is usually given along with its definition. For example, *dementia* is a cognitive function impairment marked by memory loss. The word comes from the Latin word, *demens*, which means "out of one's mind."

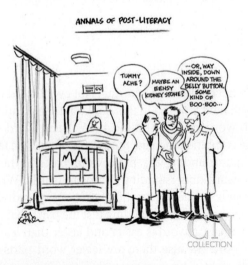

Figure 1.1 This cartoon demonstrates the value of standardized medical terms.

Acquiring and Using Language Sense

Accurate communication in any specialty field depends on *language sense*. **Language sense** is knowing what words mean and forecasting the effects their combinations will produce. This is a two-part definition. First, we must understand what the word we're using means. Second, we must trust that the person listening to what we're saying or reading what we're writing also understands the meaning of the words that we're using. While this is important in everyday language, it is especially important with medical terminology where misunderstanding can have drastic effects on patients.

Who decides what the "correct" anatomic term is? A system of anatomic naming known as *Terminologia Anatomica* is considered the international standard for terminology that deals with human anatomy. It was created by the Federative Committee on Anatomical Terminology and first published in 1998 and is updated as necessary. It is essentially an anatomy dictionary that gives the Latin base of the word along with the accepted English term. It has standardized anatomy-related terminology and is a great resource.

What does language sense have to do with learning medical terms? First, words have parts, and examining those parts forces the learner to see and hear words in a new way. That is, the person becomes conscious of words as words. You'll have to think about each part of the whole word and then put it all together to understand how the parts make up the whole. Second, the ability to use words well involves learning the phonetic and grammatical codes that make complex communication possible. This means using proper pronunciation and using medical terminology correctly in sentences. Medical terminology is probably one of your first exposures to clinical culture. So, congratulations! This is your first step toward success in the medical field!

Medical Term Parts

Nearly every medical term contains one or more *roots*. It may also contain one or more *prefixes* and one or more *suffixes*. When you start combining parts into words, you will also use a *combining form* of a root. This means a single medical term may consist of one part or several parts, but every part of a term behaves in one of three ways: root, prefix, or suffix. The good—and maybe surprising—news is that these three parts also make up all other English words. This means that you likely already know a lot of these parts, especially prefixes and suffixes.

Here is the order of word parts used in forming words: prefixes first, roots second, and suffixes last, assuming a word contains all three parts. If a prefix is present, it appears at the beginning of the term. A root is next. The root is found in the middle of the word, and roots form words by adding prefixes or suffixes to them. Suffixes are always the endings of words. A combining form is used in combination with another word part that is distinct from a prefix or suffix that adjusts the function of the word.

Let's break down the word *nontraditional*, which contains three word parts. In this word, the prefix is *non-* (not), the root is *tradition* (established customs or norms), and the suffix *-al* (makes the word an adjective meaning "relating to"). Thus, this word is an adjective that means "not relating to customs or norms."

> **Example:** There are movements that encourage women to seek *nontraditional* careers such as firefighting.

Some words contain only two parts, such as *traditionist*. Tradition is the root and *–ist* is the suffix that refers to "adhering to a system of beliefs or customs." So, a traditionist is a person with established beliefs or customs.

> **Example:** Mr. Brown, who asks young males in his classroom to remove their hats, was considered a traditionist.

Other words contain other combinations, such as *nontradionalist* (the prefix *non-* = not; the root *tradition* = established customs or norm; the suffix *-al* = adjective form meaning relating to; and another suffix *–ist* = refers to adhering to a system of beliefs or customs). So, a *nontraditionalist* is a person without established beliefs or customs.

> **Example:** Mrs. Brown, who didn't mind students wearing hats in her classroom, was considered a nontradionalist.

Here is a medical term that has two roots: *psychopath* (*psycho* and *path*). *Psychopath* is a medical term that has become a common English word. It refers to a person who has a severe psychological disorder. One might contend that *path* is a suffix because in the term psychopath, it comes last. If we consider that the word part *path* comes to us from the English word *pathos,* which means sorrow, suffering, or tragedy, then maybe we ought to identify it as a root. However, as it comes at the end of some terms, is it not also a suffix? The best answer to that question is, "Who cares?" You may call it a root or a suffix, and it doesn't really matter if you know what it means and where it goes in a particular term. The bottom line is that prefix, root, and suffix identification is a convenient way to look at and decipher terms, and most of the time, assigning the labels of prefix, root, and suffix to a word's parts leads to an acceptable definition. If the parts vary a little now and then, don't despair; the universe will go on.

Analyzing Terms

Learning to pick out prefixes, roots, and suffixes, as is done for you in **Table 1.1**, will permit you to define many, or even most, medical terms. Before going any further, we must deal with what has been traditionally referred to as a fourth word part: the **combining form**. A combining form is a root that includes one or more vowels tacked onto the end of it to make a root–suffix combination pronounceable, as in the word *psychology*. The main root is *psych* (mind), and the suffix is *-logy* (study of). But "psychlogy" doesn't flow as well as psychology; thus, we insert the "o" to create a more English-sounding word. So, as the example shows, the combining form concept is all about vowels, consonants, and pronunciation. A problem thus arises. That problem is that we remember a word or a word part in two ways: by recalling the sound it makes when we hear it spoken and by the sound a visual combination of its letters makes when we see it written. Here is an example using the prefix *iatro-*. When I asked a colleague how she pronounced the prefix *iatro-*, which means physician, she said, "eye-a-tro." Another colleague pronounced it, "eye-at-ur," and a French friend of mine insisted on, "eye-att-re" with a clipped final vowel sound, as in *Louvre*.

This book will introduce roots with their potential combining vowels added with forward slashes (/) separating them from the rest of the root.

> **Example:** card/i/o

By the way, it would make equal sense to introduce them as follows:

> **Example:** card; cardi; cardio (all three are, phonetically speaking, roots.)

You can learn a great deal from Table 1.1. To begin with, the terms *cardialgia, cardiology,* and *carditis* not only show the three forms of the root for heart (*cardi, cardio,* and *card*) but also introduce you to three important suffixes: *-algia , -logy,* and *-itis*.

- -algia = pain
- -logy = study of
- -itis = inflammation

Table 1.1 Analysis of Example Words

Term	Prefix	Root	Suffix	Term Meaning
cardialgia		cardi (heart)	-algia (pain)	pain in the heart; also, heartburn (a digestive disorder)
cardiology		cardio (heart)	-logy (study of)	study of the heart and its disorders
carditis		card (heart)	-itis (inflammation)	inflammation of the heart
diagnosis	dia- (across; through)	*gnosis* (Greek word meaning "knowledge")		discovery of signs and symptoms
iatrogenic disease		iatro (physician); gen (origin, cause)	-ic (adjective suffix)	disease caused by health care (whether an individual worker, particular institution, or the system as a whole)
psychopath		psycho (mind); path (disease)		person with a (serious) mental (mind) disease; in psychiatry it refers to antisocial personality disorder

These three suffixes occur in many medical terms. For example, when you learn a new root, such as *neur/o,* which means nerve, you will know the meanings of *neuralgia, neurology,* and *neuritis*:

- neuralgia = pain in a nerve
- neurology = the study of the nervous system; also the specialty dealing with diagnosis and treatment of nervous system disorders
- neuritis = inflammation of a nerve

QUICK CHECK

Using your knowledge of prefixes, roots, and suffixes, identify the word parts making up an example medical word. Intracranial means pertaining to the area within the skull.

Intracranial: prefix = _____ root = _____
suffix = _____

You may have noted that the suffix -logy is in the same category as the suffix -path. Although they both may be regarded as suffixes, also note that -logy is a root that comes from the Greek word *logos,* meaning "word"—not as in "a" word so much as in "the" word, that is, an explanation of things. That final meaning is why we define it as "study of" in Table 1.1. You may also recognize this root in common English words such as logic and logical.

In summary, you now know the first part of the definition of terms that end with any of the three suffixes introduced in the table. For *-algia,* the definition will begin with "pain in." It is important to note here that a second suffix, *-dynia,* also denotes pain. These two suffixes are sometimes interchangeable and

sometimes not. Eventually, you will become familiar with instances in which one or the other is appropriate or at least most common.

For *-logy,* the definition will usually begin with "study of."

For *-itis,* the definition will begin with "inflammation of."

The term *diagnosis* introduces the prefix *dia-,* which means through, between, or across. You may have noticed that *dia-* appears in common words, such as diameter, diagonal, and dialogue. Diameter is a straight line running *through* the center point of a circle; diagonal is a straight line running *between* opposite corners of a rectangle; and dialogue refers to people speaking to each other *across* a space.

The word dialogue provides an example of how words change meaning when speakers or writers misunderstand their origins. This word has also come to refer to a conversation between two people because someone mistakenly interpreted the prefix to be *di,* meaning two, and other writers and speakers followed suit.

The medical term *diagnosis* refers to identifying the nature of a disease or disorder *through* consideration of signs, symptoms, and medical test results. That definition might seem to stretch the point of the word "through" until you learn that *gnosis* is the Greek word for knowledge. In other words, diagnosis is a procedure leading to a judgment "through knowledge." The verb *diagnose* represents a departure in one respect from the etymology (word origin) of the term diagnosis. As with many back-formed verbs, clarity is easily lost. In this case, fuzziness comes about because "knowledge" (a noun) identifies something we know, whereas declaring (a verb) that we know something is slightly different.

Let's study the term, *iatrogenic*. *Iatr/o* is a root that means physician, and *gen/o* (from the Greek word *gennao*, meaning producing something) refers to origin or cause. The addition of *-ic* to *gen* forms *genic,* an adjective suffix meaning "originating from or caused by." Thus, an *iatrogenic disorder* is, literally speaking, "a disorder caused by a physician." In general use, the term *iatrogenic* refers to a disorder, disease, or ailment caused by any medical treatment or practitioner, such as a side effect from a drug or complications following surgery.

Another form of the root iatr/o is *iatr*, which may be coupled with other roots and several suffixes: *y, ic, ics, ist,* and *icial*. Here are examples of words formed from iatr, y, ic, ist, and ician:

Term	Part	Meaning
psychiatry	psych + iatr + y	specialty dealing with the study, diagnosis, and treatment of the mind (in this case, the y does not act as an adjective suffix)
psychiatric	psych + iatr + ic	adjective form of psychiatry
psychiatrist	psych + iatr + ist	physician who specializes in psychiatry
geriatrics	ger + iatr + ics	specialty dealing with the health and care of older people
pediatrician	ped + iatr + ician	physician who specializes in treating children

The root *psycho* comes from the Greek word *psyche,* which means soul or mind. The suffixes *-ist* and *-ician* mean practitioner, and the suffixes *-y* and *-ics* mean practice. The final two items in the list introduce two new roots: *ger/o* and *ped/o,* the meanings of which you may deduce from the meanings of the terms *geriatrics* and *pediatrician.* The root *ger/o* (also sometimes *ger/onto*) comes from the Greek word *geron,* which means old man. The root *ped/o* is derived from the Greek word *paedo,* which means "of children." However, orthopedics, derived from the Greek words *orthos* meaning "straight" and *paideia* meaning "rearing of children," is an exception to understanding a word by breaking it into its part. Orthopedics is a branch of medicine that deals with bones and muscles.

See **Tables 1.2**, **1.3**, and **1.4**, which list a sampling of roots, prefixes, and suffixes, respectively. Study these so you can start building and defining terms.

Table 1.2 Word Roots to Begin Building Terms

Word Root	Meaning
arthr/o	joint
card/i/o	heart
derm/o/ato	skin
gen/o	origin, cause, formation
ger/o/onto	old age
hem/a/ato	blood
iatr/o	physician
muscul/o	muscle
natal	birth, born
neur/o	nerve
os/teo	bone
path/o	disease
ped/ia	child
phren/o	diaphragm, mind
psych/o	mind
skelet/o	skeleton
tend/o, ten/o	tendon

Table 1.3 Prefixes to Begin Building Terms

Prefix	Meaning
epi-	upon, above, or in addition
micro-	small
peri-	around
post-	after
pre-	before

Table 1.4 Suffixes to Begin Building Terms

Suffix	Meaning
-al	adjective suffix
-algia	pain
-dynia	pain
-gen, -genesis	origin, cause, formation
-ic	adjective suffix denoting of
-itis	inflammation
-logy	study of
-pathy	disease
-scope	viewing, an instrument used for viewing

CASE STUDY WRAP-UP

Greta's geriatrician diagnosed arthralgia and osteoarthritis of the hip joint and referred her to an orthopedic surgeon. Dr. Nayak also recommended a series of learning and memory tests at the hospital's neuroscience laboratory.

Case Study Application Questions

1. What is a geriatrician?
2. Define *arthralgia* and its word parts.
3. Define *osteoarthritis* and its word parts.
4. Why was Greta referred to an orthopedic surgeon?
5. What is the word root in the term *neuroscience*?

END-OF-CHAPTER EXERCISES

Exercise 1.1 Defining Terms

Combine the suffix -*logy* with the proper root to indicate the following medical specialties.

1. Specialty dealing with heart disease: _____
2. Specialty that deals with the health and diseases in older people: _____
3. Specialty dealing with blood diseases: _____
4. Specialty dealing with skin ailments: _____
5. Specialty dealing with nervous system disorders: _____
6. Specialty dealing with mental (mind) disorders: _____

Exercise 1.2 Analyzing Terms

Analyze the following terms by putting the roots and suffixes in the appropriate columns. Then, write a definition for each term.

Term	Root	Suffix	Definition
1. neuropathy	_____	_____	_____
2. psychology	_____	_____	_____
3. pathogenic	_____	_____	_____
4. neuralgia	_____	_____	_____
5. systemic	_____	_____	_____
6. psychiatrist	_____	_____	_____
7. pediatrician	_____	_____	_____
8. iatrogenic	_____	_____	_____
9. cardialgia	_____	_____	_____
10. neuritis	_____	_____	_____

Exercise 1.3 Fill in the Blank

Fill in the blank with the correct answer.

1. The prefix *peri-* denotes _____.
2. The suffix *-logy* means _____.
3. The word root *derm/o* refers to _____.
4. Identify three word parts in the term *osteoarthritis*.
5. The suffix *-logy* is derived from the Greek word _____, which means _____.
6. Tendonitis refers to _____ of a _____.
7. A prenatal examination is one that occurs _____ the birth of a child.
8. _____ is indicated by the suffixes *-algia* and _____.
9. Inflammation is indicated by the suffix _____ _____.
10. The study of mental (mind) and emotional disorders is called _____.

Exercise 1.4 Reflection

1. After reading this chapter, how do you feel about learning medical terminology?
2. Identify the most interesting thing you learned in this chapter.

CHAPTER 2

Common Prefixes and Suffixes

LEARNING OUTCOMES

Upon completion of this chapter, you should be able to:

- Recognize prefixes.
- Recognize suffixes.
- Define all the prefixes and suffixes presented in this chapter.
- Analyze and define new terms introduced in this chapter.
- Pronounce, define, and spell each term introduced in this chapter.
- Apply knowledge gained to Case Study Questions.

CASE STUDY

Bear's Bad Day

His football teammates called him Bear because he was both kind like a teddy bear and fierce on the field like a grizzly bear. On Monday morning, Bear just didn't have any energy. After Friday night's game, he came directly home instead of enjoying a victory party at the coach's house. Over the weekend, he stayed in bed much of the time, ate and drank very little, and only recalled using the bathroom twice to urinate. He stayed home from school on Monday, but he was worried about missing football practice. However, as he sat on his bed, he could hear his heart thumping hard against his chest. Bear's mom called the rescue squad, and he was immediately transported to the hospital.

Introduction

Chapter 1 presented the four different word parts used in medical terminology: prefixes, roots, suffixes, and combining forms. This chapter focuses on common prefixes and suffixes.

In Chapter 1, we learned that a prefix is a word part that comes at the beginning of a word. Note that the word prefix itself contains a prefix, pre-. The second part of the word prefix is "fix," which gives us a perfect definition of prefix: something affixed (attached) to the front of or appearing before (pre-) something else. Most prefixes in medical terms are also found in everyday English. Although we have probably used many of the prefixes found in this chapter, we may have done so without realizing that they were prefixes. For example, when we are admitted to an anteroom, we may not stop to think that the prefix ante- means "before," and that it is called an anteroom because it is a room we enter before entering another room.

We also learned in Chapter 1 that a suffix is the part that comes at the end of a word. The word suffix comes from the Latin word *suffixum*, which may be translated as "to fasten to the end of." Although the suffix is located last in a medical term, it often comes first in its definition. For example, *appendicitis* means "inflammation (-itis) of the appendix." Therefore, the suffix, -itis, gives the first word of the defining phrase. The term *gastrectomy* is another example. It is defined as "removal of the stomach." The definition begins with the meaning of the suffix, *-ectomy*, which means "removal of."

Word Roots Introduced in This Chapter

Table 2.1 lists common word roots with their meanings to get you started on learning hundreds of medical terms. You may wish to memorize the roots

Table 2.1 Common Word Roots and Meanings

Word Root	Meaning
arter/i/o	artery
arthr/o	joint
card/i/o	heart
derm/at/o	skin
gen/i/o	origin, cause, formation
ger/o/onto	old age
hem/a/t/o	blood
hydr/o	water
iatr/o	physician
muscul/o	muscle
neur/o	nerve, nerve tissue
oste/o	bone
path/o	disease
ped/i/o	child
phren/o	diaphragm, mind
psych/o	mind
skelet/o	skeleton
spin/o	spine
tend/i/n/o	tendon

given in the table now, because there are just a few. Or if you prefer, just give them a quick glance now and, as you go through the chapter, refer to this table whenever you encounter a term with a root you do not recognize.

Categories of Prefixes

Not all medical terms include a prefix, but when one is present, it is important to the term's meaning. For example, hyperglycemia (high blood sugar) and hypoglycemia (low blood sugar) are conditions that are exact opposites. Confusing those two prefixes creates errors. Two other similar-sounding prefix pairs prone to creating errors are ante- and anti-. The prefix *ante-* means "before," and the prefix *anti-* means "against."

Term	Part	Meaning
hypoglycemia	prefix: hypo- = low root: glyc/o- = sugar suffix: -emia = condition	low blood sugar
antecubital	prefix: ante- = before root: cubitum = elbow	anterior to the elbow
anticoagulant	prefix: anti- = against root: coagulant = substance that causes blood to clot	preventing coagulation; preventing clotting

Dividing prefixes into functional categories makes them easier to learn. There are five logical divisions:

- Prefixes of time and speed
- Prefixes of direction
- Prefixes of position
- Prefixes of size and number
- Prefixes of negation

Seeing prefixes in words we already know helps us learn their meanings quickly and enables us to understand medical terms we encounter later. For that reason, common English words are included as examples in some of the following paragraphs and tables.

Prefixes of Time and Speed

Prefixes denoting time and speed are used in everyday English. *Prehistoric* and *postgraduate* are common words with a prefix relating to time. Prefixes denoting speed, such as tachy- (fast) and brady- (slow), are often used to describe heart rate. **Table 2.2** lists prefixes related to time and speed.

Table 2.2 Prefixes of Time and Speed

Prefix	Refers to	Example	Meaning
ante-	before	antepartum	before birth, before full development
brady-	abnormally slow rate of speed	bradycardia	abnormally slow heartbeat
neo-	new	neonate	newborn
post-	after	postscript	a written thought added after the main message
pre-	before	premature	before birth, before full development
tachy-	rapid, abnormally high rate of speed	tachycardia	abnormally fast heartbeat

Prefixes of Direction

The word *abnormal* is an example of a word containing a prefix that signifies direction. We use such prefixes in everyday life without bothering to analyze them. For example, we normally would not take the time to think about the prefix contra- (against) in the word *contradiction*, yet we understand its meaning. Prefixes related to direction are listed in **Table 2.3**.

Prefixes of Position

Infrastructure (infra- means inside or below), *interstate* (inter- means between), and *paralegal* (para- means alongside) are all words we frequently use that include prefixes of position. Having these prefix meanings already in our working vocabularies makes it easier to learn their medical uses. Prefixes of position are commonly used during diagnostic procedures and treatments. **Table 2.4** lists prefixes relating to position.

Table 2.3 Prefixes of Direction

Prefix	Refers to	Example	Meaning
ab-	away from, outside of, beyond	abnormal	not normal
ad-	toward, near to	adjective	toward a noun
con-	with, within	congenital	with (or at) birth, with feeling toward, with the same idea or purpose
contra-	against	contraband	substance against the law
dia-	across, through	diameter	a line through the middle
sym-	with	sympathetic	with; acting or considered together
syn-	with, joined together	syndesmosis	immovable joint in which the bones are joined together

Table 2.4 Prefixes of Position

Prefix	Refers to	Example	Meaning
ec-	outside	extraction	removal to the outside
ecto-	outside	ectoderm	outermost layer of embryonic cells or tissue
en-	inside	encephalopathy	disease inside the head, brain disease
endo-	within	endoscopy	visual examination of the inside of some part of the body
epi-	upon, following, above, in addition	epigastric	adjective referring to something above the stomach

(continues)

Table 2.4 Prefixes of Position   (continued)

Prefix	Refers to	Example	Meaning
ex-, exo-	outside	external	from outside
extra-	beyond	extracellular	adjective referring to something outside a cell
hyper-	above, beyond normal	hyperglycemia	high blood sugar
hypo-	low, below, below normal	hypogastric	region beneath the stomach
infra-	inside or below	infrarenal	adjective referring to something below the kidneys
inter-	between	interosseous	between bones
intra-	inside, within	intracerebral	inside the cerebrum
meso-	middle	mesothelioma	tumor arising from the mesothelium
meta-	beyond	metacarpal	the bone beyond the carpus; one of five bones in either hand
pan-	all or everywhere	pancarditis	general inflammation of the heart
para-	alongside, near, disordered function	paraplegia	paralysis of the lower half of the body
peri-	around	perivascular	in the tissues surrounding a vessel
retro-	backward, behind	retrosternal	adjective referring to something behind the sternum

Prefixes of Size and Number

A semiannual (semi- means "half," annual means "yearly") sale is one that occurs every 6 months. The unicorn (uni- means "one") is a fictitious creature that has one horn. Prefixes of size and number are very common. **Table 2.5** lists prefixes related to size and number.

Table 2.5 Prefixes of Size and Number

Prefix	Refers to	Example	Meaning
bi-	two	biannual	twice per year
di-, dipl-	two, twice	diplopia	double vision
hemi-	half	hemiplegia	paralysis of one body side
macro-	big	macrocyte	big cell
micro-	small	microscope	instrument to view small objects
mono-	one	monocyte	cell with one nucleus
olig-, oligo-	a few, a little	oliguria	small amount of urine production
pan-	all or everywhere	pancarditis	whole heart inflammation
poly-	many	polydactyly	more than five fingers or toes
quadri-	four	quadriplegia	paralysis of all four limbs
semi-	half, partial	semiannual	occurring every half year
tetra-	four	tetradactyl	having only four fingers or toes
tri-	three	triceps	three-headed muscle
uni-	one	unicellular	one-celled

Table 2.6 Prefixes of Negation

Prefix	Refers to	Example	Meaning
a-, an-	not	anuria	not able to urinate
anti-	against, opposed	antibiotic	drug that inhibits microbes
de-	without	dehumidifier	device that removes water
dis-	remove	disable	put out of action

Prefixes of Negation

Negation means without or the opposite of something. These include words like antidepressant (anti- means "against") and decriminalize (de- means "without"). **Table 2.6** lists prefixes related to negation.

QUICK CHECK

Define each prefix and state whether it refers to time, speed, position, direction, number, or negation.

1. anti- _____
2. hyper- _____
3. tachy- _____

Categories of Suffixes

Dividing suffixes into functional categories makes them easier to learn compared to keeping them as a long list. A suffix adds to or changes a root in one of four different ways. Suffixes:

- signify a medical condition;
- signify diagnostic terms, tests, and surgical procedures;
- name a medical practice or practitioner; or
- convert a noun to an adjective.

For example, the suffix -*stenosis* indicates a narrowing or blockage in a body part, which is a condition. Consider the term arteriostenosis. Because the root arter/i/o means artery, we may conclude that arteriostenosis is a narrowing of an artery. Note how this term is divided into word parts:

Term	Part	Meaning
arteriostenosis	root: arter/i/o = artery	narrowing of an artery
	suffix: -stenosis = narrowing	

Suffixes Signifying Medical Conditions

The suffix -porosis, which means porous, is added to the root oste/o, to form the term osteoporosis, which means "a porous condition of bone." See **Table 2.7** for more examples.

Table 2.7 Suffixes That Signify Medical Conditions

Suffix	Meaning of the Suffix	Example	Meaning of the Example
-algia	pain	arthralgia	joint pain
-cele	protrusion, hernia	rectocele	hernia of the rectum
-cyte	cell	leukocyte	white blood cell
-dynia	pain	arthrodynia	joint pain
-ectasis, -ectasia	expansion or dilation	angiectasis	dilation of a vessel
-edema (also a standalone word)	excessive fluid	angioedema	fluid buildup that causes swelling under the skin
-emesis	vomiting	hematemesis	vomiting of blood
-emia	blood	uremia	urea in the blood

(continues)

Table 2.7 Suffixes That Signify Medical Conditions   *(continued)*

Suffix	Meaning of the Suffix	Example	Meaning of the Example
-iasis	condition or state	cholelithiasis	stones in the gallbladder
-ism	a condition of, a process, or a state of	hypothyroidism	condition characterized by thyroid hormone deficiency
-itis	inflammation	appendicitis	inflammation of the appendix
-lith	stone, calculus, calcification	rhinolith	a stone in the nose
-lysis	disintegration, breaking down	hemolysis	rupture of red blood cells
-malacia	softening	osteomalacia	softening of the bones
-megaly	enlargement	gastromegaly	enlargement of the stomach
-oid	resembling or like	opioid	substance that resembles opium
-oma	tumor	gastroma	tumor of the stomach
-osis	abnormal condition	osteoporosis	condition of porous bones
-pathy	disease	myopathy	disease of the muscle
-penia	reduction of size or quantity	leukopenia	low number of white blood cells
-phobia	fear	carcinophobia	fear of cancer
-plasia	abnormal formation	neoplasia	abnormal growth of cells
-plegia	paralysis	hemiplegia	paralysis on one side of the body
-pnea	breathing	tachypnea	rapid breathing
-poiesis	producing	erythropoiesis	production of red blood cells
-porosis	porous condition	osteoporosis	porous
-ptosis	downward displacement	nephroptosis	downward displacement of a kidney
-rrhage	flowing forth	hemorrhage	excessive bleeding
-rrhea	discharge	rhinorrhea	discharge from the nose (runny nose)
-rrhexis	rupture	hysterorrhexis	rupture of the uterus
-sclerosis	hardness	atherosclerosis	hardening of the arteries
-spasm	muscular contraction	angiospasm	muscular contraction of a vessel
-stasis	level, unchanging	thermostasis	a constant, consistent internal body temperature
-stenosis	a narrowing	arteriostenosis	narrowed arteries

Suffixes Signifying Diagnostic Terms, Tests, and Surgical Procedures

Suffixes that form terms related to diagnoses, tests, and surgical procedures are often attached to a root that signifies a body part. The term *appendectomy* is an example. The suffix -ectomy means "removal of," and *append* is the root for appendix. Thus, the term means "removal of the appendix." **Table 2.8** lists common suffixes that signify diagnostic terms, tests, and surgical procedures.

Table 2.8 Suffixes That Signify Diagnostic Terms, Tests, and Surgical Procedures

Suffix	Refers to	Example
-centesis	surgical puncture	thoracentesis
-desis	surgical binding	arthrodesis
-ectomy	surgical removal	appendectomy
-gen, -genic, -genesis	origin, producing	osteogenic
-gram	a recording, usually by an instrument	electrocardiogram
-graph	instrument for making a recording	electrocardiograph
-graphy	act of graphic or pictorial recording	electrocardiography
-meter	instrument for measuring	audiometer
-metry	act of measuring	audiometry
-opsy	examination	autopsy
-pexy	surgical fixation	hysteropexy
-plasty	surgical repair	rhinoplasty
-rrhaphy	suture	herniorrhaphy
-scope	instrument for viewing	arthroscope
-scopy	act of viewing	arthroscopy
-stomy	artificial or surgical opening	tracheostomy
-tome	instrument for cutting	dermatome (used in skin grafts)
-tomy	incision	colotomy
-tripsy	crushing	lithotripsy

Suffixes That Signify Medical Practices and Practitioners

Some suffixes relating to medical practices and practitioners are derived from the Greek word *iatros*, which means "physician" or "medical treatment." This Greek word is the source of the root iatr/o. For practical purposes, you may consider the root iatr as an integral part of the suffixes -iatric and -iatr, as in the terms geriatrics, psychiatric, psychiatry, psychiatrist, pediatrics, and pediatrician. Although both -ician and -ist are used in referring to a specialist, the suffix -ist is perhaps the more common one. An example is gerontologist, a physician who diagnoses and treats disorders of aging.

Terms denoting a field or medical specialty may also end with the suffix, *-logy*. **Table 2.9** lists the suffixes for medical practices and practitioners.

Root, prefix, or suffix? The word part *gen* can act as a suffix or a root, but like *iatro-*, it combines nicely with several suffixes and may be considered a part of them. Terms formed with *-genic* are adjectives because of the *-ic* ending. As described later, -ic can be a suffix by itself too.

Suffixes That Denote Adjectives

As with suffixes that signify medical practices and practitioners, suffixes used to create adjective forms do not have a clear set of rules. Nevertheless, there are some rules, such as the rules of English pronunciation. For example, we replace the final letter, *x*, in the word appendix with a *c* to form the adjective *appendicitis* because "appendixitis" does not sound much like an English word.

Table 2.9 Suffixes That Signify Medical Practices and Practitioners

Suffix	Refers To	Example
-ian	specialist	pediatrician
-iatrics	medical specialty	pediatrics
-iatry	medical specialty	psychiatry
-ics	medical specialty	orthopedics
-ist	specialist in a field of study	orthopedist
-logy	study of	gynecology

In creating adjectives, we also sometimes change noun terms that name specialties. For example, *psychiatry* and *pediatrics* are the names of specialties. Removing the *y* from psychiatry and adding the adjective suffix *-ic* converts the specialty name to an adjective:

> psychiatric medicine
>
> psychiatric hospital

With pediatrics, the *s* is removed to form the adjective:

> pediatric medicine
>
> pediatric hospital

Examples of adjective suffixes are listed in **Table 2.10**.

Prefixes and suffixes presented in this chapter will become familiar as you progress through the next chapters on body systems. Review the following study tables and do the self-testing exercises.

Table 2.10 Suffixes That Denote Adjectives

Suffix	Refers to	Example
-ac, -al, -an, -aneous, -ar, -ary, -eal, -eous, -iac, -iatric, -ic, -ical, -oid, -otic, -ous, -tic, -ular	converts a root or noun to an adjective	geriatric, orthopedic, ocular

Study Table Common Prefixes		
Prefix	**Meaning**	**Example**
a-, an-	not, without	anemic
ab-	away from, outside of, beyond	abnormal
ad-	toward, near to	adduction
ante-	before	antepartum
anti-	against, opposed	antibiotic
bi-	two	bipolar
brady-	abnormally slow rate of speed	bradycardia
con-	with	conjoined
contra-	against	contralateral
de-	not	deodorant
di-, diplo-	two, double	diploid
dia-	across, through	diagnosis
dis-	remove	disinfect
dys-	painful, bad, difficult	dyspnea
ec-, ecto-	outside	ectopy

Prefix	Meaning	Example
en-	inside	endosteum
endo-	within	endoderm
epi-	upon, above, in addition	epigastric
ex-, exo-	outside	exoskeleton
extra-	beyond	extrasystole
hemi-	half	hemiplegia
hyper-	above, beyond normal	hypergastric
hypo-	below, below normal	hypogastric
infra-	inside or below	infrastructure
inter-	between	intercostal
intra-	inside	intracerebral
macro-	big	macrophage
meso-	middle	mesoderm
meta-	beyond	metacarpal
micro-	small	microscope
mono-	one	monocyte
neo-	new	neoplasm
olig-, oligo-	a few, a little	oliguria
pan-	everywhere	pandemic
para-	alongside, near	paraplegia
peri-	around	perimeter
post-	after	postsynaptic
pre-	before	premature
quadri-	four	quadriceps
retro-	backward, behind	retroperitoneal
semi-	half, partial	semiconscious
sym-	with	sympathetic
syn-	with, joined together	synarthrosis
tachy-	rapid	tachycardia
tetra-	four	tetradactyl
tri-	three	triceps
uni-	one	unilateral

(continues)

Study Table Common Suffixes		*(continued)*
Suffix	**Meaning**	**Example**
-ac, -al, -an, -aneous, -ar, -ary, -eal, -eous, -iac, -iatric, -ic, -ical, -oid, -otic, -ous, -tic, -ular	converts a root or a noun term to an adjective	geriatric, orthopedic, ocular, dental, cutaneous, cyanotic, atrial, cardiac, ureteral
-algia	pain	myalgia
-cele	protrusion, hernia	rectocele
-centesis	surgical puncture	thoracentesis
-cyte	cell	leukocyte
-desis	surgical binding	arthrodesis
-dynia	pain	urodynia
-ectasis, -ectasia	expansion or dilation	angiectasis
-ectomy	surgical removal	appendectomy
-edema	excessive fluid in intracellular tissues	angioedema
-emesis	vomiting	hematemesis
-emia	blood	uremia
-genic	origin, producing	osteogenic
-gram	a recording, usually by an instrument	electrocardiogram
-graph	instrument for making a recording	electrocardiograph
-graphy	act of graphic or pictorial recording	electrocardiography
-ian, -iatrist, -ist, -logist, -logy, -ics, -iatry, -iatrics	specialty of, study of, practice of	geriatrist, pediatrician, gynecology
-iasis	condition or state	cholelithiasis
-ism	a condition of, a process, or a state of	gigantism, hyperthyroidism
-itis	inflammation	appendicitis
-lith	stone, calculus, calcification	nephrolith
-lysis	disintegration	hemolysis
-malacia	softening	osteomalacia
-megaly	enlargement	gastromegaly
-meter	device for measuring	audiometer
-metry	act of measuring	audiometry
-oid	resembling or like	android, mucoid
-oma	tumor	gastroma
-opsy	visual examination	biopsy
-osis	abnormal condition	osteoporosis, arthrosis

Suffix	Meaning	Example
-pathy	disease	cardiopathy
-penia	reduction of size or quantity	leukopenia
-pexy	surgical fixation	hysteropexy
-phobia	fear	claustrophobia
-plasia	abnormal formation	chondroplasia
-plasty	surgical repair	rhinoplasty
-plegia	paralysis	hemiplegia
-pnea	breath, respiration	tachypnea
-poiesis	producing	erythropoiesis
-porosis	porous condition	osteoporosis
-ptosis	downward displacement	nephroptosis
-rrhage	flowing forth	hemorrhage
-rrhaphy	suture	herniorrhaphy
-rrhea	discharge	diarrhea
-rrhexis	rupture	hysterorrhexis
-sclerosis	hardness	arteriosclerosis
-scope	instrument for viewing	arthroscope
-scopy	act of viewing	arthroscopy
-spasm	muscular contraction	arteriospasm
-stasis	level, unchanging	hemostasis
-stenosis	a narrowing	arteriostenosis
-stomy	permanent opening	colostomy
-tome	instrument for cutting	osteotome
-tomy	incision	osteotomy
-tripsy	crushing	lithotripsy

CASE STUDY WRAP-UP

The medical personnel did a quick physical assessment and noted dehydration, hypotension, and oliguria. When the nurse tried to insert a needle into a vein to draw blood, she could not find a vein in his extremities that could accept the needle; she knew Bear was going into vascular collapse. She accessed his external jugular vein and began an intravenous infusion of Ringer's lactate solution. Bear fully recovered a few days later.

Case Study Application Questions

1. Define dehydration and note what the prefix *de-* and the root word *hydr* mean.
2. What does the prefix *hypo-* mean? What is hypotension?
3. Define *oliguria* and its word parts.
4. Using a reputable source, research the components of Ringer's lactate solution and name them.

END-OF-CHAPTER EXERCISES

Exercise 2.1 Adding Prefixes of Time and Speed

Form a new word by adding each prefix in the list to the word appearing next to it. Then write the meaning of the new word in the space to the right. Refer to a dictionary as needed.

Prefix	Word	New Word	Meaning
1. ante-	room	_____	_____
2. neo-	classic	_____	_____
3. post-	glacial	_____	_____
4. pre-	dominant	_____	_____
5. tacho-	meter	_____	_____

Exercise 2.2 Adding Prefixes of Direction

Form a new word by adding each prefix in the list to the word appearing next to it. Then write the meaning of the new word in the space to the right. Refer to a dictionary as needed.

Prefix	Word	New Word	Meaning
1. ab-	normal	_____	_____
2. ad-	joining	_____	_____
3. con-	centric	_____	_____
4. contra-	lateral	_____	_____
5. dia-	gram	_____	_____
6. sym-	pathetic	_____	_____
7. syn-	thesis	_____	_____

Exercise 2.3 Adding Prefixes of Position

Form a new word by adding each prefix in the list to the word or word part appearing next to it. Then write the meaning of the new word in the space to the right. Refer to a dictionary as needed.

Prefix	Word/Word Part	New Word	Meaning
1. ec-	centric	_____	_____
2. ecto-	morph	_____	_____
3. en-	slave	_____	_____
4. endo-	cardial	_____	_____
5. epi-	demic	_____	_____
6. ex-	change	_____	_____
7. exo-	sphere	_____	_____
8. extra-	terrestrial	_____	_____

Prefix	Word/Word Part	New Word	Meaning
9. hyper-	sensitive	_____	_____
10. hypo-	thesis	_____	_____
11. infra-	structure	_____	_____
12. inter-	collegiate	_____	_____
13. intra-	mural	_____	_____
14. meso-	sphere	_____	_____
15. meta-	physics	_____	_____
16. pan-	orama	_____	_____
17. para-	legal	_____	_____

Exercise 2.4 Adding Prefixes of Size and Number

Form a new word by adding each prefix in the list to the word or word part appearing next to it. Then write the meaning of the new word in the space to the right. Refer to a dictionary as needed.

Prefix	Word/Word Part	New Word	Meaning
1. bi-	annual	_____	_____
2. hemi-	sphere	_____	_____
3. macro-	cosm	_____	_____
4. micro-	scope	_____	_____
5. mono-	rail	_____	_____
6. olig-	archy	_____	_____
7. quadri-	lateral	_____	_____
8. semi-	annual	_____	_____
9. tri-	angle	_____	_____
10. uni-	cycle	_____	_____

Exercise 2.5 Combining Roots and Suffixes That Denote Medical Conditions

Build new words by combining the correct form of each root with the suffixes appearing next to it. Suffixes and their definitions may be found in the Common Suffixes Study Table in this chapter. Then write the meaning of the new word in the space to the right. Refer to a medical dictionary as needed.

Root	Suffix	New Word	Meaning
1. card/i/o	-cele	_____	_____
	-dynia	_____	_____
	-ectasia	_____	_____
	-itis	_____	_____
	-malacia	_____	_____

1. card/i/o   -megaly   _____   _____

                         -ptosis   _____   _____

                         -plegia   _____   _____

                         -rrhexis   _____   _____

                         -spasm   _____   _____

2. dermat/o   -itis   _____   _____

                         -oma   _____   _____

                         -megaly   _____   _____

                         -osis   _____   _____

3. hem/o, hemat/o   -lysis   _____   _____

                         -genesis   _____   _____

                         -oma   _____   _____

4. neur/o   -algia   _____   _____

                         -ectasis   _____   _____

                         -itis   _____   _____

                         -oma   _____   _____

5. oste/o   -dynia   _____   _____

                         -oma   _____   _____

                         -malacia   _____   _____

                         -penia   _____   _____

                         -porosis   _____   _____

                         -itis   _____   _____

6. psych/o   -osis   _____   _____

Exercise 2.6 Combining Roots and Suffixes That Denote Diagnostic Terms, Tests, and Surgical Procedures

Build new words by combining the correct form of each root with the suffixes appearing next to it. Suffixes and their definitions may be found in the Common Suffixes Study Table in this chapter. Then write the meaning of the new word in the space to the right. Refer to a medical dictionary as needed.

Root	Suffix	New Word	Meaning
1. card/i/o	-genic	_____	_____
	-gram	_____	_____
	-graph	_____	_____
	-graphy	_____	_____
	-pathy	_____	_____
	-rrhaphy	_____	_____
2. dermat/o	-plasty	_____	_____

3. hemat/o   -genesis   _____   _____

                         -metry   _____   _____

4. neur/o   -ectomy   _____   _____

                         -genic   _____   _____

                         -genesis   _____   _____

5. oste/o   -rrhaphy   _____   _____

                         -plasty   _____   _____

                         -genesis   _____   _____

                         -ectomy   _____   _____

                         -tomy   _____   _____

6. path/o   -gen   _____   _____

                         -genic   _____   _____

                         -genesis   _____   _____

7. psych/o   -genic   _____   _____

                         -genesis   _____   _____

                         -metry   _____   _____

                         -pathy   _____   _____

Exercise 2.7 Combining Roots and Suffixes Associated with Medical Practices and Practitioners

Build new words by combining the correct form of each root with the suffixes appearing next to it. Suffixes and their definitions may be found in the Common Suffixes Study Table in this chapter. Then write the meaning of the new word in the space to the right. Refer to a medical dictionary as needed.

Root	Suffix	New Word	Meaning
1. card/i/o	-logy	_____	_____
	-logist	_____	_____
2. derm/o, dermat/o	-logy	_____	_____
	-logist	_____	_____
3. ger/o/nt/o	-iatrics	_____	_____
	-logy	_____	_____
	-logist	_____	_____
4. hem/o, hemat/o	-logy	_____	_____
	-logist	_____	_____
5. neur/o	-logy	_____	_____
	-logist	_____	_____
6. oste/o	-logy	_____	_____
	-logist	_____	_____

7. path/o   -logy   _____   _____

               -logist   _____   _____

8. psych/o   -logy   _____   _____

               -iatry   _____   _____

               -iatrist   _____   _____

Exercise 2.8 Combining Roots and Suffixes That Denote Adjectives

Build new words by combining the correct form of each root with the suffixes appearing next to it. Suffixes and their definitions may be found in the Common Suffixes Study Table in this chapter. Then write the meaning of the new word in the space to the right. Refer to a medical dictionary as needed.

Root	Suffix	New Word	Meaning
1. card/i/o	-ac	_____	_____
2. hem/o, hemat/o	-toxic	_____	_____
3. derm/o, dermat/o	-al	_____	_____
	-ic	_____	_____
4. ger/o, geront/o	-iatric	_____	_____
	-al	_____	_____
5. neur/o	-al	_____	_____
	-ic	_____	_____
6. spin/o	-al	_____	_____
	-ous	_____	_____
7. oste/o	-al	_____	_____
	-oid	_____	_____

Exercise 2.9 Matching Suffixes with Meanings

Match the suffix in Column 1 with its definition in Column 2.

Column 1

1. _____ -cyte

2. _____ -edema

3. _____ -emesis

4. _____ -sclerosis

5. _____ -tome

6. _____ -ism

7. _____ -lith

8. _____ -lysis

Column 2

a. fear of or aversion to something

b. vomiting

c. a stone, calculus, calcification

d. a condition, a process or state of

e. disease

f. visual examination

g. cell

h. disintegration

9. _____ -opsy   i. excessive fluid in intracellular tissues

10. _____ -pathy   j. instrument for cutting

11. _____ -phobia   k. level, unchanging

12. _____ -poiesis   l. a narrowing

13. _____ -stomy   m. hardness

14. _____ -stasis   n. permanent opening

15. _____ -stenosis   o. producing

Exercise 2.10 Fill in the Blank

Fill in the blank with the correct answer.

1. What two suffixes mean "pain"? _____
2. *Ang/i/o* is a root meaning "blood vessel." What term means "dilation of a blood vessel"?_____
3. Angioid means "resembling blood vessels." What part of speech is angioid? _____
4. Define angiorrhaphy. _____
5. What suffix would you add to the root ang/i/o to form a term meaning "the act of making a pictorial record of blood vessels"? _____
6. What is an angioma? _____
7. What does *-plasty* mean? _____
8. What term denotes a skin specialist? _____
9. Does a gerontologist treat young or old patients? _____
10. What is the difference in meaning between *gerontology* and *geriatrics*? _____
11. The prefixes *ab-* and *ad-* are opposites; which one means "toward"? _____
12. The prefix *pre-* means "before"; what other prefix means "before"? _____
13. Write a brief definition of bradycardia _____
14. What does the prefix extra- mean in the word *extrasensory*? _____
15. What prefix would you use in a term that means "high blood pressure"? _____
16. Given the meaning of *anti-*, what would be the purpose of an anticoagulant? _____
17. Given the meaning of the prefix *tri-*, how many cusps does the tricuspid valve have? _____
18. What does the prefix *micro-* tell us about the purpose of a microscope? _____
19. Write a medical term by combining the prefix *endo-* with the root card/i/o, meaning "heart," and the suffix that means "inflammation." Using only your knowledge of these three word parts, write the best definition you can for the term _____.
20. The suffix *-pnea*, meaning "breathing" or "respiration," can follow both tachy- and dys-. Define the terms tachypnea and dyspnea: _____

Exercise 2.11 Reflection

1. After reading Chapter 2, how are you feeling about learning medical terminology?
2. Success in any course requires study, practice, and time. What study strategies do you have in place? How will you manage your time?

CHAPTER 3

Organization of the Body

LEARNING OUTCOMES

Upon completion of this chapter, you should be able to:

- Discuss the levels of body organization.
- Describe the anatomic position and cite the directional terms used in relation to the body.
- Name the body planes.
- Name the body cavities.
- Name the divisions of the abdomen and back.
- Pronounce, define, and spell each term introduced in this chapter.
- Apply knowledge gained to Case Study Questions.

CASE STUDY

Trayvon's Tibia

Trayvon is a standout college point guard with aspirations of becoming a physician. During Saturday's game, he was fouled by a player on the opposing team and fell to the basketball court, holding his left leg. The trainer rushed from the sideline and immediately began assessing the situation. After a few questions and a quick physical assessment, the trainer called for a stretcher, and Trayvon was wheeled away.

Introduction

Learning about how the human body is constructed will help you retain new medical terms by creating a mental picture of where things are. To begin, it is also useful to know the difference between these terms: *anatomy* and *physiology*. **Anatomy** comes to us from the Greek word *anatome*, which means "dissection." You may have recognized the word part "tome," which indicates that anatomy has something to do with cutting. **Physiology**, on the other hand, is one of the many "ology" words; in this case, it means study of how the body's parts work together. In short, anatomy reveals "what it is," and physiology explains "how it works."

The "what it is" begins with chemicals that act together to form cells. The cells process the food we eat and the air we breathe. Cells also reproduce themselves, each cell according to the DNA code it contains.

Word Parts Related to Body Organization

Table 3.1 lists many of the word parts that make up terms related to the body as a whole. Not surprisingly, many of them have to do with how the body is divided or where things are located.

Table 3.1 Word Parts Related to Body Organization

Word Part	Meaning
anter/o	front, anterior
cerv/o	neck
chondr/o	cartilage
cyt/o, -cyte	cell
dors/o	back
gastr/o	stomach, abdomen
inguin/o	groin
my/o	muscle
myel/o	spinal cord
neur/o	nerve, neuron
poster/o	posterior, back
proxim/o	near
super/o	superior
thorac/o	chest (thorax)
trans-	across

Word Parts Exercise

After studying Table 3.1, write the meaning of each of the word parts.

Word Part	Meaning
1. trans-	1. _____
2. dors/o	2. _____
3. proxim/o	3. _____
4. chondr/o	4. _____
5. anter/o	5. _____
6. my/o	6. _____
7. super/o	7. _____
8. cerv/o	8. _____
9. inguin/o	9. _____
10. myel/o	10. _____

Levels of Organization

The body is divided into different levels of organization, starting with the smallest level: cells, tissues, organs, organ systems (body systems), and organism, which is the body as a whole. Each level is further examined under its own heading (see **Figure 3.1**).

Cells

The adult human body is said to have nearly 40 trillion cells. This is not an exact number because people vary in size, but it is generally accepted that trillions of cells make up the body. With trillions of cells, one can appreciate the body's complexity as a functioning whole. Cells work both individually and together. Although cells differ from one another and consist of different components, they do have some common elements (see **Figure 3.2**):

- A *cell membrane* allows certain substances in and out.
- A *nucleus* directs activities within the cell.
- *Mitochondria* generate energy for the cell.
- *Cytoplasm* is a watery fluid that fills the spaces outside the nucleus.

Tissues

Cells make up tissues, which are composed of similar cells working together to perform similar functions. The four types of body tissues are muscle, connective, nerve, and epithelial.

Organs

Tissues with common functions come together to form the body's organs, which perform specialized functions. Examples of organs are the brain, stomach, and heart.

Systems

A group of organs forms an organ system, and each system has its own special purpose. Therefore, the rest of this book discusses each system in a chapter of its own.

Navigating the Body

Healthcare professionals need to be familiar with directional and positioning terms. These terms are frequently used during patient examinations, diagnostic procedures, and treatments.

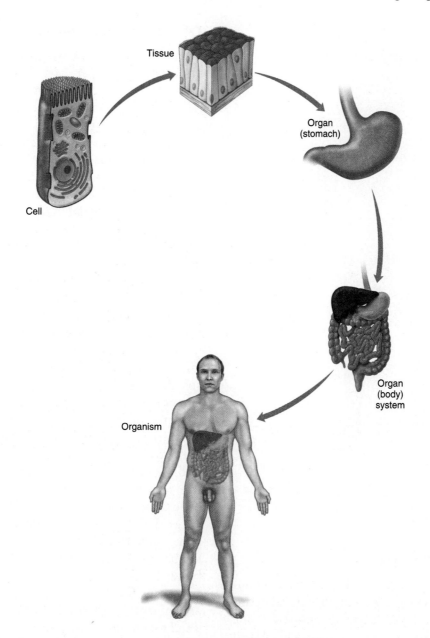

Figure 3.1 The levels of organization in the body beginning with the cell and ending with the organism.

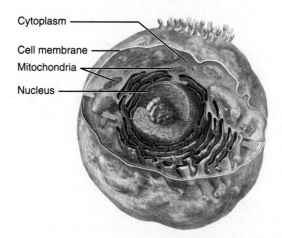

Figure 3.2 Basic structure of a cell. The basic structure of a cell includes the cell membrane, nucleus, mitochondria, and cytoplasm.

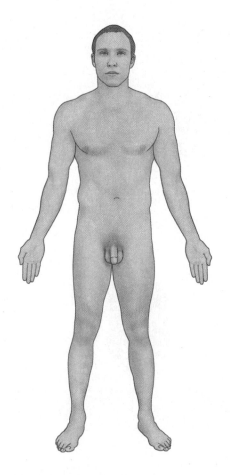

Figure 3.3 Anatomic position. In the anatomic position, the person is standing erect, and palms and body are facing forward.

Anatomic Position

Directional terms in the field of human anatomy differ from plain language because directional terms are specified relative to the anatomic position. In the **anatomic position**, the body is erect (standing) and facing forward, and the arms are at the sides with the palms of the hands facing forward (see **Figure 3.3**). Left and right are from the subject's perspective, not the observer's perspective.

The inhabitants of Pormpuraaw, a remote aboriginal community in Australia, have no words for "left" or "right." Instead, they speak of everything in terms of absolute directions (north, south, east, and west). They say things such as, "There's an ant on your southwest leg." To say hello in Pormpuraaw, one asks, "Where are you going?" An appropriate response might be, "A long way to the south-south-west. How about you?" The Pormpuraawans not only know instinctively which direction they are facing, but they also spontaneously use their spatial orientation to represent both position and time.

Directional Terms

Directional terms are words that help describe a symptom, body part, or location. These terms often have another term that is its opposite, and it is helpful to memorize these terms with their opposite to differentiate and understand them. Sometimes terms, such as *anterior* and *ventral* or *posterior* and *dorsal* can be used interchangeably. The following terms should be committed to memory. **Superior** means above or near the head. Two other words, **cranial** and **cephalic**, also mean "toward the head." For example, "The bruise is superior to the eyebrow." **Inferior** and **caudal** mean below or toward the feet, as in "The mouth is inferior to the nose." **Anterior** is a directional term that relates to the front of the body. An example of the use of *anterior* would be, "The rash covered the entire anterior of the left thigh." **Ventral**, usually used in veterinary anatomy, pertains to the front (anterior) or undersurface of an animal. **Posterior** specifies the back or toward the back of the body. **Dorsal**, generally used in veterinary anatomy, pertains to the back (posterior) or upper surface of an animal. **Medial** means toward the midline of the body, and **lateral** means away from the body's midline or toward the side. You may see the adjective *lateral* used for descriptive purposes as in, "The tumor is located on the lateral wall of the left lung." The final two directional terms are *proximal* and *distal*. **Proximal** refers to something closer to the body trunk or point of attachment to the body: The shoulder is *proximal* to the elbow. **Distal** means further from the body trunk or point of attachment: The wrist is *distal* to the shoulder and *distal* to the elbow. See **Figure 3.4** for an illustration showing directional terms.

Two terms are used for placing patients in a lying down position. Both are common English words that have been adopted by medical terminology. The two terms are *supine* and *prone*. **Supine** refers to a position in which the patient is lying face up. Noticing that the word "up" is included in the first syllable of the word "supine" will help you remember its meaning of "face up" in medical terms.

Prone is the opposite of supine and means that the patient is lying face down. Both supine and prone are frequently used in the operating room and in X-ray reports. For example, "The patient was placed in the supine position." This means that the patient was placed on the operating table on their back, lying face up. See **Table 3.2** for body position and direction terms.

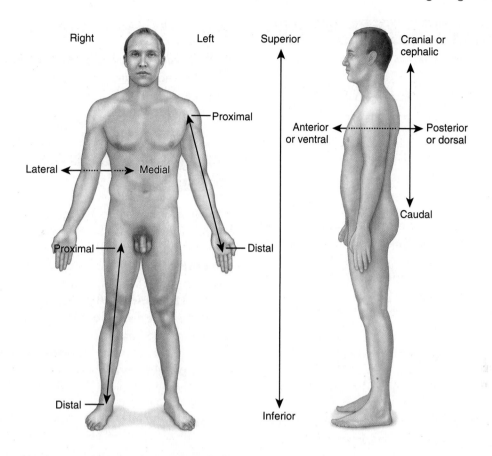

Figure 3.4 Directional terms describe the body part in relationship to another.

Table 3.2 Body Position and Directional Terms

Term	Direction	Example
anterior	toward the front	The eyes are on the anterior surface of the face.
ventral	toward the belly or undersurface	The nipples are on the ventral body surface.
posterior	toward the back	The spine is on the posterior side of the body.
dorsal	toward the back or upper surface	The vertebrae are on the dorsal surface.
superior	above; toward the head	The neck is superior to the chest.
cranial	relating to the head	The brain is in the cranial cavity.
cephalic	relating to the head	The neck is cephalic to the hips.
inferior	below; toward the soles of the feet	The knee is inferior to the hip.
caudal	pertaining to the tail	The coccyx is caudal to the sacrum.
proximal	near the point of attachment to the trunk	The elbow is proximal to the wrist.
distal	farther from the point of attachment to the trunk	The fingers are distal to the wrist.
lateral	pertaining to the side; away from the middle	The eyes are lateral to the nose.
medial	toward the middle of the body	The nose is medial to the eyes.
prone	lying flat and face downward	The patient was placed on the operating table in a prone position.
supine	lying flat and face upward	The patient was placed on the operating table in a supine position.

Body Planes

Body planes are two-dimensional flat surfaces within the body, and a **section** is a single view (slice) along a plane (see **Figure 3.5**). Planes and sections are referenced in imaging studies as done with body scans. The anatomic position is always their reference point. Three planes are frequently used to locate structural arrangements.

- **Frontal (coronal) plane**: The frontal (coronal) plane is a vertical plane that separates the front (anterior) of the body from the back (posterior).
- **Sagittal plane**: The sagittal plane is any vertical plane that divides the body or organ into left and right sides. A cut in this plane is called a *sagittal section*.
- **Transverse (horizontal) plane**: The transverse (horizontal) plane separates the body into superior (upper) and inferior (lower) planes. A cut in this plane is called a *transverse section*.

Body Cavities and Divisions

A **body cavity** is a hollow space that contains body organs. The body has several major cavities, including the cranial, spinal, thoracic, and abdominopelvic. The **cranial cavity** houses the brain, and the **spinal cavity** houses the spinal cord.

The **thoracic cavity** contains the lungs, whereas the **abdominopelvic cavity** contains digestive and reproductive organs. The abdominopelvic cavity is divided into a superior **abdominal cavity** and an inferior **pelvic cavity**. The diaphragm is the muscle of breathing that physically divides the upper thoracic cavity from the lower abdominopelvic cavity (see **Figure 3.6**).

Divisions of the Abdominopelvic Cavity

A person documenting a physical examination or a surgical procedure needs to describe incisions, procedures, and location of organs. To do this effectively,

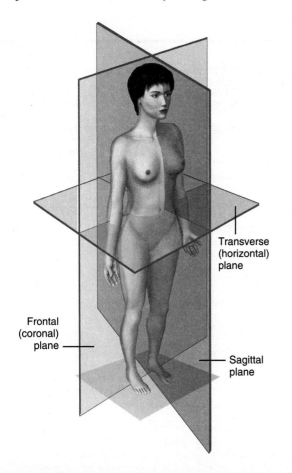

Transverse (horizontal) plane

Frontal (coronal) plane

Sagittal plane

Figure 3.5 Body planes divide the body into halves in different ways for reference purposes.

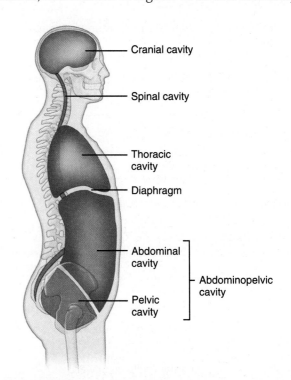

Cranial cavity

Spinal cavity

Thoracic cavity

Diaphragm

Abdominal cavity

Abdominopelvic cavity

Pelvic cavity

Figure 3.6 The major body cavities shown in lateral view.

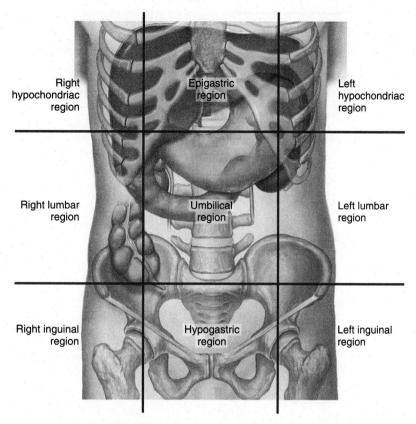

Figure 3.7 Abdominopelvic cavity. **A.** The nine regions of the abdominopelvic cavity.

the abdominopelvic cavity is divided into two different ways: either nine regions or four quadrants (see Figure 3.7A, B; Tables 3.3 and 3.4).

Nine Regions

Regions are used to describe the location of underlying organs. Note that in the following list, the number in parentheses refers to two sides within the region, a left and a right, and counts as two regions (see **Figure 3.7A** and **Table 3.3**). The regions are named as follows:

- Hypochondriac (2): There are right and left hypochondriac regions. *Chondr-* means "cartilage," and the prefix *hypo-* means "below." These areas are below the cartilage of the ribs on the left and right sides.
- Epigastric: This area is just superior to the stomach. *Epi-* is a prefix that means "above." This area is above the stomach and is between the left and right hypochondriac regions.
- Lumbar (2): There are right and left lumbar regions. They are located at waist level on either side of the umbilicus (navel).
- Umbilical: The nine regions resemble a tic-tac-toe chart; the umbilical region is the middle section. It contains the umbilicus (navel).
- Hypogastric: This is the bottom square in the middle column of the tic-tac-toe chart; the hypogastric region is inferior to the umbilical section.

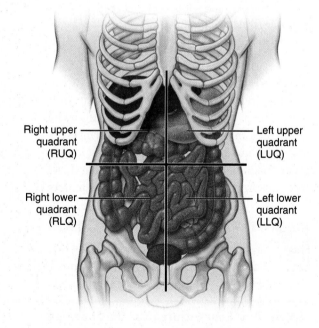

Figure 3.7 Abdominopelvic cavity. **B.** The four quadrants of the abdominopelvic cavity.

- Inguinal (2): There are right and left inguinal regions. They lie on either side of the hypogastric section. Inguinal also refers to the "groin" area.

Table 3.3 Nine Regions of the Abdomen

Region	Description
left hypochondriac region	left lateral, upper third region
left lumbar region	left lateral region of the torso
left inguinal region	left lower lateral region by the groin
epigastric region	upper central region above the umbilical region
umbilical region	middle central region surrounding umbilicus
hypogastric region	lower central region below umbilical region
right hypochondriac region	right lateral, upper third region
right lumbar region	right lateral region of the torso
right inguinal region	right lower lateral region by the groin

Doesn't the word hypochondriac have another definition? Yes. Someone with imaginary pains is called a hypochondriac, and the reason for this usage came about because the left hypochondriac region is in the area where a hypersensitive person might interpret any discomfort as a heart attack.

Four Quadrants

Clinicians typically refer to four abdominopelvic quadrants. These quadrants are shown and described in **Figure 3.7B** and **Table 3.4**. The center point is the umbilicus. The quadrants are abbreviated as follows: right upper quadrant (RUQ), left upper quadrant (LUQ), right lower quadrant (RLQ), and left lower quadrant (LLQ).

Regions of the Spinal Column

The spinal column is a series of vertebrae that extend from the head to the coccyx. The five regions include

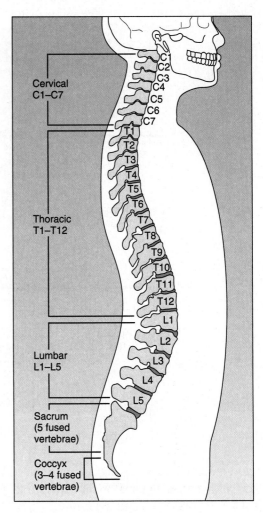

Figure 3.8 The regions of the spinal column show the locations of the vertebrae.

the cervical (C), thoracic (T), lumbar (L), sacral (S), and coccyx (Co). They are labeled with a capital letter that corresponds to the name of the region (see **Figure 3.8**; **Table 3.5**).

The terms for each region describe a part of the back. The cervical region describes the cervix (meaning neck). The thoracic region describes the thorax (meaning chest), the lumbar region describes the lumbus (meaning loin, or part of the side and back between the ribs and the pelvis), the sacral region

Table 3.4 Four Quadrants of the Abdomen

Term	Organs in Quadrant
right upper quadrant (RUQ)	right lobe of liver, gallbladder, portions of the pancreas, small intestine, and colon
left upper quadrant (LUQ)	left lobe of liver, spleen, stomach, portions of the pancreas, small intestine, and colon
right lower quadrant (RLQ)	contains portions of small intestine and colon, right ovary and uterine tube, appendix, and right ureter
left lower quadrant (LLQ)	contains portions of small intestine and colon, left ovary and uterine tube, and left ureter

Table 3.5 Regions of the Spinal Column

Region	Location
cervical	neck
thoracic	chest
lumbar	lower back
sacral	lower back inferior to lumbar
coccyx	lowermost region inferior to sacrum; tailbone

Abbreviation Table Abdominopelvic Quadrants

Abbreviation	Meaning
LLQ	left lower quadrant
LUQ	left upper quadrant
RLQ	right lower quadrant
RUQ	right upper quadrant

describes the sacrum (lower back), and the coccygeal region describes the coccyx (tailbone). It is important to recognize which word is the body part and which word is the adjective describing the region in which that body part is located.

The word *lumbar* is used to describe abdominopelvic regions and a region of the spinal column. The lumbar is "the part of the back and sides between the rib cage and the pelvis," so it makes sense that it is used to describe both these areas.

Study Table Body Position and Directional Terms

Term and Pronunciation	Analysis	Meaning
anterior (an-TEER-ee-ur)	Latin word for former; from Latin word *ante* (before)	toward the front of the body
caudal (KAW-dul)	Latin word for lower; from the Latin word *cauda* (tail of an animal)	below; toward the feet
cephalic (se-FAL-ik)	from the Latin word *cephalicus* (head)	above; toward the head
distal (DIS-tul)	from the Latin word *distantem* (distant)	farther from the point of attachment to the trunk
dorsal (dor-SUL)	from the Latin word *dorsum* (back)	toward the back of the body
inferior (in-FEER-ee-or)	Latin word for lower	below; toward the feet
lateral (LAT-er-ul)	from the Latin word *lateralis* (lateral)	away from the middle
medial (MEE-dee-ul)	from the Latin word *medialis* (middle)	toward the midline of the body
posterior (pos-TEER-ee-or)	from the Latin word *posterus* (following)	toward the back of the body
prone (PRONE)	from the Latin word *pronus* (bending down)	lying flat and face down
proximal (PROX-ih-mul)	from the Latin word *proximus* (nearest)	near the point of attachment to the trunk
superior (soo-PEER-ee-or)	from the Latin word *superus* (above)	above; toward the head
supine (soo-PINE)	from the Latin word *supinus* (bending backward)	lying flat and face up
ventral (VEN-trul)	Latin word for former; from Latin word *venter* (belly)	toward the front of the body

(continues)

Study Table Body Cavities and Divisions		(continued)
Term and Pronunciation	**Analysis**	**Meaning**
cervical (SUR-vi-kul)	from the Latin word *cervix* (neck)	adjective meaning neck
cervix (SUR-viks)	Latin for neck	noun meaning neck
coccygeal (kok-SIJ-ee-ul)	from the Greek word *kokkyx* (cuckoo)	adjective for tailbone
coccyx (KOK-siks)	from the Greek word *kokkyx* (cuckoo; because the shape resembles a cuckoo's beak)	small, fused bones at the end of the vertebral column; tailbone
epigastric (ep-ih-GAS-trik)	*epi-* (above); from the Latin *gastricus* (stomach)	area superior to the stomach
hypochondriac (high-poh-KON-dree-ak)	*hypo-* (below); from the Latin *chondriacus* (upper abdomen)	below the ribcage; also used as a noun to refer to a person whose illnesses are imaginary
hypogastric (high-poh-GAS-tric)	*hypo-* (below); from the Latin *gastricus* (stomach)	inferior to the stomach region
inguinal (IN-gwin-ul)	from the Latin word *inguinalis* (of the groin)	groin
lumbar (LUM-bar)	from the Latin word *lumbus* (loin)	adjective for lumbus
lumbus (LUM-bus)	Latin for loin	area between the ribs and pelvis
sacral (SAY-krul)	from Latin *os sacrum* (holy bone)	adjective for sacrum
sacrum (SAY-krum)	from Latin *os sacrum* (holy bone), as this was often the part of an animal that was offered as a sacrifice	five fused bones of the lower spinal column
thoracic (thor-ASS-ik)	from the Latin word *thorax* (breast)	adjective meaning chest
thorax (THOR-ax)	Latin word for breast or chest	noun meaning chest
umbilicus (um-BILL-ih-kus)	Latin word for navel or center	navel, belly button

CASE STUDY WRAP-UP

Trayvon was taken to the hospital where medical personnel physically examined him, gave him some medicine to make him comfortable, and then placed him supine on a gurney to be transported to the X-ray department. Anteroposterior (AP) and lateral X-rays of the tibia (shin bone), fibula (lateral lower leg bone), knee, and ankle were ordered for his left leg. Results showed a proximal, transverse tibial shaft fracture (break). Surgery was immediately scheduled.

Case Study Application Questions

1. Describe how you would determine which leg to correctly X-ray using only the information given.
2. What does the word *supine* mean?
3. Define *anteroposterior* and *lateral*.
4. Is Trayvon's break closer to his knee or his ankle?

END-OF-CHAPTER EXERCISES

Exercise 3.1 Matching

Insert the letter from the right-hand column that matches each numbered item in the left-hand column.

A. Planes of the Body

1. _____ frontal plane
2. _____ sagittal plane
3. _____ transverse plane

a. divides the body into upper and lower
b. divides the body into left and right
c. divides the body into anterior and posterior

B. Directional Terms

1. _____ superior
2. _____ lateral
3. _____ posterior
4. _____ medial
5. _____ distal
6. _____ prone
7. _____ supine
8. _____ inferior
9. _____ anterior
10. _____ proximal

a. lying flat and face up
b. near the point of attachment to the trunk
c. toward the front; away from the back of the body
d. below; toward the soles of the feet
e. lying flat and face down
f. above; toward the head
g. toward the side; away from the middle
h. near the back; toward the back of the body
i. farther from the point of attachment to the trunk
j. toward the middle of the body

Exercise 3.2 Fill in the Blank

Select the correct word from the list to correctly complete the sentence.

anterior   distal   dorsal   inferior   lateral
medial   posterior   proximal   superior   ventral

1. The wrist is _____ to the elbow.
2. The shoulder is _____ to the wrist.
3. The lungs are _____ to the spinal cord.
4. The nose is _____ to the eyes.
5. The head is _____ to the neck.
6. The ears are _____ to the nose.
7. The shoulder blades are on the _____ side of the body.
8. The chin is _____ to the forehead.

Exercise 3.3 Word Building

Add the correct prefix or suffix to the word root to make a new term. Select from the following word parts: *-itis*, *-ic*, *-al*, *hypo-*, *hyper-*, *epi-*, and *trans-*. The first exercise is an example.

Word Root	Add Prefix or Suffix	Meaning	Term
1. gastr/o	*hypo-* *-ic*	below the stomach	*hypogastric*
2. dors/o	_____	pertaining to the back	_____
3. chondr/o	_____	inflammation of the cartilage	_____
4. thorac/o	_____	across the chest or thorax	_____
5. neur/o	_____	inflammation of a nerve	_____
6. cardi/o	_____	pertaining to the region above or upon the heart	_____

Exercise 3.4 Short Answer

Write the answers to the following questions.

1. _____ What word describes the position of the ear in relation to the nose?
2. What does posterior mean? _____
3. What word describes the position of the elbow in relation to the wrist? _____
4. When the body is in the anatomic position, which direction are the palms of the hands facing?_____
5. What is a synonym for anterior?_____

Exercise 3.5 True or False

True or False? Circle the correct answer.

1. Prone is lying face up.	True	False
2. The left hypochondriac region is above the left lumbar region.	True	False
3. The little toe is medial to the big toe.	True	False
4. The diaphragm is a muscle.	True	False
5. There are five regions of the spinal column.	True	False
6. The sacrum is also called the tailbone.	True	False
7. The sagittal plane divides the body into right and left portions.	True	False
8. In the anatomic position, the body is horizontal.	True	False
9. The opposite of lateral is proximal.	True	False
10. The terms ventral and anterior both mean "front."	True	False

Exercise 3.6 Reflection

1. What was the most interesting thing you learned after reading this chapter?
2. Wrong-site surgeries are serious mistakes. How could they be avoided?

CHAPTER 4

The Integumentary System

LEARNING OUTCOMES

Upon completion of this chapter, you should be able to:

- Name the two main layers of the skin.
- Name the major structures and functions of the integumentary system.
- Pronounce, spell, and define medical terms related to the integumentary system and its disorders.
- Interpret abbreviations associated with the integumentary system.
- Apply knowledge gained to Case Study Questions.

CASE STUDY

Hot Tub Hives

The Kekoa Family was headed to a mountain resort for the winter holiday. Everyone was looking forward to spending the days snow skiing, sledding, and ice skating. They were thrilled that the place where they were staying had an indoor swimming pool and an outdoor hot tub, which they enjoyed using each night. By the third day of their vacation, two of the three children had broken out with skin rashes that were bumpy and itchy. Some bumps were filled with pus and resembled acne. This certainly wasn't something anybody wanted to experience, and the family wasn't sure what was causing the rash.

Introduction

The largest organ of the body is the skin, which covers more than 20 square feet on average and weighs about 24 pounds. It is the main part of the integumentary system, which also includes hair, nails, sebaceous (oil) glands, and sudoriferous (sweat) glands.

Integumentum is the Latin word for "covering" or "shelter"; thus, skin, nails, and hair that cover the body are collectively called the **integumentary system**. The adjective relating specifically to the skin is **cutaneous**.

Word Parts Related to the Integumentary System

Word parts related to hair, skin, nails, and color are presented in **Table 4.1**. It's a good idea to study those word parts, along with the others given in the table, before you go any further. That way, as you go through the text, you can practice deciphering terms using context *and* etymology (study of a word's origin).

Table 4.1 Word Parts Related to the Integumentary System

Word Part	Meaning
adip/o	fat
cutane/o	skin
-cyte, cyt/o	cell
derm/o, dermat/o	skin
-oma	tumor
onych/o	nail
pil/o	hair
seb/o	sebum (oil; fat)
sudor-	sweat

Word Part Meaning Color, Location, or Other Feature	Meaning
albin/o	white
cirrh/o	yellow
cyan/o	blue
epi-	upon, above
erythr/o	red
fer/o	to carry
ichthy/o	dry, scaly (fishlike)
jaund/o	yellow
kerat/o	horn
melan/o	black
myc/o	fungus
scler/o	hard
sub-	below
xanth/o	yellow
xer/o	dry

Word Parts Exercise

After studying Table 4.1, write the meaning of each of the word parts.

Word Part	Meaning
1. dermat/o	1. _____
2. myc/o	2. _____
3. -cyte, cyt/o	3. _____
4. sudor-	4. _____
5. erythr/o	5. _____
6. xer/o	6. _____
7. fer/o	7. _____
8. sub-	8. _____
9. seb/o	9. _____
10. epi-	10. _____
11. albin/o	11. _____
12. cyan/o	12. _____
13. ichthy/o	13. _____
14. cutane/o	14. _____
15. kerat/o	15. _____
16. derm/o	16. _____
17. onych/o	17. _____
18. melan/o	18. _____
19. pil/o	19. _____
20. scler/o	20. _____
21. cirrh/o, jaund/o, xanth/o	21. _____

Structure and Function

The skin consists of two layers: the **epidermis** and **dermis**. A layer of connective tissue called the **hypodermis** or *subcutaneous layer* lies beneath (deep to) the dermis. Although the hypodermis is not, technically speaking, part of the integumentary system, it is mentioned in this chapter because it connects the dermis to the muscles and tissues beneath it. Also found deep to the dermis is **adipose** (fat) **tissue** (see **Figure 4.1**).

The epidermis is the outside layer of skin. It is made up of epithelial tissue, which is also found in other parts of the body covering organs and body cavities. The epidermis protects the body from the outside world—this is a big job

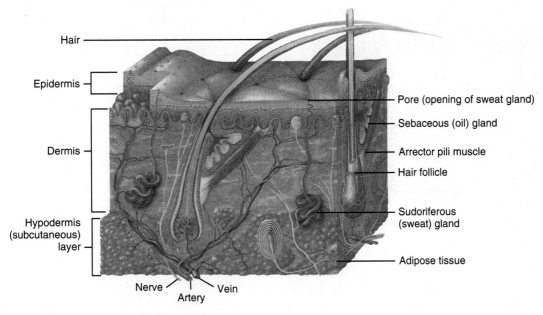

Figure 4.1 The layers of the skin with accessory structures.

for something only 0.05 mm thick on the eyelids to 1.5 mm thick on the palms of the hands and the soles of the feet. The epidermis is **avascular**, which means it does not contain blood vessels. The epithelial tissue found elsewhere in the body is also avascular.

QUICK CHECK

Fill in the **Suffix** and write the resulting word in the **Term** column. The word that appears in boldface type in the **Meaning** column is a clue.

Prefix	Root	Suffix	Term	Meaning
sub-	cutane/o	_____	_____	**adjective** meaning "below the skin"
no prefix	melan/o	_____	_____	a pigment-producing **cell**
no prefix	seb/o	_____	_____	**adjective** referring to sebum, a term meaning oil or fat

Unlike the epidermis, the dermis contains blood vessels and nerves. So, if you get a scratch that hurts and/or bleeds, you will know that you have injured the dermis. The dermis also contains accessory organs, including glands, hair, and nails. The dermis of animals is called the **corium**.

The **sebaceous glands** secrete **sebum**, which is an oily fluid, onto the hair shaft. Sebum reaches the surface of the epidermis and lubricates both the skin and hair. The **sudoriferous glands** produce sweat, a watery fluid that evaporates to help cool the body. Sweat reaches the skin surface through an opening called a **pore**. These glands are found over most of the body but are most numerous in the palms of the hands, soles of the feet, forehead, and armpits.

Hair follicles produce the hair distributed over much of the body (see Figure 4.1). Hair fibers are composed of a hard protein called **keratin**. Bundles of smooth muscle fibers known as **arrector pili muscles** pull the hairs erect, causing "goose bumps" on the skin surface. Like skin, hair color is determined by the pigment **melanin**, which is a brown–black pigment produced from special cells called **melanocytes**. These melanocytes surround

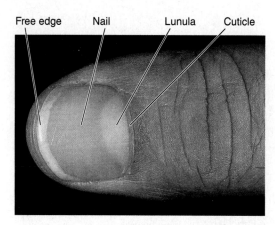

Figure 4.2 Surface view of a nail.

Table 4.2 Classification of Burns

Burn Type	Skin Layers Involved
first degree	erythema (redness); superficial damage to epidermis; no blisters
second degree	blisters; erythema
third degree	charring; damage to the epidermis, dermis, hypodermis, muscle, and bone

the hair shaft. When a small quantity of melanin is present, the hair color will be light or blonde, and as the quantity of melanin increases, the hair darkens. Gray hair occurs as melanin production decreases with age. In addition to providing color, melanin also protects the skin against ultraviolet (UV) radiation or sunlight.

Like hair, **nails** are also composed of the protein, keratin. Nail anatomy consists of the free edge, lunula, and cuticle. The **free edge** is the portion of the nail that grows beyond the tips of the fingers or toes. The **lunula** (a Latin word meaning "little moon") is the whitish crescent region of the nail. The **cuticle** is the thin band of tissue that seals the nail to the skin (see **Figure 4.2**).

Disorders Related to the Integumentary System

Because the skin is visible in its entirety, diagnosing some of its abnormalities is relatively uncomplicated. Moreover, the skin can sometimes provide clues to underlying bodily disorders, which may be signaled by changes in color, by the development of **lesions** (a vague term meaning wounds or injuries), or by the appearance of other skin rashes.

Burns

A **burn** is an injury to the skin caused by heat or chemicals. The severity of a burn is classified by the depth of the skin layers involved (see **Table 4.2**). Body surface area (BSA) is used to express the extent of skin damage.

Skin Lesions

Lesions have many different causes and appearances. They may be flat, elevated, or depressed, and each variation has its own medical term (see **Figure 4.3**).

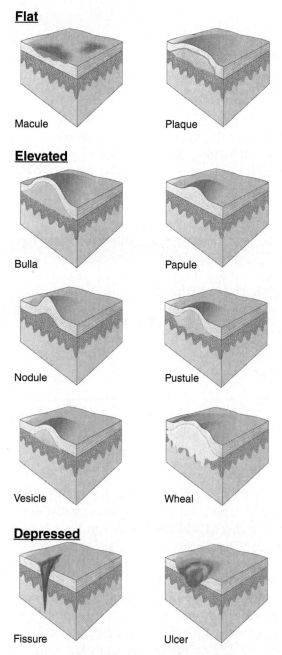

Flat

Macule   Plaque

Elevated

Bulla   Papule

Nodule   Pustule

Vesicle   Wheal

Depressed

Fissure   Ulcer

Figure 4.3 Illustrations of some of the more common skin lesions.

Flat Lesions

- **Macule**: Flat, colored spot less than 1 cm in diameter. A freckle is an example.
- **Plaque**: Flat or lightly raised lesion more than 1 cm in diameter.

Elevated Lesions

- **Bulla**: Raised, fluid-filled lesion or blister greater than 1 cm in diameter.
- **Papule**: Small, circular, solid elevation of the skin less than 1 cm in diameter. Warts and pimples are examples.
- **Nodule**: Solid, raised lesion larger than a papule, 0.6 to 2 cm in diameter.
- **Pustule**: Small, circular, pus-filled elevation of the skin, usually less than 1 cm in diameter.
- **Vesicle**: Small, circular, fluid-filled elevation of the skin less than 1 cm in diameter.
- **Wheal**: Smooth, rounded, slightly raised area often associated with itching.

Depressed Lesions

- **Fissure**: Crack or break in the skin; a slit of any size.
- **Ulcer**: An open sore or crater that extends to the dermis resulting from destruction of the skin

Inflammatory Disorders

Many skin disorders are characterized by inflammation. **Contact dermatitis** is skin inflammation and can be caused by allergen exposure or by direct contact with a chemical or plant. For example, poison ivy may be the diagnosis if the skin is **erythematous** (red), covered with tiny vesicles, and itches. The word **pruritus** means itching skin. It comes from the Latin verb *prurio*, which means "to itch." There is no corresponding root, although two other terms come from this same verb. They are **pruritic** (relating to pruritus) and **prurigo** (a chronic skin disease marked by a persistent eruption of papules that itch intensely).

    Eczema is a medical condition characterized by patches of skin that are rough and inflamed, oftentimes with blisters that cause itching and bleeding (see **Figure 4.4**). **Psoriasis** is an inherited inflammatory skin condition (see **Figure 4.5**). Neither of these terms is derived from actual roots, although the suffix *-iasis*, meaning "condition," is a common suffix. **Scleroderma** is taut, thick, leather-like skin.

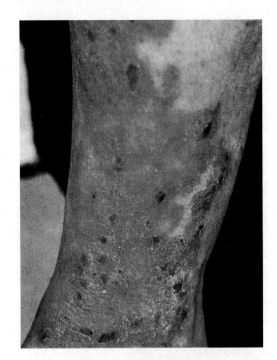

Figure 4.4 Eczema.

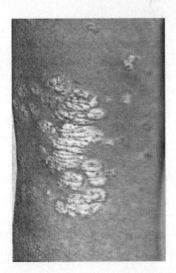

Figure 4.5 Psoriasis.

Skin Cancer

Three types of **malignant** (spreading) skin cancers are *basal cell carcinoma*, *squamous cell carcinoma*, and *malignant melanoma* (see **Figure 4.6**). The term *malignant* comes from the Latin *malignans*, meaning malicious, and is used to describe an invasive, destructive type of cancer. The suffix *-oma* means tumor. Carcinoma is a cancer derived from epithelial cells and is the most commonly occurring type of cancer. The word carcinoma comes from the Greek words *karkinos* (cancer) and *-oma* (tumor). **Malignant melanoma** (also called **melanoma**) is a serious form of skin cancer. Tumors are abnormal tissue growths that can be benign or malignant. **Benign** means nonspreading and is derived from the Latin *benignus*, meaning born well.

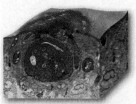
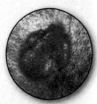

Basal cell carcinoma, the most common skin cancer, begins as a papule, enlarges, and develops a central crater. This crater usually only spreads locally.

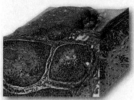

Squamous cell carcinoma begins as a firm, red nodule or scaly, crusted flat lesion. If not treated, this cancer can spread.

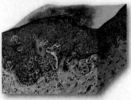

Malignant melanoma can arise on normal skin or from an existing mole. If not treated promptly, it can spread downward into other areas of the skin, lymph nodes, or internal organs.

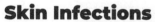

Figure 4.6 Three types of skin cancer.

Skin Infections

Skin is the protective barrier. When it breaks down, bacteria, viruses, fungi, and parasites have an opportunity to invade the body. Many infections, however, can be more annoying than they are serious. The following are examples.

- **Impetigo**: caused by bacteria (*Staphylococcus aureus*) (see **Figure 4.7**)
- **Scabies**: caused by an egg-laying mite (see **Figure 4.8**)
- **Tinea**: caused by a fungus (see **Figure 4.9**)
- **Shingles**: **(herpes zoster)**: caused by a virus; symptoms include pain and a vesicular rash that develops along the path of a nerve (see **Figure 4.10**)

Other Skin Disorders

Some skin and nail disorders do not fit previously mentioned categories. They include **decubitus** (from a Latin verb that means "to lie down") **ulcers**, also known as *bedsores*; **acne**, a disease of the sebaceous glands common in teens and young adults; **vitiligo**,

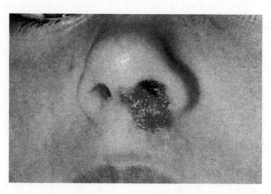

Figure 4.7 Impetigo.

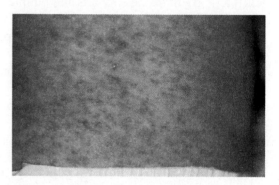

Figure 4.8 Scabies.

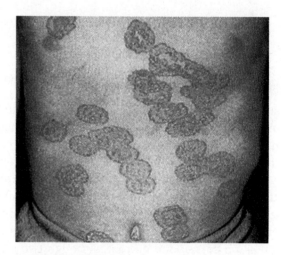

Figure 4.9 Tinea (ringworm).

depigmented blotches or macules that appear on the skin (see **Figure 4.11**); and **paronychia**, an infection of the skin around the nails (see **Figure 4.12**).

Alopecia is the medical term for hair loss or baldness. The term is derived from the Greek word *alōpekia*, meaning "fox mange." Other skin conditions include **erythema** (redness) and **ichthyosis** (dryness and skin scaling that resembles a fish). Edema means *swelling* and is a standard medical term referring to swelling that occurs anywhere in the body.

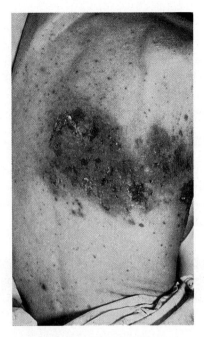

Figure 4.10 Shingles (herpes zoster).

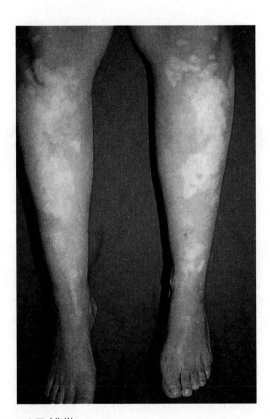

Figure 4.11 Vitiligo.

Diagnostic Tests, Treatments, and Surgical Procedures

Integumentary system surgical procedures are used for diagnosis or treatment of disorders. These procedures may include a **biopsy**, which involves the

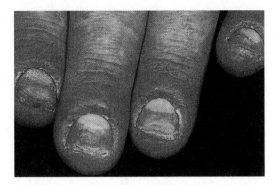

Figure 4.12 Paronychia.

surgical removal of a small piece of skin. **Cryosurgery** and **cryotherapy** use intense cold at the site to destroy tissue. The root *cry/o-* comes from the Greek word *kryos* meaning "cold." In medicine, cryogenic techniques are commonly used to destroy warts, moles, and tumors. Cryogenic surgery often involves the use of liquid nitrogen, a cryogenic liquid, which has a boiling point of –320°F. Liquid nitrogen freezes a small area of tissue quickly, and as the tissue thaws the skin cells are destroyed.

In the case of burns and some ulcerated areas, dead tissue prevents new, healthy tissue from growing. In such cases, a surgical procedure known as **debridement** may be used to remove dead tissue. Once again, the standard word parts you learned are absent from this term, which comes from a French adverb meaning "unbridled." That French word describes the purpose of debridement, which is to "unbridle" the body of dead tissue so that new, healthy tissue can replace it.

Nonsurgical treatments include medications applied to the surface of the skin. The term often used to identify this type of treatment is *topical*, meaning on top of the skin.

Doesn't topical mean "relating to a particular topic," such as a topic in the news? Occasionally, the meaning of an English word changes when a segment of the population begins using it to mean something other than its traditional meaning. The word *topical* is such a word. However, its "medical" meaning most likely came first, given that its medical use dates to the 17th century. Still, dictionaries include the notation *medical* alongside it, probably because English speakers may do a mental double take when encountering its medical use for the first time. Medical terms that fall into this category are identified throughout this book so that, as a medical professional, you will be aware of the possible confusion their use may cause, especially among patients.

Classifications of topical medications are listed as follows:

- **Antibiotics** are used to prevent bacterial infection.
- **Antifungals** are used to kill fungi.
- **Antipruritics** are used to relieve itching.
- **Antiseptics** are used to kill or inhibit bacteria.
- **Scabicides** are used to kill scabies mites.

Other treatments may include oral or injected medication. An example of an oral medication is a steroid, such as prednisone, which is used to treat many inflammatory skin conditions. A medicine that treats inflammation is called an **anti-inflammatory**. Some medications can be given in a **transdermal** manner, which is a method of administering medication through unbroken skin by a patch or topical ointment.

One surgical option is **dermatoplasty**, which uses skin grafts to repair skin. Another option is **incision and drainage (I&D)**, which involves cutting a wound open and allowing it to drain.

Nail treatments include **onychectomy**, the surgical removal of a nail, and **onychotomy**, an incision into a nail.

An antipruritic is used to relieve itching. Another medication that is easily confused with this is an antipyretic, which is used to reduce fever. Antipruritic and antipyretic are easy to mix up, but they have very different purposes.

Practice and Practitioners

The study of the skin and its related conditions is called **dermatology**. A physician who specializes in the diagnosis and treatment of skin disorders is called a **dermatologist**.

Abbreviation Table	The Integumentary System
Abbreviation	**Meaning**
BSA	body surface area
I&D	incision and drainage
SLE	systemic lupus erythematosus
UV	ultraviolet

Study Table		
Term and Pronunciation	**Analysis**	**Meaning**
Structure and Function		
adipose tissue (AD-ih-pose TISH-yoo)	from the Latin word *adiposus* (fat)	fatty tissue
arrector pili muscles (uh-REK-tor PYE-lye MUS-ulz)	from the Latin meaning "that which raises" + *pilus* (hair) + *musculus* (muscle)	bundles of smooth muscle fibers attached to hair follicles that cause the hairs to stand on end causing characteristic "goose bumps"
avascular (ay-VAS-kyuh-lur)	*a-* (without); from the Latin word *vasculum* (small vessel)	without blood vessels
corium (KO-ree-um)	Latin for skin	synonym for dermis, typically used in zoology
cutaneous (cue-TANE-ee-us)	from the Latin word *cutis* (skin)	adjective referring to the skin
cuticle (KUE-tih-kul)	from the Latin word *cutis* (skin)	the thin band of tissue that seals the nail to the skin
dermis (DUR-mis)	from the Greek word *derma* (skin)	inner layer of skin
epidermis (ep-ih-DUR-mis)	*epi-* (upon, above); *dermis* (skin)	outer layer of the skin
free edge (FREE EJ)	from German *frei* (free)	distal region at which the nail ends

Term and Pronunciation	Analysis	Meaning
Structure and Function		
hair follicles (HAIR FAWL-ih-kulz)	from the Latin word *folliculus* (a small sac)	small sacs in the skin from which hair grows
hypodermis (high-poh-DER-mis)	from the Greek word *hypo* (below); *dermis* (skin)	layer immediately beneath the epidermis; also called the subcutaneous layer
integumentary system (in-teg-yoo-MEN-tuh-ree SIS-tem)	from the Latin word *integumentum* (a covering)	the membrane covering the body, including the epidermis, dermis, hair, nails, and glands
keratin (KERR-uh-tin)	from the Greek word *keras* (horn)	protein that forms hair, nails, and the tough outer layer of skin
lunula (LOO-new-luh)	from the Latin word *luna* (moon)	white, crescent-shaped area of a nail
melanin (MEL-uh-nin)	from the Greek word *melas* (black)	dark pigment present in skin and other parts of the body
melanocytes (muh-LAN-uh-sites)	from the Greek word *melas* (black); *-cyte* (cell)	cells that produce melanin
nail (NAIL)	from Old English *naegel* (nail)	translucent plates covering the distal ends of the fingers and toes
pore (POR)	from the Greek word *poros* (passageway)	an opening
sebaceous glands (se-BAY-shus GLANDZ)	from the Latin word *sebum* (grease)	oil-producing glands
sebum (SEE-bum)	Latin for grease	oily secretion
subcutaneous (sub-kyu-TAY-nee-us)	*sub-* (beneath); *cutane* (skin); *-ous* (adjective suffix)	beneath the skin
sudoriferous glands (sue-doe-RIFF-uh-russ GLANDZ)	from two Latin words: *sudor* (sweat) and *fero* (to carry)	sweat-producing glands
Disorders		
abscess (AB-sess)	from the Latin word *abscessus* (a going away), referring to eliminating infection via pus	localized collection of pus in any body part; frequently associated with swelling and inflammation
acne (AK-nee)	from Greek *akmē* (highest point or peak)	inflammatory papular and pustular eruption of the skin
albinism (al-BUH-niz-um)	from the Latin word *albus* (white) and *-ism* (condition)	partial or total absence of pigment of the skin, hair, and eyes
alopecia (al-oh-PEE-shee-uh)	from the Greek word *alōpekia* (fox mange)	partial or complete loss of hair; baldness
benign (buh-NINE)	from the Latin word *benignus* (born well)	nonmalignant type of tumor
bulla (BOOL-uh)	Latin for bubble	raised, fluid-filled lesion greater than 1 cm in diameter
carcinoma (kar-suh-NO-muh)	from the Greek words *karkinos* (cancer) and *-oma* (tumor)	malignant neoplasm derived from epithelial cells

(continues)

Study Table		(continued)
Term and Pronunciation	**Analysis**	**Meaning**
Disorders		
comedo (KOM-eh-doh)	Latin for glutton; from *comedere* (eat up) and referring to sebaceous secretions looking like worms that can be squeezed out of blackheads	blackhead; dilated hair follicle filled with bacteria; primary lesion in acne
contact dermatitis (KON-takt dur-muh-TYE-tiss)	*dermat/o* (skin); *-itis* (inflammation)	inflammation of the skin
cyanosis (SIGH-uh-no-siss)	*cyan/o* (blue); *-osis* (abnormal condition)	abnormal condition signaled by bluish discoloration of tissue
cyst (SIST)	from the Greek word *kystis* (bladder)	closed sac or pouch in or under the skin that contains fluid or solid material
decubitus ulcers (dih-KYOO- bis-tuhs UL-surz)	from the Latin word *decumbere* (to lie down); from the Latin word *ulcus* (sore)	chronic ulcers that appear in pressure areas over a bony prominence in immobilized patients
dermatomycosis (DUR-matt-oh-MY-koh-sis)	*dermat/o* (skin); *myc/o* (fungus); *-osis* (abnormal condition)	fungal infection of the skin
diaphoresis (dy-uh-for-EE-sis)	Greek for perspiration	synonym for perspiration
ecchymosis (ek-ee-MOH-sis)	*ec-* (out); from *chymos* (Greek word for juice); *-osis* (abnormal condition)	a purple patch more than 3 mm in diameter caused by blood under the skin; see also petechiae
eczema (EK-zee-muh)	from the Greek word *eczeo* (boil over)	inflammatory condition of the skin characterized by erythema (redness), vesicles, and crusting with scales
epidermitis (ep-ih-dur-MY-tiss)	*epi-* (upon); *-dermis* (skin); *-itis* (inflammation)	inflammation of the epidermis
erythema (err-ih-THEE-muh)	from the Greek word *eruthēma* (red)	superficial skin redness
erythematous (err-ih-THEE-muh-tus)	from the Greek word *eruthēma* (red)	adjective form of erythema; superficial skin redness
excoriation (ex-KOR-ee-ay-shun)	from the Latin verb *excorio* (to skin)	scratch mark; linear break (caused most often from scratching) in the skin surface
fissure (FISH-ur)	from the Latin word *fissura* (cleft)	a break in the skin
hemangioma (hee-man-jee-OH-muh)	*hem/o* (blood); *angi/o* (vessel); *-oma* (tumor)	benign tumor of blood vessels; birthmark
herpes zoster (HER-peez ZOS-tur)	from the Greek words *herpēs* (creeping) and zoster (belt or girdle)	viral infection producing the eruption of painful vesicles that follow a nerve path; also called *shingles*
hyperhidrosis (high-per-HIGH-droh-sis)	*hyper-* (above normal); *hidr* (sweat); *-osis* (condition of)	profuse sweating; increased or excessive perspiration; may be caused by heat, menopause, or infection
ichthyosis (ik-thee-OH-sis)	*ichthy/o* (fishlike); *-osis* (abnormal condition)	abnormally dry skin; scaly; resembling fish skin
impetigo (im-puh-TYE-go)	from the Latin verb *impeto* (attack)	inflammatory skin disease with pustules that rupture and become crusted

Term and Pronunciation	Analysis	Meaning
Disorders		
keloid (KEE-loid)	from the Greek word *kelis* (tumor) and *-oid* (like)	overgrowth of scar tissue
lesions (LEE-zhunz)	from the Latin verb *laedo* (to injure)	wound, injury, or pathologic change in body tissue
macule (MAK-yul)	from the Latin word *macula* (spot)	flat, discolored area that is flush with the skin; birthmark or freckle
malignant (muh-LIG-nunt)	from the Latin word *malignant* (malicious)	invasive and destructive growth
malignant melanoma (muh-LIG-nunt mel-uh-NO-muh)	from the Latin word *malignant* (malicious) + *melan/o* (black); *-oma* (tumor)	tumor of the melanocytes; skin cancer characterized by dark-pigmented, irregular-shaped lesion; another name for *melanoma*
melanoma (mel-uh-NO-muh)	*melan/o* (black); *-oma* (tumor)	tumor of the melanocytes; skin cancer characterized by dark-pigmented, irregular-shaped lesion; another name for *malignant melanoma*
nevus (NEE-vus)	Latin for birthmark	mole; pigmented skin blemish that is usually benign but may become cancerous
nodule (NOD-yul)	from the Latin word *nodus* (knot)	a small node or circumscribed swelling
onychomalacia (ON-ih-koh-muh-LAY-shee-uh)	*onych/o* (nail); *-malacia* (softening)	softening of the nails
onychopathy (on-ih-KOP-uh-thee)	*onych/o* (nail); *-pathy* (disease)	any disease of the nails
papule (PAP-yul)	from the Latin word *papula* (pimple)	small, circumscribed solid elevation of the skin
paronychia (pair-oh-NIK-ee-uh)	*para-* (alongside); *onych/o* (nail); *-ia* (condition)	infection around a nail
petechiae (peh-TEE-kee-ee)	from the Italian word *petec-chia* (small hemorrhagic spots)	tiny hemorrhagic spots on the skin less than 3 mm in diameter; see also ecchymosis
plaque (PLAK)	from the French from the Dutch word *plak* (plate)	flat or slightly raised lesion greater than 1 cm in diameter
polyp (PAHL-ip)	from the Latin word *polypus* (a growth on a stem)	a mass of tissue that bulges outward from the skin's surface on a stem or stalk of mucous membrane
prurigo (proo-RYE-goh)	from the Latin verb *prurio* (to itch)	a chronic disease of the skin marked by a persistent eruption of papules that itch intensely
pruritic (proo-RIT-ik)	from the Latin verb *prurio* (to itch)	relating to pruritus (itching)
pruritus (proo-RYE-tis)	from the Latin verb *prurio* (to itch)	itching
psoriasis (soh-RYE-ih-sis)	Greek for being itchy	chronic skin disease characterized by itchy, red, silvery-scaled patches

(continues)

Study Table		(continued)
Term and Pronunciation	**Analysis**	**Meaning**
Disorders		
pustule (PUST-yul)	from the Latin word *pustula* (pimple)	small (up to 1 cm in diameter) circumscribed elevation of the skin containing pus
scabies (SKAY-beez)	from the Latin word *scabere* (to scratch)	contagious infection caused by a mite
scleroderma (skler-oh-DER-muh)	*scler/o* (hardness); *-derma* (skin)	chronic disease characterized by thickening and hardening of the skin
shingles (SHIN-gulz)	from the Latin word *cingulum* (girdle)	viral infection producing the eruption of highly painful vesicles that may follow a nerve path; another name for *herpes zoster*
systemic lupus erythematosus (SLE) (sis-TEM-ik LOO-pus err-ih-THEE-muh-tus)	from the Latin word *lupus* (wolf)	inflammatory autoimmune disease characterized by scaly red patches on the skin, especially the face, and affecting connective tissue in organs
tinea (TIN-ee-uh)	Latin for worm	any fungal infection of the skin (tinea barbae = beard; tinea capitis = head; tinea pedis = athlete's foot)
ulcer (UL-sur)	from the Latin word *ulcus* (a sore)	an open sore or lesion of the skin; a lesion through the skin or a mucous membrane resulting from loss of tissue
urticaria (ur-tih-KAR-ee-uh)	from the Latin word *uro* (to burn)	hives; allergic reaction of the skin characterized by eruption of pale red elevated patches
verruca (veh-ROO-kuh)	Latin for wart	wart; caused by a virus
vesicle (VES-ih-kul)	from the Latin word *vesicula* (blister)	small, fluid-filled, raised lesion; a blister
vitiligo (vit-ih-LYE-go)	from the Latin word *vitium* (blemish)	localized loss of skin pigmentation characterized by milk-white patches
wheal (WHEEL)	from the Old English verb *hwelian* (to form pus)	smooth, rounded, slightly elevated area often associated with itching
Diagnostic Tests, Treatments, and Surgical Procedures		
antibiotics (an-tee-BYE-ah-tiks)	*anti-* (against); *biotic* (organism)	medicines that kill bacteria
antifungals (an-tee-FUNG-ulz)	*anti-* (against); *fungal* (fungus)	medicines that kill fungi
anti-inflammatory (an-tee-in-FLAM-uh-tor-ee)	*anti-* (against); *inflammatory* (inflammation)	medicine that reduces inflammation
antipruritics (an-tee-pryu-RIT-iks)	*anti-* (against); *pruritic* (itching)	medicines that reduce itching
antipyretics (an-tee-PYE-ret-tiks)	*anti-* (against); *pyretic* (burning)	medicines that reduce fever
antiseptics (an-tih-SEP-tiks)	*anti-* (against); *septic* (poison)	medicines that inhibit the growth of infectious agents

Term and Pronunciation	Analysis	Meaning
Diagnostic Tests, Treatments, and Surgical Procedures		
biopsy (BYE-op-see)	from the Greek *bios* (life) + *-opsis* (sight)	process of removing tissue for diagnostic examination
cryosurgery (kry-oh-SUR-juh-ree)	*cryo-* (cold); from Old French *surgerie* (operation)	an operation using freezing temperature to destroy tissue
cryotherapy (kry-oh-THER-uh-pee)	*cryo-* (cold); from Latin *therapia* (healing, treat medically)	the use of cold in the treatment of a disease
debridement (deh-BREED-ment)	*de-* (removal); *bridement* (from the word *bridle*, the part of the riding harness by which a rider controls the horse)	removal of necrotic or dead tissue from a wound or burn
dermatoplasty (dur-MAT-oh-plass-tee)	*dermat/o* (skin); *-plasty* (surgical repair)	surgical repair of the skin using grafts
incision and drainage (I&D) (in-SIZH-en AND DRAIN-ij)	from the Latin *incidere* (cut into)	cutting open of a wound or lesion, such as an abscess, and letting out or draining the contents, such as pus
onychectomy (on-ih-KEK-toh-mee)	*onych/o* (nail); *-ectomy* (excision)	surgical removal of a nail
onychotomy (on-ih-KOT-oh-mee)	*onych/o* (nail); *-tomy* (incision)	incision into a nail
scabicides (SKAY-bih-sides)	from the Latin word *scabere* (to scratch); *-cide* (destruction)	medicines lethal to mites
transdermal (trans-DUR-mul)	*trans-* (across); *derm/o* (skin); *-al* (adjective suffix)	a method of administering medication through the unbroken skin via patch or topical ointment
Practice and Practitioners		
dermatologist (dur-MUH-tol-uh-jist)	*dermat/o-* (skin); *-logist* (specialty of)	physician who specializes in dermatology
dermatology (dur-MUH-tol-uh-jee)	*dermat/o-* (skin); *-logy* (study of)	study of the skin and diseases of the skin

CASE STUDY WRAP-UP

The resort had a nurse practitioner on staff, so the two Kekoa children saw her the next day. The nurse practitioner completed a history and physical exam and determined that the children had "hot tub rash." She diagnosed Pseudomonas folliculitis, with blisters and pruritis, and recommended an antibacterial topical cream. Hot tub rash is caused by *Pseudomonas aeuroginosa*, a common microbe that thrives in warm water, like hot tubs. These bacteria can survive in chlorinated water, so it is important that hot tubs be treated regularly and thoroughly with enough chemicals to prevent them from thriving.

Case Study Application Questions

1. Define folliculitis.
2. What caused the folliculitis?
3. Define pruritis.
4. Is the microbe, *Pseudomonas aeruginosa*, a virus or a bacterium? How do you know?

END-OF-CHAPTER EXERCISES

Exercise 4.1 Labeling: Skin

Using the following list, choose the terms to label the diagram correctly.

adipose tissue	arrector pili muscle	artery
dermis	epidermis	hair
hair follicle	hypodermis (subcutaneous) layer	nerve
pore (opening of sweat gland)	sebaceous (oil) gland	sudoriferous (sweat) gland
vein		

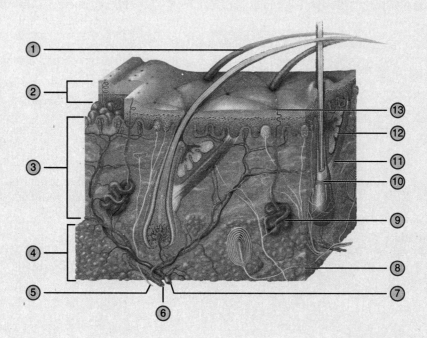

1. _____	6. _____	10. _____
2. _____	7. _____	11. _____
3. _____	8. _____	12. _____
4. _____	9. _____	13. _____
5. _____		

Exercise 4.2 Word Parts

Break each of the following terms into its word parts: prefix, root, or suffix. Give the meaning of each word part and then define the term.

Example transdermal
prefix: trans-, across
root: derm, skin
suffix: al, adjective suffix
definition: a method of administering medication through unbroken skin

1. *avascular*

   prefix: _____

   root: _____

   definition: _____

2. *epidermis*

   prefix: _____

   root: _____

   definition: _____

3. *melanocyte*

   root: _____

   suffix: _____

   definition: _____

4. *scabicide*

   root: _____

   suffix: _____

   definition: _____

5. *dermatomycosis*

   root: _____

   root: _____

   suffix: _____

   definition: _____

6. *onychectomy*

   root: _____

   suffix: _____

   definition: _____

7. *ecchymosis*

   prefix: _____

   root: _____

   suffix: _____

   definition: _____

8. *antiseptic*

prefix: _____

root: _____

definition: _____

Exercise 4.3 Word Building

Use the word parts listed to build the terms defined.

dermat/o	-ia	ichthy	-logy	sub-
-oma	-plasty	-malacia	-tomy	para-
-osis	hem/o	hyper-	-itis	
cutaneous	angi/o	hidr	onych/o	

1. _____ plastic surgical repair of the skin

2. _____ benign tumor of blood vessels

3. _____ inflammation of the skin

4. _____ beneath the skin

5. _____ incision into a nail

6. _____ the study of the skin and diseases of the skin

7. _____ softening of the nails

8. _____ infection around a nail

9. _____ dry, scaly, fishlike skin

10. _____ profuse sweating; increased perspiration

Exercise 4.4 Matching

Match the term with its definition.

1. _____ nevus   a. birthmark

2. _____ verruca   b. thickened scar

3. _____ macule   c. blackhead

4. _____ alopecia   d. mole

5. _____ keloid   e. wart

6. _____ comedo   f. baldness

7. _____ diaphoresis   g. profuse sweating; increased perspiration

8. _____ erythema   h. abrasion of upper skin layers

9. _____ excoriation   i. flat, discolored spot

10. _____ hemangioma   j. redness of the skin

11. _____ cyst   k. localized collection of pus in any part of the body

12. _____ abcess   l. a closed sac or pouch in or under the skin that contains fluid or solid material

Exercise 4.5 Multiple Choice

Choose the correct answer for the following multiple-choice questions.

1. If *myc/o* is the root for fungus, what is the term that means "condition of the nail caused by fungus"?
   a. mycosis
   b. onychomycosis
   c. trichomycosis
   d. onychomalacia
2. If *ichthy* is the root word for dry, fishlike, what is the term for a condition of being extremely dry?
   a. ichthyioma
   b. ichthyosis
   c. ichthyema
   d. ichthiitis
3. The term to describe a lesion of the skin containing pus is _____.
   a. verruca
   b. pustule
   c. bulla
   d. macule
4. A large blister filled with fluid is called a _____.
   a. hemangioma
   b. furuncle
   c. cutis
   d. bulla
5. The medical term for hair loss or baldness that may be total or partial is _____.
   a. dermoplasty
   b. alopecia
   c. urticaria
   d. transdermal
6. The term that best describes the thin band of tissue that seals the nail to the skin is _____.
   a. corium
   b. follicle
   c. cuticle
   d. epidermis
7. The term that best describes the cell that produces the pigment that provides color to the skin and hair is _____.
   a. keratocyte
   b. melanocyte
   c. erythrocyte
   d. leukocyte
8. Which term describes a fungal infection of the skin?
   a. analgesic
   b. dermatomycosis
   c. dermatitis
   d. abscess
9. A viral infection that produces the eruption of highly painful vesicles that may follow a nerve path is _____.
   a. shingles
   b. verruca
   c. herpes zoster
   d. a and c
10. An antipruritic reduces _____.
    a. fever
    b. infection
    c. inflammation
    d. itching
11. An antibiotic kills _____.
    a. fungi
    b. viruses
    c. scabies
    d. bacteria
12. The term *cyst* comes from the Greek word *kystis* meaning _____.
    a. pus
    b. bladder
    c. hill
    d. bump
13. Corium is a synonym for _____.
    a. cuticle
    b. dermis
    c. nail
    d. lunula
14. Diaphoresis is a synonym for _____.
    a. perspiration
    b. exhalation
    c. excretion
    d. inhalation
15. A macule is a _____.
    a. small node
    b. scratch mark
    c. flat, discolored area that is flush with the skin
    d. fluid-containing sac beneath the skin

Exercise 4.6 Fill in the Blank

Fill in the blank with the correct answer.

1. A firm scar that forms in the healing of a sore or wound is a(n) _____.
2. A(n) _____ is a small slit or crack-like lesion.
3. _____ is a condition with a bluish discoloration of tissue.
4. A chronic disease characterized by thickening and hardening of the skin is called _____.
5. Absence or loss of hair is a condition called _____.
6. Partial or complete absence of pigment of the skin, hair, and eyes is termed _____.
7. A loss of skin pigmentation with milk-white skin patches is a condition known as _____.
8. _____, or hives, is an allergic reaction of the skin characterized by pale red eruptions.
9. The removal of a small piece of living tissue for examination under a microscope is called a(n) _____.
10. A(n) _____ is a mass of tissue that bulges outward and grows on a stem or stalk.

Exercise 4.7 Abbreviations

Write out the term for the following abbreviations.

1. _____ BSA
2. _____ I&D

Write the abbreviation for the following terms.

3. _____ systemic lupus erythematosus
4. _____ ultraviolet

Exercise 4.8 Spelling

Select the correct spelling of the medical term.

1. _____ is the surgical removal of a nail.
   a. Onychectomie
   b. Onichektomy
   c. Onchyectomy
   d. Onychectomy

2. _____ plantaris is commonly known as a plantar wart.
   a. Verrooca
   b. Veruca
   c. Verucca
   d. Verruca

3. A _____ is a smooth, rounded, slightly elevated area often associated with itching.
   a. wheel
   b. weal
   c. wheal
   d. weel

4. _____ is characterized by eruption of pale red elevated patches.
   a. Urticaria
   b. Uticaria
   c. Uticarria
   d. Urtikaria

5. _____ is an inflammatory condition of the skin characterized by erythema, vesicles, and crusting with scales.
   a. Excema
   b. Ecksema
   c. Exzema
   d. Eczema

6. The removal of necrotic (dead) tissue from a wound or burn is called _____.
   a. debreedment
   b. dibreedment
   c. debridement
   d. dibridement

7. A chronic skin disease characterized by itchy, silvery-scaled patches is _____.
   a. soriasis
   b. psoriasis
   c. psorasis
   d. soariasis

8. A _____ is a specialist who diagnoses and treats skin diseases.
   a. dermotologist
   b. dermatologyst
   c. dermatolocist
   d. dermatologist

9. The adjective meaning *itchy* is _____.
   a. pruritic
   b. puritic
   c. pyretic
   d. pruitic

10. An _____ is an abnormal redness of the skin.
    a. erythema
    b. erathema
    c. airethema
    d. erethema

Exercise 4.9 Medical Report

Read the case and write a definition for each underlined term in the appropriate space. Think about some of the statements the dermatologist thinks are important enough to include in the report. For example, who diagnosed what? What do pets and children have to do with a diagnosis?

CHIEF COMPLAINT: Rash on the face

PRESENT ILLNESS: A 29-year-old female states that last week she started having some itching on her forehead. She went to the doctor who prescribed erythromycin, an (1) <u>antibiotic.</u> Two days later, the rash covered her entire face. The patient was diagnosed with (2) <u>impetigo</u> and was admitted to the hospital for treatment.

CONSULTATION: Dr. Smith, a (3) <u>dermatologist,</u> saw the patient. The chart was reviewed, and the patient was examined. The patient is married and has no children and no pets. She developed (4) <u>dermatitis</u> on her forehead 2 weeks ago that has spread to her entire face. The rash has become more (5) <u>erythematous,</u> and she now has (6) <u>pustules</u> on her forehead, nose, and cheeks. Facial (7) <u>edema</u> persists, and she is almost unable to open her eyes. She has been given additional antibiotics and an (8) <u>antipruritic medication.</u> She developed (9) <u>pruritus</u> on her feet, which was thought to be a reaction to the antibiotic, so the medication was changed to another antibiotic.

IMPRESSION: Impetigo; allergic response to erythromycin. Patient responds to change in antibiotic. Continue with current antibiotic regimen and continue to monitor patient. Thank you for allowing me to participate in this interesting case. I will follow patient and provide additional suggestions if necessary.

Dr. Smith

Term   **Definition**

1. _____   _____

2. _____   _____

3. _____   _____

4. _____   _____

5. _____   _____

6. _____   _____

7. _____   _____

8. _____   _____

9. _____   _____

10. Why did Dr. Smith ask about children and pets? _____

Exercise 4.10 Reflection

1. What was the most interesting thing you learned in this chapter?
2. How might you use the knowledge gained in your personal life?

CHAPTER 5

The Skeletal System

LEARNING OUTCOMES

Upon completion of this chapter, you should be able to:

- Name the major structures and functions of the skeletal system.
- Differentiate between the axial and appendicular skeleton.
- State the medical terms that name the three types of joints.
- Pronounce, spell, and define medical terms related to the skeletal system and its disorders.
- Interpret abbreviations associated with the skeletal system.
- Apply knowledge gained to Case Study Questions.

CASE STUDY

Fall in February

It was Valentine's Day, and the grandkids were excited to visit Busia. Even though they were young adults, they knew she would have decorated sugar cookies waiting. However, when they arrived at Busia's apartment, they were shocked to see her laying on the floor, conscious and talking, but unable to move. She said that she was simply walking toward the kitchen when she fell. She reports that she had only been on the floor for 5 minutes but that she had severe pain in her left hip that was radiating to her groin and down her leg. The grandkids called 911, and the emergency medical technicians (EMTs) arrived within 10 minutes and took her to the hospital.

Introduction

The skeleton forms the basic structures of the body, much like the framework of concrete and steel does in a tall building. Buildings constructed in earthquake zones are designed to move and sway so they won't fall when the earth moves beneath them. We look upon such buildings as marvels of modern engineering, perhaps without giving much thought to the human skeleton, which allows walking, running, talking, gesturing, throwing things, and even drawing up plans for tall buildings.

Word Parts Related to the Skeletal System

Many terms about the skeletal system are made up of the word parts listed in **Table 5.1**. Other word parts you have already learned are also used to make up some terms in this chapter. Prefixes you learned in Chapter 2, such as dia- (through), epi- (above), endo- (inside), and peri- (around), for example, will be evident in terms introduced under the "Structure and Function" heading. Important word parts to know for this chapter are related to the Greek word, *osteon* for bone and the Latin word *musculus* for muscle. It is also important to know that not every term has a root. The reason is simple: we borrow freely from Greek and Latin, and if you stop to think about that practice, you will realize that every word or word fragment we use is—in a narrow sense at least—a potential root. In other words, prefixes and suffixes can sometimes form the central idea of a term.

Table 5.1 Word Parts Related to the Skeletal System

Word Part	Meaning
-algia	pain
amphi-	both sides
ankyl/o	stiff, fused, closed
arthr/o	joint
brachi/o	arm
calcane/o	calcaneus, heel bone
carp/o	wrist
cervic/o	neck
chondr/o	cartilage
cost/o	rib
crani/o	cranium
dactyl/o	finger, toe
-ectomy	surgical removal
electr/o	electricity
femur/o	femur, thighbone
-gram	written record of something
humer/o	humerus, upper arm bone
-itis	inflammation
kinesi/o	movement
-kinesia	movement
kyph/o	hump
-logy	study of
lord/o	swayback, curve
lumb/o	lower back
-malacia	softening
muscul/o	muscle
my/o	muscle

Word Part	Meaning
myel/o	bone marrow
-oma	tumor
orth/o	correct, straight
os/te/o	bone
ped/o	foot, child
pelv/o	pelvis
phalang/o	bones of fingers and toes
-physis	growth
-plasty	surgical repair
-porosis	porous
-scopy	to visually examine
spondyl/o	vertebrae
syn-	joined together
thorac/o	thorax, chest
vertebr/o	vertebrae
zygo-	joined (yoked) together

Isn't it true that some people have more than 206 bones? The response 206 was deemed correct on a Jeopardy! game show, so it must be true! All joking aside, the exact number of bones can vary slightly from one person to another because some people may have extra ribs, vertebrae, or sesamoid bones that develop around joints.

Word Parts Exercise

After studying Table 5.1, write the meaning of each of the word parts.

Word Part	Meaning
1. lord/o	1. _____
2. zygo-	2. _____
3. carp/o	3. _____
4. ped/o	4. _____
5. os/te/o	5. _____
6. phalang/o	6. _____
7. -algia	7. _____
8. crani/o	8. _____
9. syn-	9. _____
10. -itis	10. _____

(continued)

Word Part	Meaning
11. my/o, muscul/o	11. _____
12. -scopy	12. _____
13. kinesi/o	13. _____
14. orth/o	14. _____
15. femur/o	15. _____
16. -malacia	16. _____
17. -plasty	17. _____
18. arthr/o	18. _____
19. pelv/o	19. _____
20. -physis	20. _____
21. brachi/o	21. _____
22. dactyl/o	22. _____
23. cost/o	23. _____
24. myel/o	24. _____
25. electr/o	25. _____
26. thorac/o	26. _____
27. humer/o	27. _____
28. -porosis	28. _____
29. ankyl/o	29. _____
30. spondyl/o, vertebr/o	30. _____
31. -gram	31. _____
32. -kinesia	32. _____
33. amphi-	33. _____
34. calcane/o	34. _____
35. kyph/o	35. _____
36. cervic/o	36. _____
37. -logy	37. _____
38. chondr/o	38. _____
39. lumb/o	39. _____
40. -ectomy	40. _____
41. -oma	41. _____

Structure and Function

The human skeleton begins to form about 6 weeks after fertilization and continues to grow and develop until the person is around 25 years old. The body's approximately 206 bones have many functions.

The skeleton serves as a rigid but articulating (movable at joints) framework for muscles and other tissues. It also protects vital organs by forming a shield against jarring and bumps. Its less obvious jobs are to store minerals and to make blood cells.

The skeleton is divided into two parts: the **axial skeleton** and **appendicular skeleton** (see **Figure 5.1**). The words axial and appendicular are adjective forms of the words, axis and appendix. Axis is derived from the Latin words for axle and pivot. Thus, axis is a common English word meaning an imaginary straight line around which something pivots, such as the one between the north and south poles of the earth. The axial skeleton has an axis running from the middle of the top of the head to the bottom of the spine. The axial skeleton therefore includes the bones on this axis: the skull, chest, and spinal column.

The appendicular skeleton comprises the arms and legs, along with the shoulder and pelvic bones. Although the appendicular skeleton has nothing to do with the appendix, which is an internal organ, these

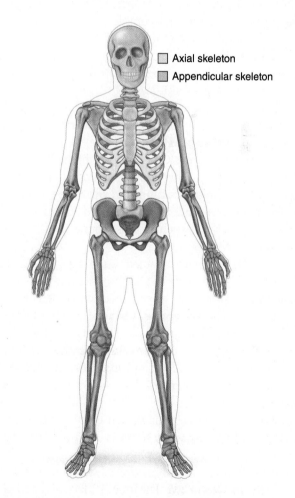

Figure 5.1 Axial and appendicular skeletons. The axial skeleton is shown in yellow, and the appendicular skeleton is shown in gray.

structures do have a common word origin: the Latin word *appendere* refers to something attached to something else. Thus, the appendicular skeleton is attached to the axial skeleton, and the appendix is attached to the large intestine.

The skeletal system depends on *ligaments*, *tendons*, and *joints* to allow for movement. Ligament comes from the Latin word *ligamentum*, meaning "a band" or "banding." **Ligaments** are bands of tissue that connect two bones together. Tendon comes from the verb *teinein*, which means to stretch, which is what tendons do. **Tendons** attach muscles to bone. The difference between these two connective tissues is that ligaments connect two bones, whereas tendons connect a muscle to a bone. Strictly speaking, of course, these two terms belong to the muscular system, but they are mentioned here because their function is essential to the skeleton. **Joints**, also called *articulations*, are the places where bones come together.

Ossification is bone formation, and it begins early in fetal development when the skeleton is composed mostly of cartilage. During the second and third months of fetal development, cartilage hardens and turns into bone, but complete ossification takes place after birth until about age 25. Bone is made up of **osseous tissue**, a form of connective tissue with mature bone cells called **osteocytes**. As a living tissue, bone undergoes a process of *remodeling* throughout life. This means that there is a delicate balance between bone break down by **osteoclasts** and bone build up by **osteoblasts**.

The bones of the skeleton are of different shapes, sizes, and makeup. They may be essentially flat, such as those found in the cranium and ribs. They may also be short, such as those in the wrist and ankles. Or the bones may be long, such as those found in the arms, legs, hands, and feet.

Long bones have named subparts. The term **diaphysis** is the shaft of a long bone, and the term **epiphysis** is the name given to each expanded end of a long bone. The **epiphyseal plate** (growth plate) is the growth area of a long bone. The term for the interior of the diaphysis is **medullary cavity**. Because it is a cavity, it is hollow, and *medullary* means that the cavity contains marrow. *Marrow* is the tissue that produces blood cells.

Compact bone is hard, dense bone and makes up the diaphysis. **Spongy bone** is mesh-like bone tissue and is found in the epiphyses (*epiphysis*, singular).

Most bone surfaces are covered with a membrane called the **periosteum**. The inner surface of the medullary cavity is lined with a thin layer of cells called the **endosteum** (see **Figure 5.2**).

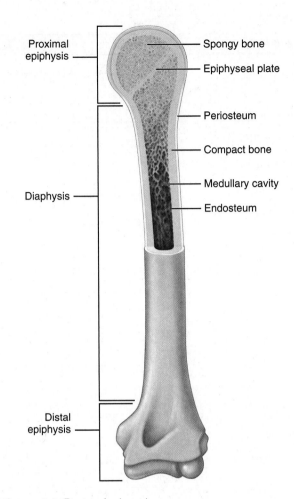

Figure 5.2 Parts of a long bone.

By now, you are probably familiar with the prefixes, *peri-* and *endo-*. But if you didn't automatically identify those prefixes as meaning around and inside, you may benefit from a review of Chapter 2, Table 2.8.

The Axial Skeleton

The axial skeleton comprises the bones of the **cranium** (head), thorax, and **vertebral column** (series of vertebrae from the cranium to the coccyx). Cranial bones enclose and protect the brain. The six main cranial bones include the **frontal bone**; two **parietal bones**, one on each side; two **temporal bones**, on the sides of the head; and the **occipital bone** (see **Figure 5.3**).

Facial bones protect entrances to the digestive and respiratory tracts. The main paired facial bones are the *nasal bone*, *zygomatic bone*, the *maxilla*, and the *mandible*. The **nasal bone** forms the bridge of the nose, and the two **zygomatic bones** form the cheeks. The **maxilla** is the immovable upper jawbone, and the **mandible** is the movable lower jawbone.

Lateral view

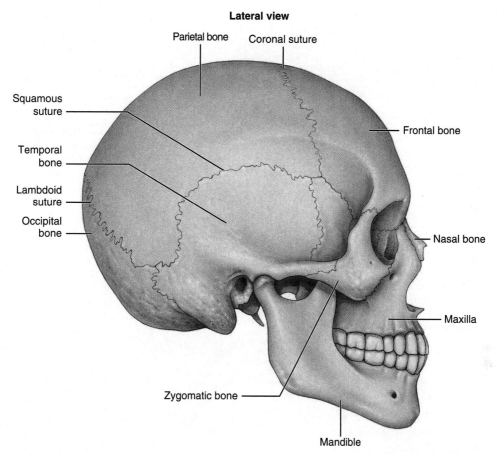

Parietal bone   Coronal suture

Squamous suture

Temporal bone

Lambdoid suture

Occipital bone

Frontal bone

Nasal bone

Maxilla

Zygomatic bone

Mandible

Figure 5.3 The bones of the cranium, face, and the associated sutures.

The cranial bones are joined by **cranial sutures**, which are fibrous membranes that join them. These include the *coronal suture*, *squamous suture*, and *lambdoid suture* (see Figure 5.3).

> Isn't *maxilla* Latin for jaw? Yes. So where does the word mandible come from if we already have a Latin word for jaw? Mandible comes from the Latin word *mandibula*, which means "to chew," and the mandible moves while chewing.

The skeleton of the **thorax** (*thorax*, breastplate) is known as the **thoracic cage** (rib cage). The thoracic cage includes the 12 thoracic vertebrae, 12 ribs, costal (rib) cartilages, and the sternum. Parts of the flat **sternum** are the manubrium, body, and xiphoid process. The major organs inside the thoracic cage are the heart and lungs (see **Figure 5.4**).

Rib pairs are attached to their corresponding numbered **vertebrae** (back bones). Ribs 1 to 7 are called *true ribs* or *vertebrosternal ribs* because their cartilages attach directly to the sternum. Ribs 8 to 12 are the five lower ribs that do not attach directly to the sternum. Ribs 8 to 10 are called *false ribs* or *vertebrochondral* ribs. The last two rib pairs (11 and 12) "float," which

means that they are attached only to the vertebrae (see Figure 5.4).

The spinal column includes five sections of vertebrae (*vertebra*, singular). The naming of a vertebra consists of a prefix letter (C for cervical, T for thoracic, and L for lumbar), followed by a number indicating the placement on the column. There are 7 cervical vertebrae (C1–C7), 12 thoracic vertebrae (T1–T12), and 5 lumbar vertebrae (L1–L5). At the base of the spinal column are the sacrum and coccyx. The **sacrum** is formed by five fused sacral vertebrae, and the **coccyx** contains three to five fused coccygeal vertebrae (see **Figure 5.5**).

> Isn't the cervix part of the female reproductive system? The word *cervix* is Latin for "neck." The words cervix and cervical refer not only to the "neck" of the uterus, which is a part of the female reproductive system (see Chapter 15), but also to the neck to which the head is attached.

The Appendicular Skeleton

Recall that the appendicular skeleton consists of the body's appendages (upper limbs and lower limbs)

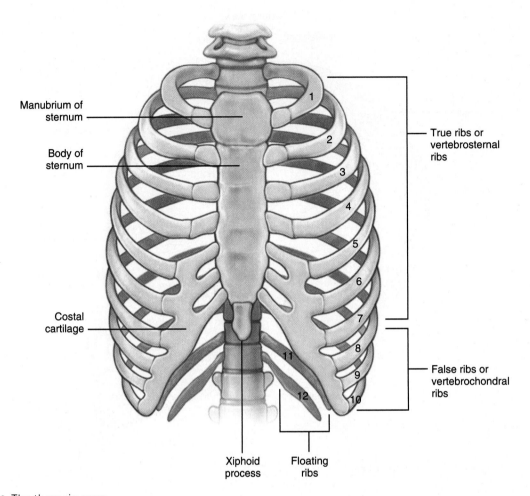

Manubrium of sternum

Body of sternum

Costal cartilage

True ribs or vertebrosternal ribs

False ribs or vertebrochondral ribs

Xiphoid process

Floating ribs

Figure 5.4 The thoracic cage.

and the areas to which these appendages are attached: *shoulder girdle* and *pelvic girdle*. An upper limb is also called an *upper extremity*, and a lower limb is also called a *lower extremity*. The shoulder girdle is also called the *pectoral girdle*. Shoulder girdle bones include the **clavicle** (collarbone) and the **scapula** (shoulder blade) (see **Figure 5.6**).

The long arm bone extending from the shoulder and ending at the elbow is called the **humerus**, not because it is the "funny bone" but because *humerus* is the Latin word for "shoulder." However, there is a connection with the word "humorous." The phrase "funny bone" was most probably coined as a joke because the ulnar nerve, which causes the pins-and-needles sensation when it is struck, is located where the humerus joins the elbow (see **Figures 5.6** and **5.7**).

The forearm consists of the **ulna** and **radius**, which extend from the elbow to the wrist (see Figure 5.7). The wrist includes eight bones, arranged in two rows, called **carpal bones** (*karpos*, wrist). These bones are the *scaphoid, lunate, triquetrum, pisiform, trapezium, trapezoid, capitate,* and *hamate*. The five

metacarpals are the hand bones connecting the wrist to the fingers. The 14 **phalanges** are the bones that make up the fingers. The term *phalanges* is the plural form of *phalanx*, which is Greek for "line of soldiers." The bones of the wrist and hand are shown in **Figure 5.8**.

The pelvic girdle, so named because it surrounds and protects the pelvic organs, consists of the two hip bones (right and left), joined anteriorly at the pubic symphysis and posteriorly at the sacrum. The **hip bone**, also called the *coxal bone*, is a fusion of three bones: the **ilium**, the **ischium**, and the **pubis**.

The **femur**, Latin for "thigh," is a long bone that extends from the hip to the knee, and the **tibia** and **fibula** are long bones that extend from the knee to the ankle. The femur attaches to the pelvic girdle (hip) at the *acetabulum* (see **Figures 5.9** and **5.10**). The tibia, Latin for "shin," is the shin bone or heavy bone of the lower leg. The fibula, from the Latin word *figibula*, meaning "fastener," does not bear the body's weight, but together with the tibia, it is connected to the **talus** (ankle bone) (see **Figure 5.11**). The **patella** (kneecap) is a "floating" bone that is imbedded in the tendon of

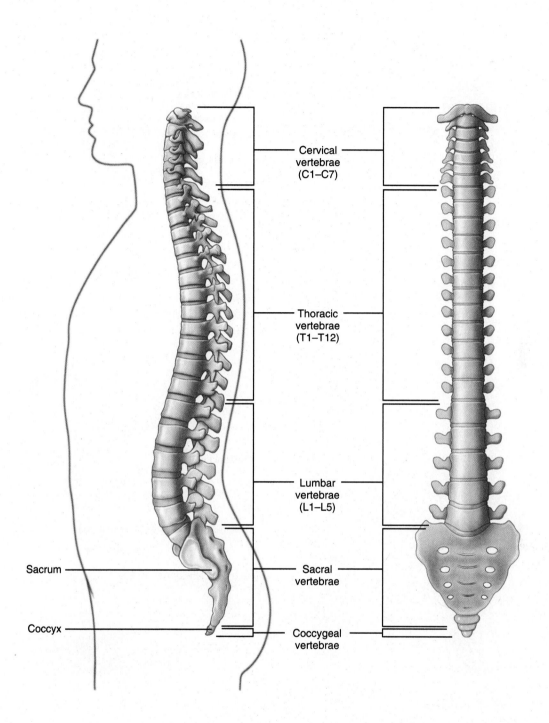

Figure 5.5 The vertebral column in sagittal (anteroposterior) and anterior views.

the thigh muscle. It offers protection to the knee joint (see Figure 5.10).

Tarsus (from the Greek *tarsos*, meaning "flat of the foot") is sometimes used as a technical name for the ankle. The seven **tarsal bones** of the ankle and the five **metatarsals** of the foot correspond with the carpal bones and metacarpals of the wrist and hand. The tarsal bones are the *talus; calcaneus;*

navicular; medial, lateral, and intermediate cuneiforms; and *cuboid.* Just like the fingers, the bones making up the toes are also called **phalanges**. The bony protrusion at the distal end of the fibula is called the **lateral malleolus**; the bony process on the tibia is the **medial malleolus**. The heel bone, or **cal-caneus**, is the largest bone in the foot. Figure 5.11 shows the bones of the ankle and foot.

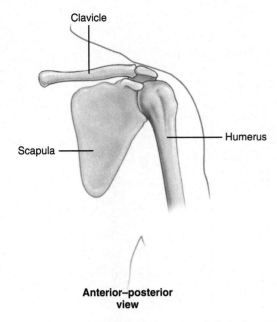

Anterior–posterior view

Figure 5.6 The bones of the shoulder girdle show the articulation with the humerus.

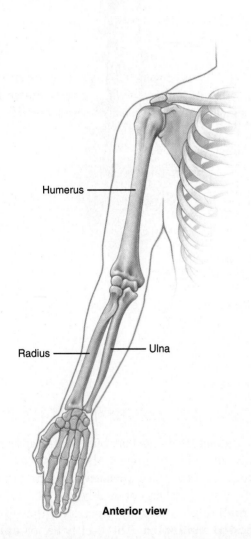

Anterior view

Figure 5.7 Bones of the upper limb. The arm contains the humerus, and the forearm is made up of the radius and ulna.

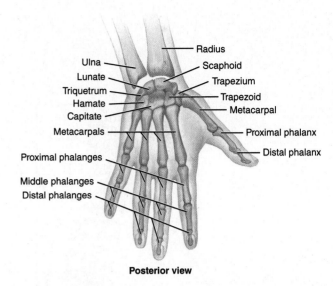

Posterior view

Figure 5.8 Wrist and hand bones. Eight carpal bones form the wrist. Five metacarpals and 14 phalanges form the hand. The pisiform is not visible in this view.

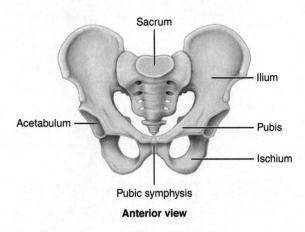

Anterior view

Figure 5.9 The bones of the pelvic girdle.

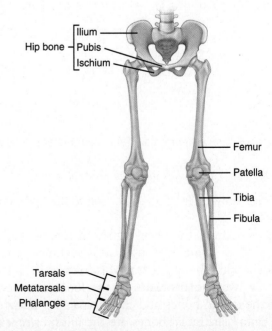

Figure 5.10 Bones of the pelvic girdle and lower limb.

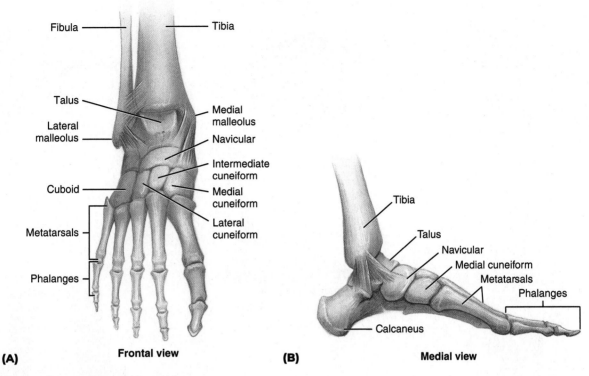

Figure 5.11 Bones of the ankle and foot.

Joints

A **joint**, or *articulation,* is the place where bones come together. Some joints, such as the shoulder and hip, are highly movable, and some have little or no movement. A joint with no movement is called a **synarthrosis**. Any of the suture joints in the cranium would be a good example of a synarthrosis. A joint with little movement is called an **amphiarthrosis**. The joint between the pubic bones, called the pubic symphysis, is an example of an amphiarthrosis. A joint that is freely movable is called a **diarthrosis** or a **synovial joint**. Examples of diarthroses are the shoulder, knee, and ankle.

The spaces within each synovial joint are filled with a viscous liquid called **synovial fluid**. Although the spaces in a large joint are so small that less than 1/100th of an ounce of synovial fluid fills it, the fluid is needed to lubricate the joint as it moves and to cushion it against jolts. Synovial joints permit a variety of movements and are further classified based on *how* they move. The knee and elbow joints, for example, are "hinge joints" that allow *flexion* (decreasing the angle at a joint causing bending of the limb) and *extension* (increasing the angle at a joint causing straightening of the limb). The "ball-and-socket joint" of the shoulder provides the greatest range of motion (ROM) including rotation.

Cartilage, a precursor of bone tissue, is classified as connective tissue, but it is mentioned here because cartilage enables movement in the synovial joints.

Bursae (*bursa*, singular) are found wherever tendons or ligaments impinge on other tissues. Bursae are spaces within connective tissue filled with synovial fluid.

Figure 5.12 shows the various movements at synovial joints, and **Table 5.2** describes their various movements.

QUICK CHECK

Fill in the blank with the correct answer.

1. Osseous tissue consists of special mature bone cells called _____.
2. A diarthrosis is a joint that has free movement. It is also called a(n) _____ joint.
3. The paired facial bones include the nasal bone, zygomatic bone, the maxilla, and the _____.

Disorders Related to the Skeletal System

A **sprain** is a tear in a ligament or the fibrous tissue that connects bones. A **fracture** (Fx) is a broken bone. However, not all fractures are the same. If the fracture is a **simple fracture** (**closed fracture**), there is no open skin. If the broken bone protrudes through the skin, it is called a **compound fracture** (**open fracture**).

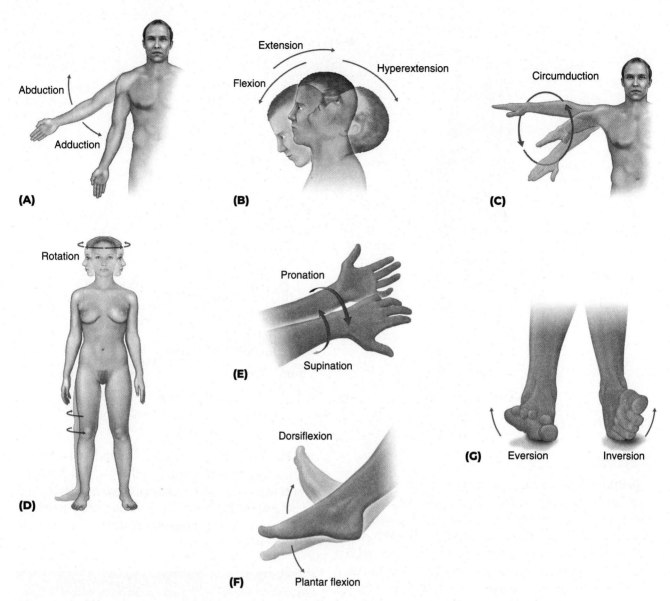

Figure 5.12 Movements at synovial joints.

Table 5.2 Movements of Synovial Joints

Movement	Description
abduction	movement away from the midline of the body
adduction	movement toward the midline of the body
flexion	decreasing the angle of a joint; movement that bends a limb
extension	increasing the angles of a joint; movement that straightens a limb
hyperextension	excessive extension beyond the normal anatomical position; movement could not be done without incurring damage, such as whiplash
circumduction	movement in a circular direction from a central point
rotation	turning a body part on its own axis
pronation	turning the palm posteriorly
supination	turning the palm anteriorly

Table 5.2 Movements of Synovial Joints *(continued)*

Movement	Description
dorsiflexion	bending the sole foot upward toward the shin
plantar flexion	bending the sole of the foot downward or pointing the toes downward
eversion	turning the sole of the foot outward
inversion	turning the sole of the foot inward

Common Types of Fractures

Fracture	Description	Example
Simple (closed)	break in which there is no open skin	**Simple (closed)**
Compound (open)	broken bone protrudes through the skin	**Compound (open)**
Comminuted	break in which the bone is crushed or splintered	**Comminuted**

Common Types of Fractures

Fracture	Description	Example
Spiral	break is S-shaped, usually caused by a twisting injury	**Spiral**
Transverse	break is straight across the shaft of the bone, at a right angle to the long axis	**Transverse**
Greenstick	incomplete break in which the bone bends	**Greenstick**

Bone disorders arising from disease include conditions such as **osteomyelitis**, an inflammation caused by bacteria. **Osteoporosis** is a bone disorder characterized by a decrease in bone density and mass. Two other bone disorders are **rickets**, causing bowed legs in children, and **osteomalacia**, which is bone softening in adulthood. These two conditions result from vitamin deficiency and lack of calcium absorption. **Neoplasms** or tumors of the bone may be primary (originating at the site) or secondary (originating from other sites in the body). **Osteosarcoma** is a bone tumor. **Chondrosarcoma** is a tumor that originates in cartilage.

Joint disorders include **arthritis**, a general term used for joint inflammation. Joint degeneration from wear and tear over time results in **osteoarthritis**. **Rheumatoid arthritis** (RA) also results in inflammation, but it has a different cause than osteoarthritis. Rheumatoid arthritis is a long-term autoimmune disorder that results in inflammation with subsequent tissue destruction (see **Figure 5.13**).

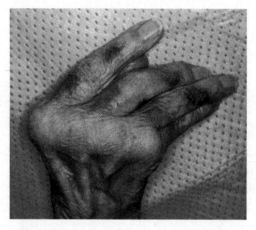

Figure 5.13 Advanced rheumatoid arthritis. These hands show joint swelling and finger deformity.

The spine has several conditions that affect it. A disc that protrudes into the vertebral canal and puts pressure on the spinal nerve is called a **herniated disc**. Compression fractures of the vertebrae may produce **kyphosis** (humpback) and loss of height. **Lordosis** is curvature in the lumbar region. **Scoliosis** is a sideways curvature of the spine that may occur in any region of the spine (see **Figure 5.14**).

Diagnostic Tests, Treatments, and Surgical Procedures

Treatment of a fracture consists of **reduction** (realignment) of the broken bone. In some cases, **traction** (Tx) (using elastic bands or pulley and weights to maintain alignment) may be needed. Casts and splints are used to immobilize a broken bone during the healing process.

Symptomatic treatments (just treating the symptoms but not the problem) are also common with skeletal system conditions. For osteoarthritis, treatment may include medication for pain and inflammation and/or physical therapy. For conditions like rheumatoid arthritis, treatments consist of medication, rest, and physical therapy. Another option is **arthrocentesis**, which drains fluid and relieves the pressure in the joint.

Practice and Practitioners

Many specialists work in **orthopedics**, the branch of medicine dealing with the musculoskeletal

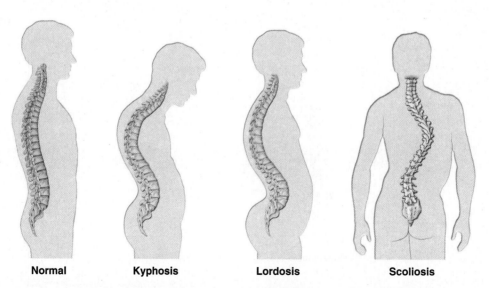

Normal   **Kyphosis**   **Lordosis**   **Scoliosis**

Figure 5.14 Abnormal curvatures of the spine can cause pain and disfigurement.

system. **Orthopedic surgeons** coordinate patient care with **physical therapists** (professionals who treat disorders with physical methods), **occupational therapists** (professionals who rehabilitate through performance of activities of daily living), **kinesiologists** (professionals who aid by studying body movements), or other practitioners in sports medicine. A **rheumatologist** is a physician who specializes in the treatment of infectious or inflammatory joint disorders and other conditions of the musculoskeletal system.

What is the difference between occupational therapy and physical therapy? The goal of occupational therapy is for the individual to be able to take care of themselves and complete activities of daily living, such as getting in and out of the car, getting dressed, or being able to push a grocery cart in the store. This type of therapy is common for people who recently had a stroke or surgery, such as total hip replacement (THR) or total knee arthroplasty (TKA). Physical therapy focuses on muscle groups to help the individual improve strength, balance, and range of motion. Physical therapy is common after sports injuries, like an anterior cruciate ligament (ACL) tear.

Abbreviation Table The Skeletal System

Abbreviation	Meaning
ACL	anterior cruciate ligament
C (C1–C7)	cervical
CT	computed tomography
Fx	fracture
L (L1–L5)	lumbar
MRI	magnetic resonance imaging
NSAID	nonsteroidal anti-inflammatory drug
RA	rheumatoid arthritis
ROM	range of motion
S	sacral
T (T1–T12)	thoracic
THR	total hip replacement
TKA	total knee arthroplasty
TKR	total knee replacement
Tx	traction

Study Table The Skeletal System

Term and Pronunciation	Analysis	Meaning
Structure and Function		
amphiarthrosis (AM-fee-ar-THROW-sis)	*amphi-* (both sides); *arthr/o* (joint); *-osis* (abnormal condition)	joint with little movement
appendicular skeleton (APP-en-DIK-yu-lur SKEL-uh-tun)	adjective referring to something that is added or attached	bones of the limbs, including the shoulder girdle and pelvic girdle
axial skeleton (AX-ee-ul SKEL-uh-tun)	adjective form of axis, a common English word	articulated bones of the head, vertebral column, and thorax
brachial (BRAY-kee-ul)	*brachi/o* (arm); *-al* (adjective suffix)	having to do with an arm
bursae; bursa (singular) (BUR-see; BUR-suh)	a Latin word meaning "bag or purse"	saclike connective structure found in some joints that contains synovial fluid; protects moving parts from friction
calcaneus (kal-KAY-nee-us)	Latin word for heel	the heel bone
carpal bones (KAR-pull BONZ)	adjective form of carpus (wrist)	wrist bones
cartilage (CAR-tih-lij)	from the Latin word *cartilago* (gristle)	dense, flexible connective tissue
cervical (SUR-vih-kul)	*cervic/o* (neck); *-al* (adjective suffix)	adjective describing the vertebrae (C1–C7) in the neck region; also used in connection with the uterus, which is part of the female reproductive system

(continues)

Study Table The Skeletal System		(continued)
Term and Pronunciation	**Analysis**	**Meaning**
Structure and Function		
cervix (SUR-vix)	Latin word for neck	neck (also the neck of the uterus)
clavicle; clavicular (adjective) (KLAV-ih-kul; kluh-VIK-yu-lur)	from the Latin word *clavicula* (a small key)	the collarbone
coccyx; coccygeal (adjective) (KOK-six; kok-sih-JEE-ul)	from the Greek word *kokkyx* (cuckoo; because the bone shape resembles the cuckoo's bill)	the tailbone, made up of the four fused vertebrae at the base of the spinal column
compact bone (KOM-pakt BONE)	common English word	type of dense bone
coxal bone (COX-ul BONE)	*coxa* (Latin for hip)	hip bone
cranial bones (KRAY-nee-ul BONZ)	*crani/o* from the Greek word *kranion* (skull); *-al* (adjective form)	collectively, and along with other minor bones, the frontal bone, two parietal bones, two temporal bones, and the occipital bone
cranial sutures (KRAY-nee-ul SOO-churz)	from the Latin word *sutura* (seam)	fibrous membrane forming an immovable joint that joins the skull bones
cranium (KRAY-nee-um)	from medieval Latin, *kranion* (skull)	the bones of the head
diaphysis (dye-AFF-ih-sis)	a Greek word (growing between)	shaft of the long bone
diarthrosis (dye-ar-THRO-sis)	a Greek word (articulation)	synonym for synovial joint
endosteum (en-DOS-tee-um)	*endo-* (inside); *oste/o* (Greek word for bone)	inner membrane layer of the bone
epiphyseal plate (ep-ih-FIZ-ee-ul PLATE)	relating to an epiphysis (bone end)	disk of cartilage between the metaphysis and epiphysis of an immature long bone; growth plate
epiphysis (eh-PIFF-ih-sis)	*epi-* (upon; above); *-physis* (growth)	end of the long bone (proximal, distal)
extension (ex-TEN-shun)	a common English word	to straighten a joint
femur (FEE-mur)	a Latin word (thigh)	thighbone
fibula (FIB-yu-luh)	a Latin word (clasp)	the lateral leg bone
flexion (FLEX-shun)	from the Latin verb *flectere* (to bend)	bending a joint
frontal bone (FRUN-tul BONE)	frontal (adjective form of English noun: front)	one of the six main cranial bones
hip bone (HIP BONE)	from the Old English, *hype*	large flat bone formed by the fusion of the ilium, ischium, and pubis
humerus (HUE-muh-rus)	Latin for shoulder	the long bone extending from the shoulder to the elbow

Term and Pronunciation	Analysis	Meaning
Structure and Function		
ilium (IL-ee-um)	Latin for flank	one of the three bones fused together to form the hip bone
ischium (IS-kee-um)	Latin for hip	one of the three bones fused together to form the hip bone
Joint (JOINT)	from the Latin word *jungere* (to join)	place where two bones come together
lateral malleolus (LAT-er-ul mahl-ee-OH-lus)	from the Latin words, *lateralis* (side) and *malleus* (hammer)	projection on the lateral side of the lower end of the fibula
ligaments (LIG-uh-ments)	from the Latin word *ligamentum* (a tie or binding)	tissue that connects two bones
lumbar (LUM-bar)	from the Latin word *lumbus* (loin); *-ar* (adjective suffix)	adjective describing the vertebrae (L1–L5) in the lower vertebral column
mandible; mandibular (adjective) (MAN-dih-bul; man-DIB-yu-lur)	from the Latin verb *mandere* (to chew)	the lower jawbone
maxilla; maxillary (adjective) (MAX-ih-luh; MAX-ih-lair-ee)	Latin for jawbone	the bone above the upper teeth
medial malleolus (mee-DEE-ul mahl-ee-OH-lus)	from the Latin words *medialis* (middle) and *malleus* (hammer)	projection on the medial side of the lower end of the tibia
medulla (MUH-dull-uh)	Latin for marrow	soft, marrow-like structure
medullary cavity (MED-yu-lair-ee KAV-ih-tee)	an adjective form of *medulla* (Latin for marrow)	bone marrow cavity
metacarpals (MET-uh-KAR-pulz)	*meta-* (beyond); carp from *carpus* (wrist); *-al* (adjective suffix)	the five bones extending from the wrist to the first knuckle in each hand
metatarsals (MEH-uh-TAR-sulz)	*meta-* (beyond); tarsal from *tarsos* (flat surface); *-al* (adjective suffix)	the bones between the tarsals and the phalanges (toes) of the foot
nasal bone (NAY-zuhl BONE)	*nas/o* (nose); *-al* (adjective suffix)	a facial bone (nose)
occipital bone (ox-SIP-it-ul BONE)	*occiput* (Latin for back of the head); *-al* (adjective suffix)	one of the six main cranial bones
osseous tissue (OSS-ee-us TISH-yu)	from the Latin word *osseus* (bony); *-ous* (adjective suffix)	bone tissue
ossification (OSS-ih-fih-KAY-shun)	*os* (bone); *facio* (Latin verb for make)	bone formation
osteoblast (OSS-tee-oh-blast)	*osteo-* (bone); *blastos* (Greek for germ, sprout)	bone cell that secretes bone matrix
osteoclast (OSS-tee-oh-klast)	*osteo-* (bone); *klastēs* (Greek for breaker)	bone cell that destroys bone matrix
osteocyte (OSS-tee-oh-sight)	*oste/o* (bone); *-cyte* (cell)	mature bone cells
osteogenesis (oss-tee-oh-JEN-uh-sis)	*oste/o* (bone); *-genesis* (origin)	formation of bone
parietal bones (puh-RYE-uh-tul BONZ)	from a Latin word *paries* (wall) and *-al* (adjective suffix)	two of the six main cranial bones

(continues)

Study Table The Skeletal System		*(continued)*
Term and Pronunciation	**Analysis**	**Meaning**
Structure and Function		
patella (puh-TELL-uh)	Latin for small plate	kneecap
pectoral girdle (pek-TOR-ul GIR-dul)	from *pectus*, a Latin word (chest); -*al* (adjective suffix)	the shoulder girdle
periosteum (pair-ee-OS-tee-um)	*peri-* (around); *oste/o* (bone)	membrane that surrounds the outside of the bone
phalanges (FUH-lan-jeez)	plural of the Greek word *phalanx* (a line of soldiers)	fingers (singular form is phalanx)
pubis (PYU-bis)	short for "os pubis"; from the Latin word *os pubes* (bones of the pubes)	one of the three bones fused together to form the hip bone
radius; radial (adjective) (RAY-dee-us; RAY-dee-ul)	a Latin word (staff, spoke, ray)	one of the two bones (the other is the ulna) extending from the elbow to the wrist
sacrum; sacral (adjective) (SAY-krum; SAK-rul)	from Latin *os sacrum* (sacred bone; from the belief that the soul resided there)	bone formed from five vertebrae fused together near the base of the vertebral column
scapula; scapulae (plural); scapular (adjective) (SKAP-yu-luh; SKAP-yu-lay; SKAP-yu-lur)	Latin for shoulder blade	the shoulder blade
synarthrosis (syn-ARE-throw-sis)	*syn-* (together); *arthr/o* (joint); -*osis* (condition)	joint with no movement
synovial joint (sigh-NO-vee-ul JOINT)	*syn-* (together); Latin *ovum* (egg); -*al* (adjective suffix)	freely movable joint; diarthrosis
talus (TAY-lus)	Latin for ankle	the bone in the ankle that articulates with the tibia and fibula
tarsal bones (TAR-sul BONZ)	from the Greek word *tarsos* (a flat surface, sole of the foot)	the bones of the sole of the foot
tarsus (TAR-sus)	from the Greek word *tarsos* (flat of the foot)	ankle
tendons (TEN-dunz)	from the verb *teinein* (to stretch)	connective tissue that connects muscle to bone
temporal bones (TEM-por-ul BONZ)	from the Latin *tempus* (time, temple)	two of the six main cranial bones; located on the side of the head near the ears
thoracic cage (thor-ASS-ik CAGE)	from the Greek word *thorax* (breastplate, chest)	skeleton of the thoracic consisting of the thoracic vertebrae, ribs, costal (rib) cartilages, and sternum
thorax (THOR-ax)	from the Greek word *thorax* (breastplate, chest)	chest
tibia; tibial (adjective) (TIH-bee-uh; TIH-bee-ul)	Latin for shin bone	shin bone
ulna; ulnar (adjective) (ULL-nuh; ULL-nur)	From Latin related to *ell* (denoting the humerus)	one of the two bones (the other is the radius) extending from the elbow to the wrist

Term and Pronunciation	Analysis	Meaning
Structure and Function		
vertebrae; vertebrae (plural) (VUR-tuh-bray; VUR-tuh-bruh)	from the Latin verb *vertere* (to turn)	one of the 33 bones making up the vertebral column
vertebral column (VER-tee-brul KOL-um)	from the Latin verb *vertere* (to turn)	series of vertebrae extending from the cranium (head) to the coccyx (tailbone)
xiphoid process (ZIGH-foyd PRO-cess)	from the Greek word *xipho* (sword), *-oid* (resemblance to)	bony, dagger-like structure at the lower end of the sternum
zygomatic bones (ZI-go-MAT-ik BONZ)	from the Greek word *zygoma* (bolt or bar); *-tic* (adjective suffix)	a facial bone (cheek, one of two)
Disorders		
arthralgia (ar-THRAL-jee-uh)	*arthr/o* (joint); *-algia* (pain)	pain in a joint
arthritis (ar-THRIGH-tis)	*arthr/o* (joint); *-I* (inflammation)	inflammation of a joint
arthrochondritis (AR-throw-kon-DRY-tis)	*arthr/o* (joint); *chondr/o* (cartilage); *-I* (inflammation)	inflammation of joint cartilage
arthropathy (ar-THROP-uh-thee)	*arthr/o* (joint); *-pathy* (disease or disorder)	any disorder of a joint
arthrosis (ar-THROW-sis)	*arthr/o* (joint); *-osis* (abnormal condition of)	degenerative joint changes
brachialgia (BRAY-kee-AL-jee-uh)	*brachi/o* (arm); *-algia* (pain)	pain in the arm
bursitis (burr-SIGH-tis)	*burs/o* (bursa); *-I* (inflammation)	inflammation of a bursa
carpal tunnel syndrome (KAR-pul TUN-ul SIN-drum)	*carp/o* (wrist); *-al* (adjective suffix); *syn-* (together); from the Greek *dromos* (a running)	condition characterized by wrist pain, caused by chronic entrapment of the median nerve within the carpal tunnel
chondromalacia (konn-droh-muh-LAY-she-uh)	*chondr/o* (cartilage); *-malacia* (softening)	softening of cartilage
chondropathy (kon-DROP-uh-thee)	*chondr/o* (cartilage); *-pathy* (disease or disorder)	disease of cartilage
chondrosarcoma (KONN-droh-sar-KOH-muh)	*chondr/o* (cartilage); *sarc/o* (flesh); *-oma* (tumor)	malignant tumor arising from the cartilage
closed fracture (CLOSED FRAK-chur)	from the Latin word *fractura* (to break)	break in the bone in which the skin is intact at the site; also called simple fracture
compound fracture (KOM-pound FRAK-chur)	from the Latin word *fractura* (to break)	break in the bone where the bone comes through the skin; also called open fracture
costalgia (koss-TAL-jee-uh)	*cost/o* (rib); *-algia* (pain)	rib pain
costochondritis (KOSS-toh-kon-DRY-tis)	*cost/o* (rib); *chondr/o* (cartilage); *-I* (inflammation)	inflammation of rib cartilage
dactylalgia (DAK-til-AL-jee-uh)	*dactyl/o* (finger, toe); *-algia* (pain)	pain in the fingers

(continues)

Study Table The Skeletal System		(continued)
Term and Pronunciation	**Analysis**	**Meaning**
Disorders		
dactylodynia (DAK-til-oh-DINN-ee-uh)	*dactyl/o* (finger, toe); *-dynia* (pain)	pain in the fingers
fracture (FRAK-chur)	from the Latin word *fractura* (break)	break in a bone
herniated disc (HER-nee-ay-ted DISK)	from the Latin word *hernia* (rupture); *disc/o* (disk)	protrusion of a fragmented intervertebral disc in the intervertebral foramen with potential compression of a nerve
kyphosis (kye-FOE-sis)	*kyph/o* (humped); *-sis* (condition)	humpback; anteriorly concave curvature of the thoracic and sacral region of the spine
lordosis (lor-DOE-sis)	from the Greek word *ordosis* (bent backwards)	swayback; abnormal anteriorly convex curvature of the lumbar part of the spine
megadactyly (meg-uh-DAK-tuh-lee)	*mega-* (enlargement); *dactyl/o* (finger, toe)	enlargement of one or more fingers or toes
neoplasms (NEE-oh-plaz-umz)	neo- (new); *plasma* (anything formed)	abnormal tissue that grows rapidly
open fracture (OH-pen FRAK-chur)	*open* (exposed)	bone break in which the skin is lacerated and there is an open wound; also called compound fracture
ostealgia (oss-tee-AL-jee-uh)	*oste/o* (bone); *-algia* (pain)	pain in a bone; also called osteodynia
osteitis (oss-tee-EYE-tis)	*oste/o* (bone); *-l* (inflammation)	inflammation of bone
osteochondritis (OSS-tee-oh-konn-DRY-tis)	*oste/o* (bone); *chondr/o* (cartilage); *-l* (inflammation)	inflammation of bone and associated cartilage
osteodynia (oss-tee-oh-DINN-ee-uh)	*oste/o* (bone); *-dynia* (pain)	pain in a bone; also called ostealgia
osteomalacia (OSS-tee-oh-muh-LAY-she-uh)	*oste/o* (bone); *-malacia* (softening)	softening of bone
osteomyelitis (OSS-tee-oh-my-eh-LYE-tis)	*oste/o* (bone); *myel/o* (marrow); *-l* (inflammation)	inflammation of bone marrow
osteopenia (oss-tee-oh-PEEN-ee-uh)	*oste/o* (bone); *-penia* (deficiency)	abnormally low bone density
osteoporosis (OSS-tee-oh-puh-RO-sis)	*oste/o* (bone); *por/o* (porous); *-sis* (condition)	atrophy and thinning of bone tissue
osteosarcoma (OSS-tee-oh-sar-KOH-muh)	*oste/o* (bone); *sarc/o* (fleshlike); *-oma* (tumor)	highly malignant tumor of the bone
rheumatoid arthritis (ROO-muh-toid ar-THRIGH-tis)	from the Greek word *rheuma* (flux); *-oid* (resemblance of)	systemic autoimmune disease occurring more often in women that affects the connective tissue; involves many joints, especially those of the hands and feet
rickets (RICK-ets)	common English word; might be an alteration of the Greek word *rhakhitis*	disease due to vitamin D deficiency characterized by deficient calcification and soft bones associated with skeletal deformities

Term and Pronunciation	Analysis	Meaning
Disorders		
scoliosis (skoh-lee-OH-sis)	*scoli/o* (twisted); *-sis* (condition)	lateral curvature of the spine; S-shaped curvature
simple fracture (FRAK-chur)	from the Latin word *fractura* (break)	break in the bone in which the skin is intact at the site; also called closed fracture
sprain (SPRAIN)	common English word; unknown origin	injury to a ligament
syndrome (SIN-drum)	*syn-* (together); from the Greek *dromos* (running)	collection of signs and symptoms occurring together and characterizing a medical condition
Diagnostic Tests, Treatments, and Surgical Procedures		
analgesics (an-al-GEE-ziks)	*an-* (absence); from the Greek word *gesis* (sensation)	medication used to relieve pain
anti-inflammatory (AN-tie-in-FLAMM-uh-tor-ee)	*anti-* (against); inflammatory (common English word)	medication used to reduce inflammation (e.g., used to reduce joint inflammation in arthritis)
arthrectomy (ar-THREK-tuh-mee)	*arthr/o* (joint); *-ectomy* (surgical removal)	excision of a joint
arthrocentesis (arth-roh-sen-TEE-sis)	*arthr/o* (joint); *-centesis* (surgical puncture for aspiration)	removing fluid from a joint through a needle puncture
arthrogram (ARTH-roh-gram)	*arthr/o* (joint); *-gram* (record or picture)	imaging of a joint after injecting a contrast dye to aid visualization
arthrometry (arth-ROM-uh-tree)	*arthr/o* (joint); *-metry* (process of measuring)	measurement of the amount of movement in a joint
arthroplasty (ARTH-roh-plass-tee)	*arthr/o* (joint); *-plasty* (surgical repair)	surgical repair of a joint
arthroscope (ARTH-roh-skope)	*arthr/o* (joint); *-scope* (instrument for viewing)	device used in arthroscopy
arthroscopy (ar-THROS-koh-pee)	*arthr/o* (joint); *-scopy* (use of instrument for viewing)	examination of the interior of a joint
arthrotomy (ar-THROT-uh-mee)	*arthr/o* (joint); *-tomy* (cutting operation)	surgical incision into a joint
carpectomy (kar-PEK-tuh-mee)	*carp/o* (wrist); *-ectomy* (surgical removal)	excision of part of the wrist
chondroplasty (KON-droh-plass-tee)	*chondr/o* (cartilage); *-plasty* (surgical repair)	surgical repair of cartilage
computed tomography scan; CT scan (com-PYOOT-ed TOH-mog-ruh-fee SKAN)	from the Greek *tomos* (slice, section) and *graphy* (image)	noninvasive imaging test; imaging anatomical information from a cross-sectional plane of the body
costectomy (koss-TEK-tuh-mee)	*cost/o* (rib); *-ectomy* (surgical removal)	excision of a rib
magnetic resonance imaging (MRI) (mag-NET-ik REZ-uh-nens IM-ih-jing)	from Latin *resonantia* (echo)	a diagnostic radiograph in which the magnetic nuclei of a patient are aligned in a magnetic field; these signals are converted into tomographic images

(continues)

Study Table The Skeletal System		(continued)
Term and Pronunciation	**Analysis**	**Meaning**
Diagnostic Tests, Treatments, and Surgical Procedures		
myelogram (MY-el-oh-gram)	*myel/o* (bone marrow); *-gram* (record or picture)	X-ray of the spinal column using contrast medium
narcotic (nar-KOT-ik)	*narc/o* (sleep)	drug derived from opium with potent analgesic effects; potential effects of dependency through prolonged use
nonsteroidal anti-inflammatory drug (NSAID) (non-STAIR-oid-ul an-tye-in-FLAM-uh-tor-ee DRUG)	from the Greek *stereos* (solid lipid)	medication that exerts analgesic and anti-inflammatory actions
ostectomy (os-TECK-tuh-mee)	*oste/o* (bone); *-ectomy* (surgical removal)	surgical removal of bone
osteoplasty (OS-tee-oh-plass-tee)	*oste/o* (bone); *-plasty* (surgical repair)	surgical repair of bone
osteorrhaphy (OS-tee-or-uh-fee)	*oste/o* (bone); *-rrhaphy* (surgical suturing)	suturing together the parts of a broken bone
osteotomy (os-tee-OT-uh-mee)	*oste/o* (bone); *-tomy* (cutting operation)	surgical cutting of bone
reduction (ree-DUK-shun)	common English word	correcting a fracture by realigning the bone pieces
traction (TRAK-shun)	common English word	using elastics or pulley and weights to maintain alignment; a pulling or dragging force exerted on a limb in a distal direction
vertebrectomy (ver-tuh-BREK-tuh-mee)	from the Latin word *vertere* (to turn); *-ectomy* (surgical removal)	excision (resectioning) of a vertebra
Practice and Practitioners		
kinesiologist (kih-nee-see-ol-UH-jist)	*kinesis* (Greek for movement); *-logist* (one who studies a certain field)	practitioner who studies movement and the involved structures
occupational therapist (ock-YOU-pay-shun-ul THER-uh-pist)	*occupationem* (Latin for business); *therapia* (Latin for curing the sick)	practitioner who works to increase independent function through therapy
orthopedics (or-thoh-PEE-diks)	*orth/o* (straight or correct); *ped-* (child); *-ic* (adjective suffix)	the medical specialty concerned with the development, preservation, restoration, and function of the musculoskeletal system
orthopedic surgeon (or-thoh-PEE-dik SUR-juhn)	*orth/o* (straight or correct); *ped-* (child); *-ic* (adjective suffix)	a physician in the field of orthopedics (can be MD or DO)
physical therapist (FIZ-ih-kul THER-uh-pist)	*physicalis* (Latin for nature); *therapia* (Latin for curing the sick)	practitioner who works to restore correct muscle movement and ability
rheumatologist (ROO-muh-tal-oh-gist)	*rheumat/o* (flux); *-logist* (one who studies a certain field)	physician who treats joint and connective tissue disorders such as arthritis
rheumatology (ROO-muh-tal-oh-jee)	*rheumat/o* (flux); *-logy* (the study of)	field of specialty that deals with joints and connective tissue disorders

CASE STUDY WRAP-UP

Healthcare personnel conducted a complete history and physical examination along with diagnostic X-rays. Busia, age 86, was diagnosed with a left hip fracture secondary to osteoporosis. The orthopedic surgeon, Dr. Bein, explained that the proximal portion—specifically the femoral neck—of Busia's femur was fractured so she was being prepped for immediate THR surgery.

Case Study Application Questions

1. What bone is broken?
2. Where does the femur attach to the hip?
3. Describe osteoporosis.
4. Dr. Bein used the medical abbreviation THR. What surgery is this?

END-OF-CHAPTER EXERCISES

Exercise 5.1 Labeling: Skeleton

Using the following list, choose the terms to label the diagram correctly.

calcaneus	femur	metacarpals	phalanges	sternum
carpal bones	fibula	metatarsals	radius	tarsal bones
clavicle	humerus	patella	ribs	tibia
costal cartilage	ilium	pubis	sacrum	ulna
cranium	mandible	phalanges	scapula	vertebral column
facial bones				

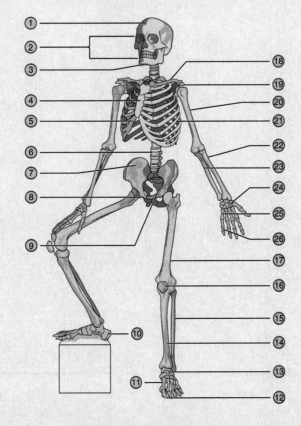

1. _____   7. _____   13. _____   19. _____   25. _____

2. _____   8. _____   14. _____   20. _____   26. _____

3. _____   9. _____   15. _____   21. _____

4. _____   10. _____   16. _____   22. _____

5. _____   11. _____   17. _____   23. _____

6. _____   12. _____   18. _____   24. _____

Exercise 5.2 Labeling: Long Bone

Using the following list, choose the terms to label the diagram correctly.

compact bone   endosteum   periosteum

diaphysis   epiphyseal plate   proximal epiphysis

distal epiphysis   medullary cavity   spongy bone

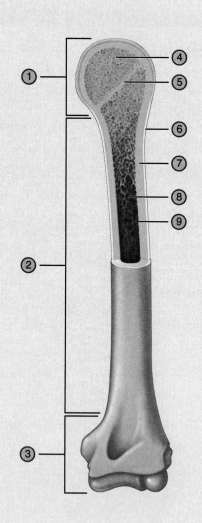

1. _____   4. _____   7. _____

2. _____   5. _____   8. _____

3. _____   6. _____   9. _____

Exercise 5.3 Word Parts

Break each of the following terms into its word parts: prefix, root, or suffix. Give the meaning of each word part and then define the term.

1. *osteorraphy*

   root: _____

   suffix: _____

   definition: _____

2. *arthrocentesis*

   root: _____

   suffix: _____

   definition: _____

3. *brachialgia*

   root: _____

   suffix: _____

   definition: _____

4. *osteochondritis*

   root: _____

   root: _____

   suffix: _____

   definition: _____

5. *carpectomy*

   root: _____

   suffix: _____

   definition: _____

6. *chondrosarcoma*

   root: _____

   suffix: _____

   definition: _____

7. *dactylomegaly*

   root: _____

   suffix: _____

   definition: _____

Exercise 5.4 Word Building

Use the word parts listed to build the defined terms.

-algia	-dynia	-itis	myel/o sarc/o
arthr/o	-ectomy	kinesi/o	-oma -scopy
cardi/o	electr/o	-logy	oste/o
chondr/o	-gram	-malacia	-plasty
cost/o	inter-	my/o	-porosis

1. _____ inflammation of the bone and bone marrow

2. _____ visual examination of a joint

3. _____ abnormal softening of cartilage

4. _____ imaging of a joint

5. _____ pain in a joint

6. _____ the study of movement of body parts

7. _____ surgical repair of cartilage

8. _____ pertaining to the area between the ribs

9. _____ inflammation of the bone

10. _____ a highly malignant tumor of the bone

11. _____ surgical repair of a joint

12. _____ X-ray of the spine

13. _____ inflammation of the cartilage

14. _____ bones with diminished density; porous

15. _____ pain in the ribs

Exercise 5.5 Matching

Match the term in the first column with its definition in the second column.

1. _____ abduction   a. backward bending of hand or foot

2. _____ rotation   b. bending the foot toward the ground

3. _____ plantar flexion   c. straightening a limb

4. _____ extension   d. motion around a central axis

5. _____ dorsiflexion   e. motion away from the body

6. _____ flexion   f. bending motion

7. _____ adduction   g. motion toward the body

Exercise 5.6 Multiple Choice

Choose the correct answer for the following multiple-choice questions.

1. The formation of a bone is called _____.
   a. osteoporosis
   b. osteology
   c. orthogenesis
   d. osteogenesis

2. The bony structure that forms the upper part of the sternum is the _____.
   a. manubrium
   b. mandible
   c. temporomandibular joint
   d. maxilla

3. An outward curvature of the thoracic spine is called _____.
   a. spondylosis
   b. lumbago
   c. lordosis
   d. kyphosis

4. The cartilaginous lower portion of the sternum is called the _____.
   a. xiphoid process
   b. sacroiliac
   c. olecranon process
   d. pelvic girdle

5. The collar bone is the _____.
   a. ischium
   b. ulna
   c. clavicle
   d. zygomatic

6. The bones of the hands are the _____.
   a. tarsals
   b. metacarpals
   c. metatarsals
   d. calcaneus

7. The bones of the fingers and toes are the _____.
   a. metatarsals
   b. carpal
   c. phalanges
   d. fibulas

8. The heel bone is the _____.
   a. ilium
   b. zygomatic
   c. ulna
   d. calcaneus

9. The bones of the spine are the .
   a. vertebrae
   b. temporals
   c. maxilla
   d. scapula

10. The shoulder blade is the _____.
    a. scapula
    b. sternum
    c. maxilla
    d. scoliosis

11. Which term does not belong with the others?
    a. scoliosis
    b. rickets
    c. rheumatoid arthritis
    d. diaphysis

12. Which term does not belong with the others?
    a. humerus
    b. fibula
    c. radius
    d. ulna

13. Which term does not belong with the others?
    a. deltoid muscle
    b. patella
    c. sternum
    d. carpal bone

14. Which term does not belong with the others?
    a. sclerosis
    b. kyphosis
    c. scoliosis
    d. lordosis

15. Which term does not belong with the others?
    a. cervical
    b. parietal
    c. thoracic
    d. lumbar

Exercise 5.7 Fill in the Blank

Fill in the blank with the correct answer.

1. The word that means "inflammation of a joint" is _____.
2. Aspiration of fluid from a joint by a needle puncture is a(n) _____.
3. The physician who treats disorders of the skeletal system is called a(n) _____.
4. A break in the bone where the bone comes through the skin is called an open fracture or a _____ fracture.
5. Bone marrow can be found in the _____ cavity.

6. A(n) _____ connects tissue to bone.

7. A(n) _____ is the protrusion of a fragmented intervertebral disc in the intervertebral foramen and can cause compression of a nerve.

Exercise 5.8 Abbreviations

Write out the term for the following abbreviations.

1. _____ ACL

2. _____ CT

3. _____ C1

4. _____ TKA

5. _____ L5

6. _____ RA

7. _____ NSAID

8. _____ MRI

Write the abbreviation for the following terms.

9. _____ total hip replacement

10. _____ fracture

11. _____ traction

12. _____ range of motion

13. _____ thoracic vertebra

14. _____ total knee replacement

15. _____ magnetic resonance imaging

Select the correct spelling of the medical term.

1. A practitioner who studies movement and the involved structures is a _____.
   a. kinesiologist
   b. kinisiologist
   c. kynesiologist
   d. kiniseologist

2. Suturing together the parts of a broken bone is called _____.
   a. osteorhaphy
   b. osteorrhaphy
   c. osteorafy
   d. osteoraphy

3. The measurement of the amount of movement in a joint is _____.
   a. athrometery
   b. arthrometry
   c. athrometry
   d. arthrometery

4. _____ are used to relieve pain.
   a. Analjesics
   b. Analgisics
   c. Analgezics

5. Analgesics
   a. RA stands for _____.
   b. rhumatoid arthritis
   c. rhuematoid arthritis
   d. rheumatoid arthritis
   e. rheumitoid arthritis

6. _____ is an adjective that means having to do with an arm.
   a. Brakial
   b. Breakial
   c. Braychial
   d. Brachial

7. _____ is a condition where the bone tissue atrophies and thins.
   a. Osteoporosis
   b. Ostioporosis
   c. Osteopourosis
   d. Osteoporosys

8. The long bone that extends from the shoulder to the elbow and is Latin for "shoulder" is the _____.
   a. humerous
   b. humeres
   c. humerus
   d. humeris

9. The posterior part of the hip bone is the _____.
   a. ischium
   b. ishium
   c. ichium
   d. ischiem

10. Another name for the kneecap is the _____.
    a. patela
    b. patella
    c. pattela
    d. pattella

Exercise 5.9 Medical Report

The underlined medical terms refer to a physician, a condition, or a treatment. Replace the underlined terms with a description.

Mrs. Smith, an 82-year-old woman, was out walking her dog on a cold day. She slipped on a patch of ice, fell, and incurred painful injuries. In the emergency room, Dr. Farley Burrows, an <u>orthopedic surgeon</u> (1), examined her. Mrs. Smith had limited <u>ROM</u> (2) in her right wrist and was experiencing pain in her left hip. Dr. Burrows ordered X-rays, which revealed a <u>comminuted fracture</u> (3) in the wrist and <u>compression fracture</u> (4) in the hip. He then performed a <u>reduction</u> (5) of the wrist bone and ordered that Mrs. Smith be admitted to the hospital and placed in <u>traction</u> (6) to maintain realignment of her hip.

Write your descriptions of each of the underlined terms in the spaces.

1. _____

2. _____

3. _____

4. _____

5. _____

6. _____

Exercise 5.10 Reflection

1. After reading this chapter, what are you most curious to learn more about?
2. What were the most and least interesting things that you learned?

CHAPTER 6

The Muscular System

LEARNING OUTCOMES

Upon completion of this chapter, you should be able to:

- Name the three types of muscle tissue.
- Define terms related to muscle names and functions.
- Describe the types of muscle movement.
- Pronounce, spell, and define medical terms related to the muscular system and its disorders.
- Interpret abbreviations associated with the muscular system.
- Apply knowledge gained to Case Study Questions.

CASE STUDY

Nushi is a 32-year-old female who enjoys being outdoors, walking her Siberian husky dog, and watching movies. She always considered herself to be an active person, but she and her husband have noticed that she is having trouble walking upstairs to go to bed at night or walking downstairs to let the dog outside. At first, they didn't think anything of it and attributed it to the winter "blahs." As the weeks went on, Nushi could no longer raise her arms over her head to pull a sweater on. In fact, holding her head up was challenging because it was too heavy. When she started having trouble swallowing and choked frequently while drinking water, she decided it was time to call her family physician for a wellness exam.

Introduction

In the preceding chapter, you learned that there are approximately 206 bones in the human body. The total number of muscles is harder to calculate because of the various ways to distinguish them. A fair approximation is that there are three times as many muscles as there are bones. Moreover, muscles make up about half of the total body weight.

We may think of muscles as necessary for lifting objects, running, jumping, throwing a ball, or swinging a golf club. Even though that is true, muscles are also needed for seeing, talking, eating, digesting, breathing, smiling, frowning, blinking, and so on. And let's not forget the heart, which is a muscle that pumps blood through the body. The heart is discussed in Chapter 10 because its function is better related to the cardiovascular system than to the muscular system.

Word Parts Related to the Muscular System

The word parts presented in **Table 6.1** are often found in terms related to the muscular system. Two main word parts that mean muscle are my/o and muscul/o. Other word roots refer to muscle movement, such as kine- and kinesi/o.

Table 6.1 Common Word Parts Related to the Muscular System

Word Part	Meaning
fasci/o	fibrous membrane
fibr/o	fiber
hemi-	half
kine-, kinesi/o	movement
ligament/o	ligament
muscul/o	muscle
my/o	muscle
para-	alongside, near
-paresis	partial or incomplete paralysis
-plegia	paralysis
quadri-	four
sthen/o	strength
tend/o, tendin/o	tendon
ton/o	tone

Word Parts Exercise

After studying Table 6.1, write the meaning of each of the word parts.

Word Part	Meaning
1. ligament/o	1. _____
2. tend/o, tendin/o	2. _____
3. ton/o	3. _____
4. -plegia	4. _____
5. muscul/o	5. _____
6. kine-, kinesi/o	6. _____
7. -paresis	7. _____
8. sthen/o	8. _____
9. my/o	9. _____
10. quadri-	10. _____
11. fasci/o	11. _____
12. fibr/o	12. _____
13. hemi-	13. _____
14. para-	14. _____

Structure and Function

Muscles are characterized by their location, cell characteristics (striated or nonstriated), and control of movement (voluntary or involuntary). The three types of muscle tissue are skeletal, smooth, and cardiac (see **Figure 6.1**).

Skeletal Muscle

Of the three types, **skeletal muscle** is the largest group, comprising more than 600 separate muscles. Skeletal muscles attach to bones (the skeleton). These voluntary muscles are made up of **muscle fibers**, which is another name for *muscle cells*. Muscle tissue has a rich blood vessel network. A bundle of muscle fibers is called a **fascicle**. **Fascia** encloses muscle. **Tendons** are made of connective tissue that connect muscle to bone (see **Figure 6.2**). **Ligaments** are bands of fibrous connective tissue that connect bones to bones or bones to other structures to support muscles.

Contractions of skeletal muscles pull on bones at joints to produce movement. The muscle that is responsible for the main movement is the **prime mover** or **agonist**. The muscle that opposes the movement is the **antagonist**. For example, in the arm, the biceps brachii (anterior arm muscle) is the prime mover, and the triceps brachii (posterior arm muscle) is its antagonist. After contracting, muscle tension lessens, and muscles then relax.

Skeletal muscle is also known as **striated muscle** because the dark and light bands in the muscle fibers create a striated (striped) appearance. Skeletal muscle is unlike smooth or cardiac muscle because skeletal muscle is voluntary. A by-product of normal skeletal muscle contraction is heat; when the body is cold, heat is generated by shivering, which is rapid, small contractions. Skeletal muscles also contract to maintain posture (see **Figure 6.3**).

Smooth Muscle

Smooth muscle, which acts involuntarily, lines blood vessels, respiratory passageways, the digestive tract, and walls of hollow internal organs (see Figure 6.3). In blood vessels, smooth muscle contractions regulate

Comparison of the different types of muscle			
	Skeletal	Smooth	Cardiac
Location	Attached to bones	Wall of hollow organs, vessels, respiratory passageways	Wall of heart
Cell characteristics	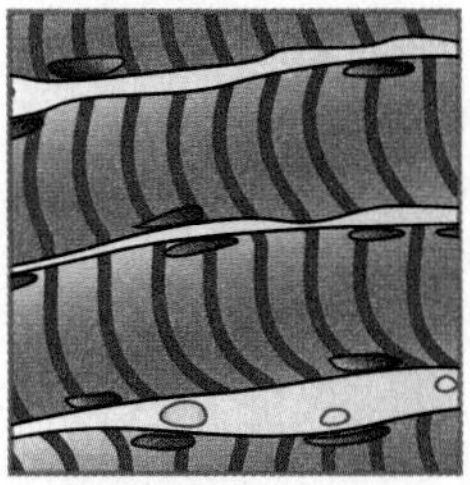 Long and cylindrical, multinucleated, heavily striated	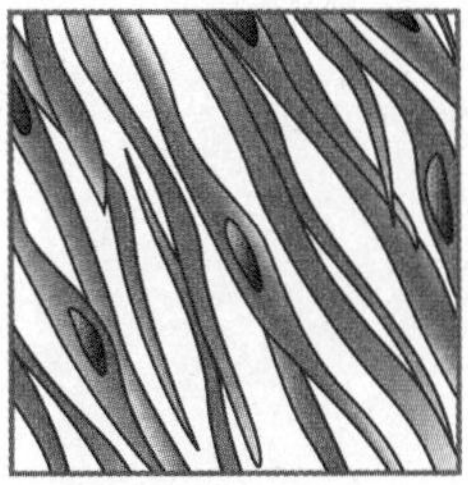 Tapered at each end, single nucleus, nonstriated	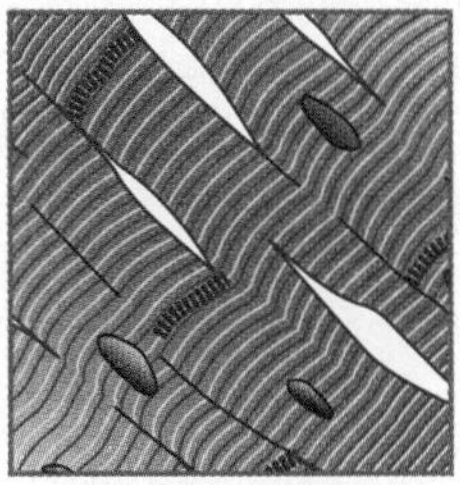 Branching networks, single nucleus, lightly striated
Control	Voluntary	Involuntary	Involuntary

Figure 6.1 A comparison of the three types of muscle tissue.

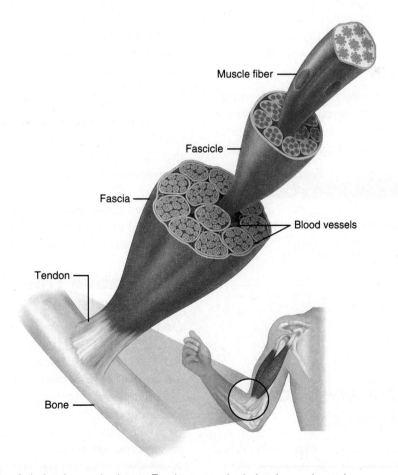

Figure 6.2 Components of skeletal muscle tissue. Tendons attach skeletal muscles to bones.

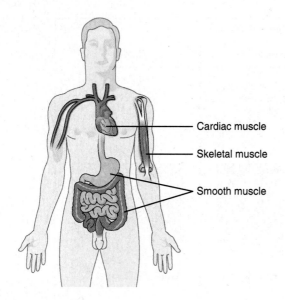

Figure 6.3 The three types of muscle tissue and their locations.

the diameter of the vessels to help control blood flow. In respiratory passageways, smooth muscle regulates air flow; in the digestive tract, smooth muscle contracts to move substances through passageways with wavelike motions. Smooth muscle is also known as **nonstriated muscle** because it lacks the striped appearance that skeletal muscle has.

Cardiac Muscle

Cardiac muscle, also known as heart muscle, forms the wall of the heart. It acts involuntarily and has a lightly striated appearance. Cardiac muscle is responsible for the heart's pumping action (see Figure 6.3).

QUICK CHECK

Name the three types of muscle tissue and give an example of where each type might be located.

Muscle Tissue Type	Location
1. _____	_____
2. _____	_____
3. _____	_____

Disorders Related to the Muscular System

Disorders of the muscular system often involve other systems. However, the terms introduced in the following discussion are specific to the muscular system.

Many muscle disorders are caused by physical trauma, such as those occurring in sports or accidents, and others are chronic. We begin with chronic disorders.

Chronic Disorders

Muscular dystrophy (MD) is a hereditary, progressive degenerative disorder that causes skeletal muscle weakness. The most common childhood muscular dystrophy is **Duchenne dystrophy**, which mostly affects males.

Myasthenia gravis (MG) is an immunologic disorder characterized by fluctuating weakness, especially of the facial and external eye muscles. Signs and symptoms can include drooping eyelids, double vision, difficulty talking, and **dysphagia** (difficulty swallowing).

> Two commonly confused words are dysphagia and dysphasia. Considering the words are only one letter apart, it's easy to do. The root word of dysphagia is the Greek word *phage*, meaning "eater." So, dysphagia is difficulty swallowing. The root word of dysphasia is the Greek word *phase*, meaning "to speak." So, dysphasia is difficulty speaking.

Fibromyalgia is a disorder characterized by widespread aching and stiffness of muscles and soft tissues, fatigue, tenderness, and disordered sleep. The cause of fibromyalgia is unknown, and it may coexist with other chronic diseases.

Amyotrophic lateral sclerosis (ALS), also called *Lou Gehrig's disease*, is a neuromuscular disease that affects both the nervous and muscular systems. As nerve cells that control the body's muscles die, the person's ability to control their muscles vanishes. It is a fatal, progressive degeneration of the nerve tracts of the spinal cord leading to muscular **atrophy**, which is muscle shrinking and wasting.

Cumulative Trauma and Sports Injuries

Cumulative trauma disorders (CTDs) are often caused by repetitive, work-related motions that damage muscles, tendons, joints, or nerves. A common one is **carpal tunnel syndrome**, which is a painful condition of the hand and fingers caused by compression of the median nerve in the wrist (see **Figure 6.4**).

The rotator cuff of the shoulder is formed by four muscles and reinforcing tendons of the shoulder joint. When these muscles become inflamed and swollen from overuse, a **rotator cuff injury** occurs.

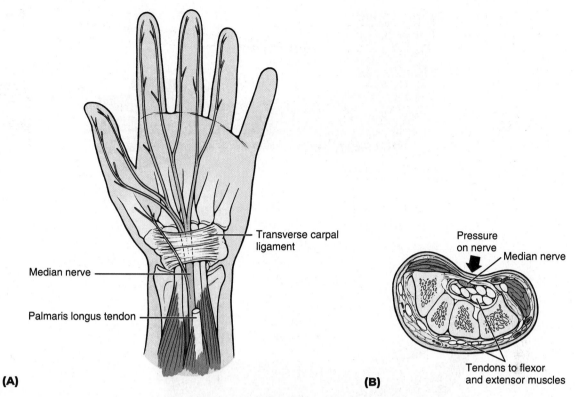

- Transverse carpal ligament
- Median nerve
- Palmaris longus tendon

(A)

- Pressure on nerve
- Median nerve
- Tendons to flexor and extensor muscles

(B)

Figure 6.4 Carpal tunnel syndrome. **A.** Pressure on the median nerve as it passes through the carpal (wrist) bones causes numbness and weakness in the areas of the hand supplied by the nerve. **B.** Cross-section of the wrist shows pressure on the median nerve.

Epicondylitis is an inflammation of an epicondyle, a bony projection on the distal humerus. When the lateral epicondyle is affected, it is termed "tennis elbow" because it is common in tennis players. When the medial epicondyle is affected, it is known as "golfer's elbow" because it is common in golfers (see **Figure 6.5**).

Plantar fasciitis is an inflammation of the plantar fascia (connective tissue in the arch of the foot) that can cause intense pain when walking or running. It may be caused by long periods of weight bearing, sudden changes in activity, or obesity.

Sports injuries often occur to overstressed or poorly conditioned muscles. However, injuries can occur in professional athletes in good physical condition. Two examples are *hamstring injuries* and *shin splints*. A **hamstring injury** is a strain or tear in one of the hamstring muscles (group of three posterior thigh muscles). This injury is common among sprinters, track hurdlers, baseball players, and football players. **Shin splints** refers to pain and tenderness in the lower leg muscles along the shin bone (tibia) following athletic overexertion. It may include a stress fracture (Fx) (small crack in the bone) of the tibia or an inflammation of the periosteum. Shin splints is a collective term describing the pain rather than the condition.

Paralysis and Paresis

Paralysis is the loss of voluntary muscle movement caused by injury or disease. **Paresis** is partial or incomplete paralysis. Following are examples.

- **Hemiparesis**: weakness or paralysis affecting one side of the body
- **Hemiplegia**: total paralysis of one side of the body
- **Paraplegia**: paralysis of both legs and generally the lower trunk
- **Quadriplegia**: paralysis of all four extremities (both arms and both legs)

Diagnostic Tests, Treatments, and Surgical Procedures

Tests used to diagnose disorders of the muscular system include blood and urine tests, electromyogram (EMG), magnetic resonance imaging (MRI), muscle

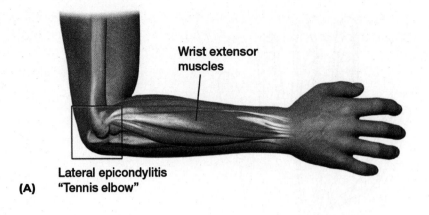

Wrist extensor muscles

Lateral epicondylitis "Tennis elbow"

(A)

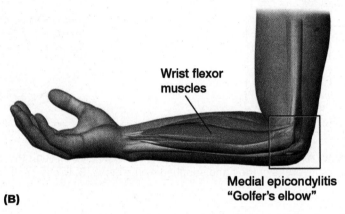

Wrist flexor muscles

Medial epicondylitis "Golfer's elbow"

(B)

Figure 6.5 Epicondylitis. **A.** Tennis elbow (lateral epicondylitis). **B.** Golfer's elbow (medial epicondylitis).

biopsy, nerve conduction studies, and spinal tap (lumbar puncture). For many of the chronic muscle conditions, there is no cure, only treatment of symptoms. For muscular dystrophy, steroids are used to reduce inflammation.

Like muscular dystrophy, there is no cure for myasthenia gravis. Treatment consists of antiacetylcholinesterase medications to keep the neurotransmitter, acetylcholine, at certain body sites to continue activating muscles. Steroids can reduce muscle inflammation in myasthenia gravis as well. Because there is also an autoimmune component to this disease, immunosuppressant agents (drugs that reduce the body's immune response to itself) can be used to suppress immune reactions.

Current treatments for amyotrophic lateral sclerosis (ALS) cannot reverse the disorder so treatments are only to slow disease progression and to make the person more comfortable. Riluzole (Rilutek) is an oral medication that increases life expectancy by 3 to 6 months. Edaravone (Radicava) is an intravenous infusion that helps improve daily functioning. Other treatments consist of breathing therapy as the muscles

needed to breathe start atrophying; occupational, physical, and speech therapy to address mobility issues and to provide adaptive techniques; nutritional support to find foods that are easier to swallow while providing adequate nutrition; and psychological and social support to address personal and emotional well-being.

Treatment of sports injuries commonly consists of rest, ice, compression (bandaging), and elevation, abbreviated "RICE." Intramuscular (IM) injections for pain are sometimes given.

Practice and Practitioners

Myology is the branch of science concerned with study of muscles and their accessory structures, including tendons, bursae, and fasciae. The medical specialists who treat disorders of the muscular system are similar to (and in some cases the same as) the specialists who treat disorders of the skeletal system, as discussed in Chapter 5. Specialists include **orthopedic surgeons**, **kinesiologists**, **occupational**

therapists, and **physical therapists**. Many conditions involve joints as well as muscles, and orthopedic physicians diagnose and treat patients with musculoskeletal disorders.

What is the difference between an abbreviation and an acronym? We speak each letter of an abbreviation, like ALS, and we pronounce an acronym from the sound its letter combination makes. Because RICE spells a common word, it is often pronounced. Most acronyms do not start out as common English words. So, is RICE an acronym? Even though many healthcare workers treat it as an acronym, it remains an abbreviation, and its pronunciation as a word includes the potential for confusion. AIDS is another example of an acronym because it is generally pronounced as a word.

Abbreviation Table The Muscular System

Abbreviation	Meaning
ALS	amyotrophic lateral sclerosis
EMG	electromyography; electromyogram
Fx	fracture
IM	intramuscular
MD	muscular dystrophy
MG	myasthenia gravis
MRI	magnetic resonance imaging
NSAID	nonsteroidal anti-inflammatory drug
PT	physical therapy
RICE	rest, ice, compression, elevation
ROM	range of motion

Study Table The Muscular System

Term and Pronunciation	Analysis	Meaning
agonist (AG-uh-nist)	from the Greek, *agon* (contest)	muscle that moves a body part when it contracts
antagonist (an-TAG-oh-nist)	a common English word	something (or in common use, someone) opposing or resisting the action of another
cardiac muscle (KAR-dee-ak MUS-ul)	*cardi/o* (heart); *-ac* (adjective); from the Latin word *musculus* (muscle)	involuntary, striated heart muscle
fascia (FASH-ee-uh)	Latin word for *band*	fibrous sheath of connective tissue that covers a muscle
fascicle (FAS-ih-kul)	from the Latin, *fasciculus (bundle)*	bundle of muscle fibers
ligament (LIG-uh-ment)	from the Latin noun *ligament* (string)	a fibrous connective tissue connecting bones, cartilage, or other tissue structures
muscle fiber (MUS-ul FIGH-bur)	from the Latin, *fibra* (fiber)	the term for a muscle cell
nonstriated muscle (non-STRIGH-ay-ted MUS-ul)	non- (adjective); from the Latin verb *striare* (to groove)	muscle that lacks the overlapping myofilaments (muscle proteins) that are found in striated (skeletal) muscles
prime mover (PRIME MOOV-ur)	two common English words; from the Latin *primus*, meaning first	muscle that has the principal responsibility for a given movement
smooth muscle (smooth MUS-ul)	common English word; from the Latin word *musculus* (muscle)	involuntary, nonstriated muscle of the internal organs and blood vessels
skeletal muscle (SKEL-uh-tul MUS-ul)	*sceleton* (modern Latin for skeleton); *-al* (adjective); *musculus* (Latin word for muscle)	voluntary, striated muscle connected to the bony framework of the body

(continues)

Study Table The Muscular System		*(continued)*
Term and Pronunciation	**Analysis**	**Meaning**
striated muscle (STRIGH-ay-ted MUS-ul)	from the Latin verb *striare* (to groove)	muscle with overlapping myofilaments (muscle proteins); also called skeletal muscle
tendon (TEN-dun)	from the Latin verb *tendo* (stretch)	a nonstretching fibrous cord that is part of the muscle complex, such as the Achilles tendon, associated with appendicular muscles
tone (TONE)	from the Greek word *tonos*	tension present in resting muscles
tonicity (TOE-nis-ih-tee)	from the Greek word *tonos*	muscle tone
Disorders		
amyotrophic lateral sclerosis (ALS) (ay-my-oh-TROH-fik LAT-er-ul SKLER-oh-sis)	*a-* (deficient); *my/o* (muscle); lateral (side); *scler/o* (hard); *-osis* (abnormal condition)	a progressive degeneration of the nerve tracts of the spinal cord, causing muscular atrophy; also called Lou Gehrig's disease
asthenia (as-THEE-nee-uh)	*a-* (deficient); *sthenos* (Greek word for strength)	weakness
atonia (AY-toh-nee-uh)	*a-* (deficient); *tonia* (tone)	flaccidity; lack of muscle tone; relaxation of muscle
atrophy (a-TROH-fee)	*a-* (deficient); *-trophy* (from the Greek word *trophé* meaning "nourishment")	wasting of the muscles
carpal tunnel syndrome (KAR-pul TUN-ul-SIN-drum)	carpal (a wrist bone); tunnel (common English word); syndrome (a Greek word meaning "running together")	entrapment of the median nerve in the wrist with chronically swollen and inflamed tendons
dysphagia (dis-FAY-juh)	*dys-* (Greek for bad); *-phage* (Greek word for eater)	difficulty swallowing
epicondylitis (EP-ih-KON-dih-LYE-tis)	*epi-* (around); *condyl* (rounded end surface of a bone); *-itis* (inflammation)	inflammation of the tissues around the elbow; golfer's or tennis elbow
fibromyalgia (FIGH-broh-MY-al-jee-uh)	*fibr/o* (fiber); *my/o* (muscle); *-algia* (pain)	a chronic disorder characterized by widespread aching and stiffness of muscles and soft tissues, accompanied by fatigue
hamstring injury (HAM-string IN-juh-ree)	Three muscles make up the hamstrings: biceps femoris, semitendinosis, and semimembranosus; group of muscles that resemble the cut of meat known as ham	strain or tear of the hamstring muscle group (posterior femoral muscle group)
hemiparesis (hem-ee-PUH-ree-sis)	*hemi-* (half); *-paresis* (paralysis)	weakness affecting one side of the body
hemiplegia (hem-ee-PLEE-jee-uh)	*hemi-* (half); *-plegia* (paralysis)	total paralysis of one side of the body
muscular dystrophy (MUS-kyu-lur DIS-troh-fee)	muscular (common English word); *dys-* (difficult); *-trophy* (from the Greek word *trophé* meaning "nourishment")	group of inherited muscle disorders that cause muscle weakness without affecting the nervous system
myalgia (my-AL-juh)	*my/o* (muscle); *-algia* (pain)	muscle pain

Term and Pronunciation	Analysis	Meaning
myasthenia gravis (MY-as-THEE-nee-uh GRA-viss)	*my/o* (muscle); asthenia (from the Greek word *astheneia* meaning "weakness")	an immunologic disorder characterized by fluctuating weakness, especially of the facial and external eye muscles
myocele (MY-oh-seel)	*my/o* (muscle); *-cele* (hernia)	hernia of a muscle
myalgia (my-AL-jee-uh)	*my/o* (muscle); (pain); *-algia* (pain)	muscle pain
myoma (my-OH-muh)	*my/o* (muscle); *-oma* (tumor)	benign neoplasm of muscle tissue
myopathy (my-OP-uh-thee)	*myo* (muscle); *-pathy* (suffering, feeling)	disease of muscle tissue
myositis (my-oh-SIGH-tis)	*my/o* (s) (muscle); *-itis* (inflammation)	inflammation of muscle
myospasm (MY-oh-spaz-um)	*my/o* (muscle); *-spasm* (involuntary motion)	involuntary contraction of a muscle
paralysis (puh-RAL-ih-sis)	*para-* (beside); *-lysis* (loosening)	loss of voluntary muscle movements caused by an injury or disease
paraplegia (PAR-uh-PLEE-jee-uh)	*para-* (beside); *-plegia* (paralysis)	paralysis of both legs and the lower trunk
paresis (puh-REE-sis)	*para-* (beside); *hienai* (let go)	partial or incomplete paralysis
periostitis (PAIR-ee-os-TYE-tis)	*peri-* (around); *oste/o* (bone); *-itis* (inflammation)	inflammation of the periosteum or the covering that surrounds the bone
plantar fasciitis (PLAN-tar FASH-ee-eye-tis)	plantar (sole of the foot); fasci- (from *fascia*, Latin for band); *-itis* (inflammation)	inflammation of the plantar fascia causing foot and heel pain
polymyositis (pol-ee-my-oh-SIGH-tis)	*poly-* (many); *myo-* (muscle); *-itis* (inflammation)	widespread inflammation and degeneration of muscle tissue
quadriplegia (kwah-druh-PLEE-jee-uh)	*quadri* (four); *-plegia* (paralysis)	paralysis of all four extremities
rotator cuff injury (ROH-tay-tur KUFF IN-jur-ee)	four muscles in the shoulder: supraspinatus, infraspinatus, teres minor, subscapularis	inflammation of the muscles and associated structures in the shoulder (rotator cuff) caused by overuse
shin splints (SHIN SPLINTS)	from Old English *scinu* meaning *narrow or thin piece* and Middle low German *splinte* meaning *metal plate or pin*	term given to describe pain in the anterior portion of the lower leg during running, walking, and other similar activities
tendonitis or tendinitis (ten-doh-NYE-tis; TEN-dih-NYE-tiss)	*tendon/o* (tendon); *-it is* (inflammation)	inflammation of a tendon

Diagnostic Tests, Treatments, and Surgical Procedures

blood test (BLOOD TEST)	*blut* (blood)	laboratory analysis of blood
electromyogram (EMG) (ee-LEK-troh-MY-oh-gram)	*electr/o* (electricity); *my/o* (muscle); *-gram* (something written or recorded)	record produced by electromyography

(continues)

Study Table The Muscular System		*(continued)*
Term and Pronunciation	**Analysis**	**Meaning**
electromyography (ee-LEK-troh-my-OG-ruh-fee)	*electr/o* (electricity); *my/o* (muscle); *-graphy* (process of writing)	records the strength of muscle contractions by means of electrical stimulation
lumbar puncture (LUM-bar PUNK-shur)	*lumbus* (loin); *puncture* (puncture)	done under local anesthesia, the removal of a sample of cerebrospinal fluid using a small needle inserted between two lumbar vertebrae for laboratory testing; also called spinal tap
magnetic resonance imaging (MRI) (mag-NET-ik REZ-uh-nence im-ih-JING)	*magneta* (magnet); *resonantia* (echo); *imago* (imitate)	uses radio waves and a strong magnetic to produce detailed images of body structures
muscle biopsy (MUS-ul BYE-op-see)	from Latin m*usculus* and the diminutive of *mus* (mouse, as some muscles were thought to be shaped like a mouse); *bios* (life) + *opsis* (sight)	removal of a small piece of muscle tissue for laboratory analysis
myectomy (my-EK-tuh-mee)	*my/o* (muscle); *-ectomy* (excision)	excision of part of a muscle
nerve conduction study (NURV kon-DUCK-shun STUD-ee)	*nervus* (nerve); *conduction* (safe passage); *stadium* (zeal, painstaking application)	test that measures transmission of nerve impulses to muscles; used to detect nerve damage, nerve disease, or muscle disease
physical therapy (FIZZ-ih-kul THER-uh-pee)	common English phrase	treatment to prevent disability and restore function using heat, exercise, and massage to improve circulation, strength, flexibility, and muscle strength
skeletal muscle relaxants (SKEL-ih-tul MUS-ul REE-LAX-unts)	*skelet/o* (skeleton); *-al* (adjective suffix); relaxant: that which relaxes	medications used to reduce muscle spasm
spinal tap (SPY-nul TAP)	*spina* (spine)	done under local anesthesia, the removal of a sample of cerebrospinal fluid using a small needle inserted between two lumbar vertebrae for laboratory testing; also called lumbar puncture
tendinoplasty (TEN-dih-no-plass-tee)	*tendin/o* (tendon); *-plasty* (surgical repair)	surgical repair of a tendon
tenorrhaphy (TEN-or-aff-ee)	*ten/o* (tendon); *-rrhaphy* (suturing)	suturing of a tendon
tenotomy (ten-OT-uh-mee)	*ten/o* (tendon); *-tomy* (incision)	incision into a tendon
urine test (YOOR-en TEST)	*urina* (urine)	laboratory analysis of urine
Practice and Practitioners		
kinesiology (kih-nee-see-OL-uh-jee)	*kinesi/o* (movement); *-logy* (study of)	study of muscle motion
kinesiologist (kih-nee-see-OL-uh-jist)	*kinesi/o* (movement); *-logist* (one who studies)	a specialist in kinesiology
myology (my-OL-uh-jee)	*my/o* (muscle); *-logy* (study of)	study of muscles

Term and Pronunciation	Analysis	Meaning
occupational therapist (odk-YOU-pay-shun-ul THER-uh-pist)	*occupationem* (Latin for business); *therapia* (Latin for curing the sick)	practitioner who works to increase independent function through therapy
orthopedic (or-thoh-PEE-dik)	*orth/o* (straight); *pedics* (child); note: the word was coined in the 18th century, originating with the study of skeletal disorders in children	pertaining to orthopedics or the study of the musculoskeletal system
orthopedic surgeon (or-thoh-PEE-dik SUR-jin)	*orth/o* (straight); *pedics* (child); surgeon (common English word)	a physician in the field of orthopedics (can be MD or DO)
physical therapist (FIZZ-ih-kul THER-uh-pist)	*physicalis* (Latin for nature); *therapia* (Latin for curing the sick)	practitioner who works to restore correct muscle movement and ability
rheumatologist (roo-muh-TOL-oh-jist)	*rheuma* (bodily fluid); *-ologist* (person who practices a particular subject)	physician who deals with inflammatory and infectious conditions of the musculoskeletal system

CASE STUDY WRAP-UP

At the wellness examination, the doctor was concerned that Nushi had lost weight, her walking gait was abnormal, she had bilateral asthenia and atrophy, and she ate very little because of her dysphagia. Her grip strength was poor, and her head ptosis (drooping) was so severe that she could not look forward. She was referred to a rheumatologist, who conducted diagnostic tests over several weeks, including blood tests, an EMG, nerve conduction studies, and a muscle biopsy. The results of the tests indicated a diagnosis of polymyositis, an autoimmune, inflammatory myopathy. The doctor began an immediate course of corticosteroids for muscle inflammation and advised her that immunosuppressive medications may be necessary in the future. Physical and speech therapy were also recommended.

Case Study Application Questions

1. Describe the scope of practice for a rheumatologist.
2. What is dysphagia?
3. What disorder does Nushi have?
4. Define myopathy.
5. Explain "bilateral asthenia and atrophy."

END-OF-CHAPTER EXERCISES

Exercise 6.1 Word Parts

Break each of the following terms into its word parts: prefix, root, or suffix. Give the meaning of each word part and then define the term.

1. *fibromyalgia*

   root: _____

   root: _____

   suffix: _____

   definition: _____

2. *periostitis*

    prefix: _____

    root: _____

    suffix: _____

    definition: _____

3. *tendinoplasty*

    root: _____

    suffix: _____

    definition: _____

4. *myology*

    root: _____

    suffix: _____

    definition: _____

5. *electromyography*

    root: _____

    root: _____

    suffix: _____

    definition: _____

6. *epicondylitis*

    prefix: _____

    root: _____

    suffix: _____

    definition: _____

7. *hemiplegia*

    prefix: _____

    root: _____

    definition: _____

8. *paralysis*

    prefix: _____

    suffix: _____

    definition: _____

Exercise 6.2 Word Building

Use the word parts listed to build the terms defined.

-algia	-cele	fasci/o	fibr/o
hemi-	-itis	kinesi/o	-logist
-logy	muscul/o	my/o	neur/o
para-	-paresis	-pathy	-plegia
tendin/o	ten/o	-tomy	-trophy

1. _____ incision into a tendon

2. _____ physician who diagnoses and treats diseases of the nervous system

3. _____ paralysis of both legs and the lower part of the body

4. _____ hernia of a muscle

5. _____ slight paralysis of one side of the body

6. _____ inflammation of the fascia

7. _____ pain resulting from movement

8. _____ a chronic disorder characterized by widespread aching

9. _____ any disease of the muscle

10. _____ inflammation of a muscle

Exercise 6.3 Matching

Match the term with its definition.

1. _____ antagonist   a. fibrous sheath of connective tissue that covers a muscle

2. _____ myoma   b. surgical repair of a tendon

3. _____ tenorrphapy   c. hernia of a muscle

4. _____ tenontoplasty   d. something opposing or resisting the action of another

5. _____ myocele   e. flaccidity; lack of muscle tone; relaxing of muscle

6. _____ atonia   f. suturing of a tendon

7. _____ fascia   g. involuntary contraction of a muscle

8. _____ myospasm   h. a type of muscle structure associated with appendicular muscles

9. _____ atrophy   i. benign neoplasm of muscle tissue

10. _____ tendon   j. a type of muscle tissue connecting bones, cartilage, or other tissue structures

11. _____ prime mover   k. wasting of the muscles

12. _____ ligament   l. muscle that has the principal responsibility for a given movement

Exercise 6.4 Multiple Choice

Choose the correct answer for the following multiple-choice questions.

1. The three types of muscle tissue are _____.
   a. smooth, cardiac, deltoid
   b. cardiac, epicardium, skeletal
   c. cardiac, skeletal, smooth
   d. skeletal, trapezius, deltoid

2. _____ Physicians in which of the following medical specialty(ies) take care of muscular disorders?
   a. neurology
   b. orthopedic
   c. neurology and orthopedics
   d. chiropractic and orthopedics

3. Kinesiology is the study of _____.
   a. dance
   b. movement
   c. aerobics
   d. athletics

4. A person who is quadriplegic is paralyzed in _____ limbs.
   a. one
   b. two
   c. three
   d. four

5. Carpal tunnel syndrome affects the _____.
   a. wrist
   b. knee
   c. elbow
   d. ankle

6. A muscle antagonist is _____.
   a. a muscle that resists the action of another
   b. a muscle that has the principal responsibility for a given movement
   c. a type of muscle that connects one muscle to another
   d. none of the above

7. Which muscular disease is usually diagnosed in childhood and typically affects only males?
   a. MG
   b. multiple sclerosis
   c. MD
   d. paraplegia

8. This is a progressive degeneration of the nerve tracts of the spinal cord, causing muscular atrophy, also known as Lou Gehrig's disease.
   a. ALS
   b. asthenia
   c. multiple sclerosis
   d. paraplegia

9. This type of muscle has fibers with noticeable overlapping myofilaments and is involuntary.
   a. cardiac
   b. nonstriated
   c. smooth
   d. skeletal

10. This is an immunologic disorder characterized by fluctuating weakness, especially of the facial and external eye muscle.
    a. MG
    b. fibromyalgia
    c. MD
    d. paraplegia

Exercise 6.5 Fill in the Blank

Fill in the blank with the correct answer.

1. _____ is the medical term for tennis elbow.
2. The term, which is also the Latin word for string, that names what connects bones to bones to support muscles is _____.
3. Pointing the toes downward is called _____.
4. _____ is the term for weakness.
5. A hernia of a muscle is called _____.
6. _____ causes intense pain in the heel region and sole of the foot upon walking.
7. A(n) _____ records the strength of muscle contractions.
8. The surgical repair of a tendon is called _____.
9. _____ is the study of muscles.
10. Muscle pain is called _____.

Exercise 6.6 Abbreviations

Write out the term for the following abbreviations.

1. ._____ MD

2. _____ RICE

3. _____ CTD

4. _____ MG

Write the abbreviation for the following terms.

5. _____ electromyography

6. _____ amyotrophic lateral sclerosis

7. _____ intramuscular

8. _____ fracture

9. _____ muscular dystrophy

Exercise 6.7 Spelling

Select the correct spelling of the medical term.

1. _____ means weakness.
   a. Athenia
   b. Athena
   c. Asthenia
   d. Asthena

2. _____ is a chronic disorder characterized by widespread aching and stiffness of muscles and soft tissues, accompanied by fatigue.
   a. Fibromyalgia
   b. Fibromylgia
   c. Fibromyalga
   d. Fibomyalgia

3. The name of this disorder comes from the root word meaning *muscle* and the Greek word meaning *weakness*.
   a. myathenia gravis
   b. myasthenia gravis
   c. myasthenia graviss
   d. myathenia graviss

4. _____ means difficulty swallowing.
   a. Disphagia
   b. Disfagia
   c. Dysfagia
   d. Dysphagia

5. _____ is also known as Lou Gehrig's disease.
   a. Amotrophic lateral sclerosis
   b. Amyotrophic lateral sklerosis
   c. Amotrophic lateral sclarosis
   d. Amyotrophic lateral sclerosis

6. The muscle movement that closes the angle of a joint is called _____.
   a. flextion
   b. flexsion
   c. flexion
   d. flexon

7. Cardiac muscle is considered lightly _____, and skeletal muscle is considered heavily _____.
   a. stryated
   b. striatted
   c. striated
   d. strieted

8. _____ describes paralysis of all four extremities.
   a. Quadraplegia
   b. Quadriplegia
   c. Quadraplesia
   d. Quadriplesia

9. An _____ surgeon is a physician who specializes in the musculoskeletal system.
   a. orthopedic
   b. orthapedic
   c. orthopaedik
   d. orthopedik

10. A _____ is the connective tissue connecting bones and cartilage.
    a. ligament
    b. ligument
    c. legament
    d. liguhment

Exercise 6.8 Medical Report

PHYSICAL THERAPY PROGRESS NOTE

CHIEF COMPLAINT: Cervical neck pain with limited movement and right shoulder pain with limited ROM.

PROGRESS: The patient states that he is the same as he was the last time he was in for therapy.

AGGRAVATING FACTORS: Working.

PAIN/DISCOMFORT LEVEL: The patient states that the pain is 5/10.

TREATMENT: Treatment today consisted of moist heat and ultrasound of the cervical spine; therapeutic exercise to the neck and shoulder for 45 minutes.

PATIENT'S PROGRESS: The patient is doing well with his cervical spine exercises. His neck flexion and neck extension and rotation are relatively improved. His radiating pain is reduced. His right shoulder is very painful. He has pain on flexion and abduction. He has pain on resisted abduction. He has rotator cuff tendonitis, probably caused by impingement.

The patient was put on a four-step treatment approach to decrease pain and increase neck and shoulder movement. He was advised to limit the use of his right arm as much as possible for 2 weeks, use ice and NSAIDs for pain, and keep his arm in a sling. He demonstrated improved ROM following his therapy. He was advised to use the exercise program on a regular basis.

QUESTIONS

1. What medical terms are associated with the patient's limited neck movements? Define each one. _____
2. What does "tendonitis" mean?_____
3. Explain what ROM is._____
4. What does NSAID stand for?_____

Exercise 6.9 Reflection

1. Identify the most interesting thing you learned after working through this chapter.
2. Put yourself in Nushi's situation. How do you think a person would feel if they could not hold their head up?

CHAPTER 7

The Nervous System

LEARNING OUTCOMES

Upon completion of this chapter, you should be able to:

- Name the major structures and functions of the nervous system.
- Name the parts of a neuron.
- Name the major divisions of the nervous system.
- Pronounce, spell, and define medical terms related to the nervous system.
- Interpret abbreviations associated with the nervous system.
- Apply knowledge gained to Case Study Questions.

CASE STUDY

Pierce Can No Longer Play

Pierce was a 40-year-old male police officer who enjoyed playing guitar in a band. As an active father of three small children, he noticed that he couldn't open juice containers as easily anymore. He didn't think much of that because he had been practicing at the law enforcement firing range and thought his hands were just tired. However, during the band's last practice session, his hands weren't moving easily across the guitar strings. His wife noticed that when he walked across the kitchen floor his left foot slapped on the tile. When his gait seemed to be getting worse, Pierce made an appointment with his physician at the clinic.

Introduction

The nervous system is one of the most complex systems in the body, coordinating both involuntary and voluntary actions. It works in conjunction with the endocrine system to maintain **homeostasis**, a term that means a state of equilibrium. The nervous system also works with the muscular system to control the body's voluntary and involuntary muscles.

The nervous system has two main divisions: the **central nervous system (CNS)** and the **peripheral nervous system (PNS)**. The central nervous system consists of the brain and spinal cord. The peripheral nervous system consists of all the nerves outside the CNS, including the cranial nerves and spinal nerves (see **Figure 7.1**). The PNS is further divided into the *somatic nervous system* and the *autonomic nervous system*. The autonomic nervous system is then subdivided into the *sympathetic nervous system* (fight or flight responses) and the *parasympathetic nervous system* (rest and digest responses), depending on the involuntary functions it controls (see **Figure 7.2**).

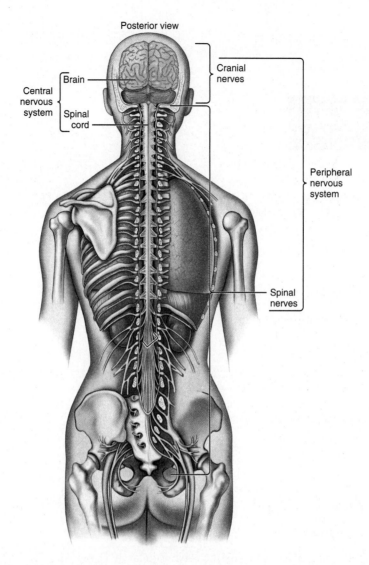

Figure 7.1 A posterior view of the nervous system. The central nervous system consists of the brain and spinal cord, and the peripheral nervous system consists of the cranial nerves and spinal nerves.

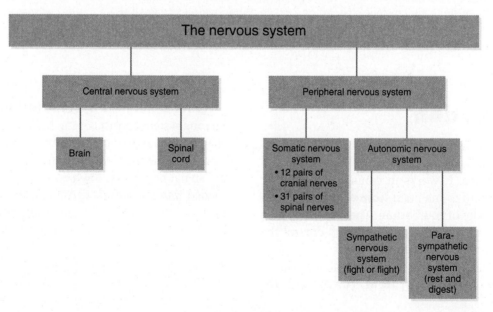

Figure 7.2 The divisions of the nervous system. The chart shows the divisions and subdivisions but all components work together.

Word Parts Related to Nervous System

The central nervous system control center is the brain, so many of the word parts used to describe nervous system structures pertain to the head. For example, cephal/o is the word root for head, and encephal/o is the word root for brain. Another word root for brain is cerebr/o, which refers specifically to the cerebrum (the largest part of the brain). Both psych/o and ment/o refer to the mind, the part of the brain responsible for consciousness and higher functions. **Table 7.1** lists word parts that make up nervous system terms. Some suffixes that you already learned are also listed.

Table 7.1 Word Parts Related to the Nervous System

Word Part	Meaning
arachn/o	spider
cephal/o	head
cerebell/o	cerebellum
cerebr/o	cerebrum; also, the brain in general
cortic/o	outer layer or covering
crani/o	cranium, skull
encephal/o	brain
gangli/o	swelling or knot
ganglion/o	swelling or knot
gli/o	glue
hydr/o	water
iatr/o	physician; to treat
-mania	mental abnormality or obsession
meningi/o	membrane
ment/o	referring to the mind
-mnesia	memory
myel/o	in connection with the nervous system, refers to the spinal cord and medulla oblongata
neur/o	nerve, nerve tissue
-oid	resembling
-paresis	slight paralysis
-phasia	speech
-phobia	fear

Word Part	Meaning
-plegia	paralysis
psych/o	mind
schiz/o	to split
spin/o	spine

Word Parts Exercise

After studying Table 7.1, write the meaning of each of the word parts.

Word Part	Meaning
1. –paresis	1. _____
2. cortic/o	2. _____
3. ment/o	3. _____
4. –plegia	4. _____
5. –mnesia	5. _____
6. iatr/o	6. _____
7. –phobia	7. _____
8. encephal/o	8. _____
9. cerebr/o	9. _____
10. hydr/o	10. _____
11. meningi/o	11. _____
12. gangli/o	12. _____
13. –mania	13. _____
14. myel/o	14. _____
15. neur/o	15. _____
16. arachn/o	16. _____
17. schiz/o	17. _____
18. cephal/o	18. _____
19. psych/o	19. _____
20. –oid	20. _____
21. cerebell/o	21. _____
22. spin/o	22. _____
23. –phasia	23. _____
24. gli/o	24. _____

Structure and Function

Nerve tissue, together with its associated connective tissue and blood vessels, makes up both the CNS and the PNS. Nerve tissue is composed of fundamental units called **neurons** (nerve cells), which are separated, supported, and protected by specialized cells called **neuroglia**. Neurons carry electrical messages that coordinate the exchange of information between the body's internal and external environments, and the neuroglia offer protection and support to the nerve tissue. Neurons are grouped together to carry out the highly complex sensing and processing actions required for everything humans do.

The three main parts of a neuron are its *cell body*, *dendrites*, and *axon*. The **cell body** contains the nucleus and receives electrical messages in the form of nerve impulses (action potentials) from other cells through the dendrites. The **nucleus** is an organelle found in the central region of the cell body that contains genetic material. The **dendrites**, which project outward from the cell body, act as antennae that receive and transmit messages between the neuron and muscles, skin, other neurons, or glands. The cell body passes these messages to the **axon**, which conducts nerve impulses away from the cell body. Axons are covered by **myelin**, a white fatty material that protects and insulates (see **Figure 7.3**). The connecting points for these message transfers are called **synapses**. Synaptic connections can occur between two neurons. A chemical called a **neurotransmitter** stimulates the transfer of the nerve impulse from the neuron to another neuron, muscle fiber, or other structure. For example, acetylcholine, dopamine, norepinephrine, and serotonin are typical neurotransmitters.

Groups of neuron cell bodies within the peripheral nervous system are called **ganglia** (*ganglion*, singular). Groups of neuron cell bodies within the central nervous system are called **nuclei** (*nucleus*, singular). Groupings of axons are called **nerves** wherever they occur in the body.

Central Nervous System (CNS)

The central nervous system is the body's control center. All messages originate or terminate either in the brain or in the spinal cord. The brain and spinal cord also interpret the messages and determine the body's responses.

The brain is a large organ that plays a role in many activities, both mental and physical. For example, regions of the brain control bodily functions, such as thinking, breathing, and temperature regulation, whereas other regions influence walking and other deliberate activities.

The brain is separated into left and right hemispheres each with four lobes: **frontal lobe**, **parietal lobe**, **occipital lobe**, and **temporal lobe** (see **Figure 7.4**). The names of the lobes relate to their location relative to the skull and the overlying skull bones. For example, *frontal* relates to the front part of the head, *parietal* refers to the sides of the head, *occipital* identifies the back of the head, and *temporal* refers to the temples or the flat sides of the head between the forehead and each ear.

The major parts of the brain include the following (see Figures 7.4 and **7.5**):

- **Cerebrum** The cerebrum, the largest part of the brain, is where memories and conscious thoughts are stored. It also directs some voluntary bodily

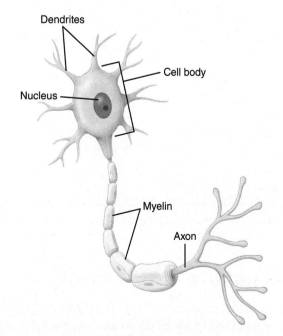

Figure 7.3 Structure of a typical neuron.

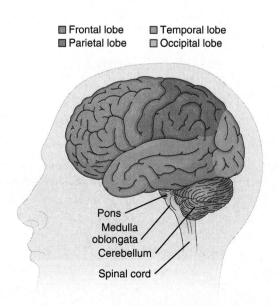

Figure 7.4 Lateral view of the four brain lobes and pons, medulla oblongata, cerebellum, and spinal cord.

Anterior

Posterior

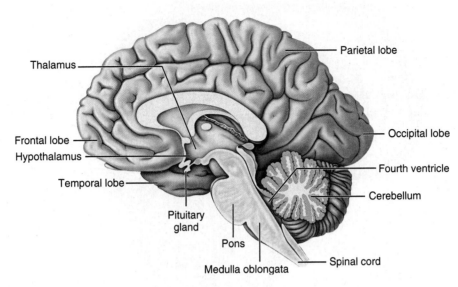

Thalamus

Parietal lobe

Frontal lobe

Occipital lobe

Hypothalamus

Fourth ventricle

Temporal lobe

Cerebellum

Pituitary gland

Pons

Spinal cord

Medulla oblongata

Figure 7.5 A sagittal section of the brain showing important structures.

movements. An outer layer of gray matter called the **cerebral cortex** controls higher mental functions.

- **Cerebellum** The cerebellum is located at the back of the skull. It coordinates voluntary muscles and maintains balance.
- **Diencephalon** The diencephalon is the link between the cerebral hemispheres and the brainstem. It contains both the *thalamus* and the *hypothalamus*. The **thalamus** processes sensory information. The **hypothalamus** coordinates the autonomic nervous system and the pituitary gland. The diencephalon releases hormones, controls body temperature, and regulates mood.
- **Brainstem** The brainstem connects the brain to the spinal cord. It is made up of the *midbrain*, *pons* (Latin for *bridge*), and *medulla oblongata*. The **midbrain** processes visual and audible sensory information. Visual tracking, such as moving the eyes to read or follow a moving object, is an example of a midbrain function. It also transmits hearing impulses to the brain. The **pons** passes information to the cerebellum and the thalamus to control subconscious activities such as regulating breathing. The **medulla oblongata** sends sensory information to the thalamus to direct the autonomic functions of the heart, lungs, and other body organs. The interconnected cavities within the brain are the **ventricles**. The fourth ventricle is shown in Figure 7.5.

The **spinal cord** is the portion of the CNS found within the vertebrae. It conducts nerve impulses to and from the brain and the body. The brain and spinal cord are surrounded by membranes called **meninges**, which absorb physical shocks that could otherwise damage nerve tissue (see **Figure 7.6**). The outer layer is the **dura mater**, a dense collection of collagen fibers. The middle layer is the **arachnoid mater**, which is thin, delicate, and weblike. The inner layer, called the **pia mater**, is in direct contact with nerve tissue. Together, the arachnoid and pia mater are two layers making up the **leptomeninx**. **Cerebrospinal fluid (CSF)** is the colorless liquid that circulates in and around the brain and spinal cord that transports nutrients.

Peripheral Nervous System (PNS)

The peripheral nervous system includes 12 pairs of cranial nerves and 31 pairs of spinal nerves that run along the periphery of the body (see Figure 7.1). The cranial and spinal nerves carry information via impulses from the CNS to the PNS and carry information from the PNS back to the CNS. The PNS controls skeletal muscles via the cranial and spinal nerves.

Recall that the PNS is divided into the somatic nervous system and the autonomic nervous system. The **somatic nervous system** controls voluntary movement, whereas the **autonomic nervous system** controls involuntary muscles (smooth muscle and cardiac muscle) and glands. Remember that the autonomic nervous system is made up of sympathetic and parasympathetic divisions. The **sympathetic nervous system** controls quick responses and is

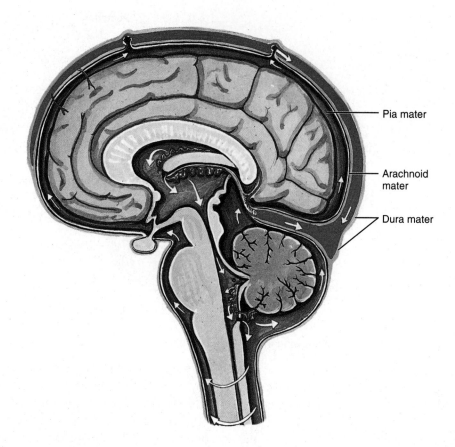

Figure 7.6 The meninges protect the brain and spinal cord. Arrows indicate the flow of cerebrospinal fluid.

often called the "fight or flight" division because this system increases heart rate and dilates airways during times of stress. The **parasympathetic nervous system** controls responses that do not need to be fast and is often called the "rest and digest" division. The parasympathetic nerves counterbalance sympathetic changes and return the body to homeostasis when the danger has passed (see Figure 7.2).

These two divisions of the autonomic nervous system are complementary. The sympathetic nervous system can be thought of as the gas pedal, and the parasympathetic nervous system can be thought of as the brake pedal.

QUICK CHECK

Fill in the blanks.

1. The CNS consists of the _____ and the _____.
2. The nervous system works in conjunction with the endocrine system to maintain _____, a term that means a state of equilibrium.
3. The major parts of the brain include the cerebrum, cerebellum, diencephalon, and _____.

Disorders Related to the Nervous System

Disorders of the nervous system can result from trauma, vascular insults, tumors, systemic degenerative diseases, and seizures. Behavioral disorders are treated as a separate category.

Trauma

Head injuries can cause skull fractures, hemorrhage, swelling, and direct damage to the brain itself. Brain injury may be relatively mild, involving bruises to brain tissues, or it can be severe, causing tissue destruction and massive swelling. Common types of brain trauma include the following:

- **Concussion** is an injury to the brain resulting from violent shaking or a hit to the head. A concussion may cause temporary loss of consciousness followed by a short period of amnesia (loss of memory). Dizziness, nausea, and headache are common with a concussion.
- **Epidural hematoma** occurs when blood collects between the dura mater and the skull, causing pressure on the blood vessels and

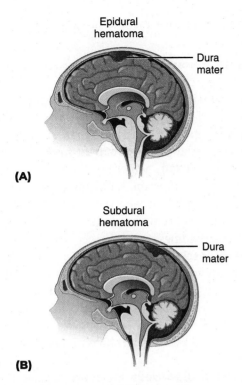

Figure 7.7 Hematoma. **(A)** Epidural hematoma occurs with a traumatic brain injury when blood accumulates between the dura mater and the skull. **(B)** Subdural hematoma occurs between the dura mater and arachnoid mater.

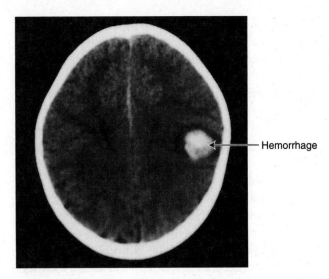

Figure 7.8 Cerebrovascular accident. Computed tomography (CT) scan of the brain shows a large hemorrhage in the brain of a 4-year-old boy.

interrupting blood flow to the brain. This condition is caused by a skull fracture or a hit to the head (see **Figure 7.7A**).

- **Subdural hematoma** is a collection of blood trapped in the subdural space, the area beneath the dura mater. It may result from a hit to the front or back of the head (see **Figure 7.7B**).

Vascular Insults

A vascular insult is an injury to blood vessels.

- **Cerebrovascular accident (CVA)** Also known as a stroke, a cerebrovascular accident results from an interruption of oxygen caused by blood vessel blockage or rupture, causing hemorrhage (bleeding) (see **Figure 7.8**).
- **Transient ischemic attack (TIA)** A transient ischemic attack is a temporary interruption in the blood supply to the brain. This is sometimes called a "mini-stroke" but can indicate serious problems and be a forewarning of a stroke.
- **Cerebral aneurysm** An aneurysm is a localized dilation (widening) of an artery caused by weakness in the vessel wall.

Doesn't the word "insult" refer to a verbal attack, such as when someone calls someone else a name that causes hurt feelings? Yes, it does, but in the phrase "vascular insult," it means something else. The Latin verb *insulto* literally means "to physically jump on." So, a vascular insult is a physical event related to that Latin meaning.

Tumors

Tumors are **lesions** (regions in an organ that are damaged) or neoplasms that may cause localized dysfunction, producing an increase in intracranial pressure (ICP). It is important for the pressure within the cranium to stay within its normal range, because a high ICP usually leads to death if it is not relieved. Tumors may be benign or malignant. Two examples of tumors occurring in the nervous system include *astrocytomas* and *meningiomas*. An **astrocytoma** is a tumor derived from a star-shaped type of neuroglia called an astrocyte. A **meningioma** is a tumor derived from the meninges surrounding the brain and spinal cord.

Systemic Degenerative Diseases

Degenerative diseases develop slowly over time. A progressive deterioration may start out affecting individual body functions and end up involving other body systems. Examples of systemic degenerative diseases include *Alzheimer's disease* (AD), *amyotrophic lateral sclerosis* (ALS), *multiple sclerosis* (MS), and *Parkinson's disease* (PD).

- **Alzheimer's disease (AD)** is a degenerative, eventually fatal condition involving atrophy of the cerebral cortex, producing a progressive loss of intellectual function.
- **Amyotrophic lateral sclerosis (ALS)** is a degenerative disease that destroys motor neurons, which are the specific neurons that control voluntary movement. It is also known as *Lou Gehrig's disease*, after New York Yankee baseball player, Lou Gehrig (1903–1941), who died from ALS. The fatal disease causes progressive weakness and muscle atrophy because of gradual motor neuron destruction.
- **Multiple sclerosis (MS)** is a progressive degenerative disease with symptoms caused by **demyelination**, a patchy loss of the myelin sheath.
- **Parkinson's disease (PD)** usually develops after age 60 and occurs with the loss of the neurotransmitter **dopamine (DA)**, which inhibits nerve impulse transmission. When these nerve impulses are no longer inhibited by dopamine, signs such as tremors and muscle rigidity occur. This can affect posture, balance, speech, and other activities of daily living.

Seizures

A **seizure** occurs when there is an abnormal, uncontrolled burst of electrical activity in the brain. Seizures may result from trauma, tumors, fevers, medications, or other causes. Some seizures go unnoticed when the signs are very subtle. Other seizures can cause loss of consciousness or involuntarily body movements.

Epilepsy is a chronic disorder characterized by recurrent seizures that result from excessive discharge of brain neurons. Two basic types of epileptic seizures are *grand mal seizures* and *absence seizures*. A **grand mal seizure**, also called a *generalized tonic–clonic seizure*, is severe and characterized by alternating contraction and relaxation of muscles, which produces jerking movements of the face, trunk, and/or extremities. An **absence seizure** (formerly called a *petit mal seizure*) is a milder form of seizure that lasts only a few seconds and does not include convulsive movements. The term *mal* comes from the French language and means sickness.

Behavioral Disorders

Some behavioral disorders are related to the nervous system. They may be caused by physical changes, substance abuse, medications, or any combination

thereof. The categories include anxiety, mood, and psychotic disorders.

- **Anxiety disorders** are characterized by feelings of apprehension or uneasiness, sometimes associated with the anticipation of danger. Common examples include **obsessive–compulsive disorder (OCD)**, which may be signaled by repetitive behaviors; **posttraumatic stress disorder (PTSD)**, which is the development of long-term symptoms following a psychologically traumatic event; and the various **phobias**, which are persistent, irrational fears of specific situations or things.
- **Mood disorders** are a group of mental disorders involving a disturbance of internal emotional states. They include **depression**, which is characterized by loss of interest or pleasure in activities, and **bipolar disorder**, which is characterized by unusual shifts in mood, energy, and activity.
- **Psychotic disorders** are more serious than anxiety or mood disorders because they feature a loss of contact with reality and a deterioration of normal social functioning. An example of a psychosis is **schizophrenia**, which is characterized by abnormal thoughts, hallucinations, delusions, and withdrawal. **Paranoia** is another example characterized by jealousy, delusions of persecution, or perceptions of threat or harm.

Diagnostic Tests, Treatments, and Surgical Procedures

When evaluating the health of a person's nervous system, medical professionals use various procedures. Sometimes, a patient's mental health is determined by a qualified professional observing and talking with the patient. Other times, diagnostic tests evaluate the condition of the brain and its function. Some examples of diagnostic tests and procedures are listed next.

- **Computed tomography (CT)** is a noninvasive radiologic test that uses a computer to produce cross-sectional images of the soft-tissue structures of the brain and spinal cord. This procedure can reveal problems such as brain tumors and aneurysms.
- **Electroencephalography (EEG)** is the measurement of electrical activity in the brain and the visual trace (electroencephalogram) of that

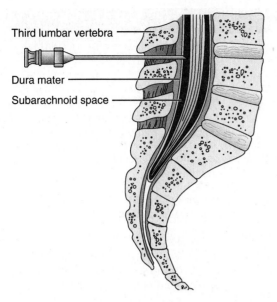

- Third lumbar vertebra
- Dura mater
- Subarachnoid space

Figure 7.9 Shows the location for a lumbar puncture between L3 and L4.

spinal cord, spinal column, and peripheral nerves. **Psychiatrists** are physicians who treat behavioral and mental health disorders. The healthcare professional with an advanced academic degree who treats mental and behavioral disorders is a **psychologist**.

What's the difference between a psychiatrist and a psychologist? Using word parts, we can break each word up: psych-olog-ist and psych-iatr-ist. Remember that -logy means "study of" and iatro means "physician." The degrees that each profession receives are different: a psychologist has a doctorate degree in the form of a PhD, PsyD, or EdD, whereas a psychiatrist has an MD or a DO and is a medical doctor, meaning they can prescribe medications (unlike a psychologist). This is a key difference and means the two practitioners are not interchangeable; however, they often work together to treat patients.

activity. It is used to document increased electrical events of the brain caused by seizures.

- **Nerve conduction study (NCS)** measures how fast electrical impulses move through a nerve. Also called a *nerve conduction velocity* (NCV) test, it evaluates nerve function of motor nerves to determine nerve damage or disease.
- **Magnetic resonance imaging (MRI)** uses radio waves and a very strong magnetic field to produce images of the neural soft tissues. It is used to visualize disease-related changes in the brain or spinal cord that conventional X-ray procedures cannot detect. For example, MRI can isolate damaged areas of the brain caused by multiple sclerosis.
- **Lumbar puncture (LP)** requires the insertion of a needle into the subarachnoid space (the area between the arachnoid mater and pia mater) between the third and fourth or fourth and fifth lumbar vertebrae to withdraw cerebrospinal fluid for analysis (*see* **Figure 7.9**).

Practice and Practitioners

Medical specialists who diagnose and treat the nervous system are *neurologists*, *neurosurgeons*, *psychiatrists*, and *psychologists*. **Neurologists** are medical specialists trained in the diagnosis and treatment of neuromuscular disorders. **Neurosurgeons** are physicians specialized in operations on the brain,

Abbreviation Table	The Nervous System
Abbreviation	**Meaning**
AD	Alzheimer's disease
CNS	central nervous system
CSF	cerebrospinal fluid
CP	cerebral palsy
CT	computed tomography
CVA	cerebrovascular accident
DA	dopamine
ECT	electroconvulsive therapy
EEG	electroencephalography
ICP	intracranial pressure
LP	lumbar puncture
MG	myasthenia gravis
MRI	magnetic resonance imaging
MS	multiple sclerosis
OCD	obsessive–compulsive disorder
PD	Parkinson's disease
PNS	peripheral nervous system
PTSD	posttraumatic stress disorder
TIA	transient ischemic attack

Study Table The Nervous System

Term and Pronunciation	Analysis	Meaning
Structure and Function		
autonomic nervous system (ANS) (aw-toh-NOM-ik NERV-us SIS-tum)	autonomy (self-sufficiency); -ic (adjective suffix)	the parts of the peripheral nervous system (PNS) that carry messages between the central nervous system (CNS) and organs that function autonomously
arachnoid mater (uh-RAK-noyd MAY-tur)	from the Greek word *arachne* (spider, cob- web); -oid (resembling)	delicate weblike layer of the meninges; middle layer
axon (AX-on)	*axo-* (axis); -n noun ending	the part of a neuron that conducts electrical impulses away from the cell body
brainstem (BRAIN-stem)	related to Dutch word, *brein* (brain)	the part of the brain that controls functions, such as heart rate, breathing, and body temperature; includes midbrain, pons, and medulla oblongata
cell body (SELL BOD-ee)	cell means a small room	the main part of a neuron that contains the nucleus
central nervous system (CNS) (SEN-trul NERV-us SIS-tum)	from the Latin words, *centrum* (center), *nervosus* (nerve), and *systema* (system)	the division of the nervous system that includes the brain and spinal cord
cerebellum (SERR-uh-bell-um)	*cerebr/o* (brain)	the part of the brain that controls the skeletal muscles
cerebral cortex (seh-REE-brul KOR-tex)	*cerebr/o* (brain); -al (adjective suffix)	the gray matter surrounding the cerebrum
cerebrospinal fluid (CSF) (seh-REE-broh-SPY-nul)	*cerebr/o* (brain); from Latin word *spina*; fluid (common English word)	the fluid in and around the brain and spinal cord
cerebrum (seh-REE-brum)	*cerebr/o* (brain)	the largest part of the brain; controls conscious thought and stores memories
dendrite (DEN-dryte)	from the Greek word *dendrites* (relating to a tree)	process extending from a neuron cell body
diencephalon (dye-en-SEFF-uh-lon)	*di-* (two); *encephal/o* (of or relating to the brain); -on (noun suffix)	the part of the brain containing both the thalamus and the hypothalamus
dura mater (DOO-ruh MAY-tur)	Latin words meaning "hard mother"	the outer meninx, the fibrous membrane protecting the CNS
frontal lobe (FRUN-tul LOBE)	common English words	the front part of the brain from which voluntary muscle movements and other sensory and motor (movement) tasks are directed
ganglion; ganglia (plural) (GANG-lee-on); (GANG-lee-uh)	a Greek word meaning "swelling" or "knot"	a group of neuron cell bodies grouped together in the PNS
homeostasis (hoh-me-oh-STAY-sis)	*homos* (Greek for "same"); *stasis* (Greek for "existence")	tendency toward equilibrium; remaining normal
hypothalamus (HIGH-po-thal-uh-mus)	*hypo-* (below, deficient); from the Greek word *thalamus* (a bed, a bedroom)	the hormone and emotion center of the brain that controls autonomic functions
leptomeninx (LEPP-toh-MEN-inks)	*lepto-* (light, slender, thin frail); meninx is the singular form of meninges (membranes)	collective term for the arachnoid mater and pia mater

Term and Pronunciation	Analysis	Meaning
Structure and Function		
medulla oblongata (meh-DUH-luh ob-long-GAH-tuh)	a Latin word (marrow); from the Latin *oblongatus* (oblong)	the part of the brainstem that sends sensory information to the thalamus to direct the autonomic functions of the heart, lungs, and other organs
meninges (meh-NIN-jeez)	*mening/o* (membrane)	three-layer membrane surrounding the brain and spinal cord
mesencephalon (mez-en-SEFF-uh-lon)	*mes/o* (middle); *encephal/o* (brain); *-on* (noun suffix)	the middle part of the brain between the diencephalon and the pons; also called the midbrain
midbrain (MID-brain)	*mid* = middle	the middle part of the brain between the diencephalon and the pons; also called the mesencephalon
myelin (MY-eh-lin)	*myel/o-* (bone marrow; spinal cord)	a fatty white wrapper on cells providing protection and electrical insulation to neurons
nerve (NERV)	*nervus*, Latin for nerve; common English word	a whitish, cordlike structure composed of one or more bundles of nerve fibers outside the CNS, together with their connective tissues and nourishing blood vessels
neuroglia (new-ROG-lee-uh)	*neur/o* (nerve); from the Greek *glia* (glue)	cells within both the CNS and PNS, which, although they are external to neurons, form an essential part of nerve tissue
neuron (NUR-on)	*neur/o* (nerve); *-on* (noun suffix)	a nerve cell, including the cell body and its axon
neurotransmitter (NOO-roh-TRANS- mitt-ur)	*neur/o* (nerve); from the Latin *trans* (across); *mittere* (to send)	chemical released by the presynaptic cell (cell before the synapse) that is then picked up by the postsynaptic cell (cell after the synapse) to affect an action
nucleus; nuclei (plural) (NEW-klee-us); (NEW-klee-eye)	From the Latin word meaning "kernel"	central region of neuron cell body that contains genetic information; a group of neuron cell bodies grouped together in the CNS
occipital lobe (AWK-sip-ih-tul LOBE)	from Latin word *occiput* (back of the head)	the part of the brain that processes information from the sense of sight and other sensory and motor (movement) tasks
parasympathetic nervous system (pair-uh-sim-puh-THET-ik NERV-us SIS-tum)	*para-* (beside); *sympatheia* (Greek meaning community of feeling); *-ic* (adjective)	division of the ANS responsible for rest and digest responses
parietal lobe (pah-RYE-uh-tul LOBE)	from the Latin adjective *parietalis* (walls); *-al* (adjective suffix)	the part of the brain that processes information from the sense of touch and other sensory and motor (movement) tasks
peripheral nervous system (PNS) (puh-RIFF-uh-rul NERV-us SIS-tum)	*peri-* (surrounding); from the Greek word *pherein* (to carry); nervous system (common English words)	made up of neurons, neuroglia, and associated tissue, including the cranial and spinal nerves and the sensory and motor (movement) nerves that extend throughout the body
pia mater (PEE-uh MAY-tur)	Latin words meaning "tender mother"	inner layer of the meninges

(continues)

Study Table The Nervous System		*(continued)*
Term and Pronunciation	**Analysis**	**Meaning**
Structure and Function		
pons (PONS)	a Latin word meaning "bridge"	the part of the brainstem that passes information to the cerebellum and the thalamus to regulate subconscious somatic activities
psychomotor (SIGH-koh-moh-tur)	*psych/o* (of the mind); from the Latin word *motor* (mover)	an adjective used to indicate the relation between psychic activity and muscular movement
somatic nervous system (so-MAT-ik NURV-us SIS-tum)	*somat/o* (body, bodily); *-ic* (adjective suffix)	the parts of the PNS that carry nerve impulses for conscious activity rather than habitual activity
sympathetic nervous system (sim-puh-THET-ik NERV-us SIS-tum)	*sympatheia* (Greek meaning community of feeling); *-ic* (adjective)	division of the ANS responsible for fight or flight responses
spinal nerves (SPY-nul NURVZ)	from the Latin word *spina* (spine)	the 31 pairs of nerves located along the spinal cord
synapse (SIN-aps)	*syn-* (together); from the Greek word *hapto* (clasp)	the connecting point between neurons or between a neuron and a receptor or effector cell
temporal lobe (TEM-por-ul LOBE)	from the Latin word *temporalis* (time, temple)	the part of the brain that processes information from the senses of hearing, smell, and taste, and other sensory and motor (movement) tasks
thalamus (THAL-uh-mus)	from the Greek word *thalamus* (bed, bedroom)	part of the brain that processes sensory information
ventricles (VEN-tri-kulz)	from the Latin word *ventriculus*, dim. of *venter* (belly)	cavities within the brain
Disorders		
absence seizure (AB-sens SEE-zhur)	from the Latin word *absentia*, absent	seizure characterized by impaired awareness; milder form of seizure lasting only a few seconds and does not include convulsive movements; formerly known as *petit mal seizures;* French words meaning little sickness
Alzheimer's disease (AD) (ALZ-high-murz de-ZEEZ)	named after German physician Alois Alzheimer, who first described it in 1906	a disease that may begin in late middle life, characterized by progressive mental deterioration that includes loss of memory and visual and spatial orientation
amnesia (am-NEE-zuh)	*a-* (without); *-mnesia* (memory)	loss of memory
amyotrophic lateral sclerosis (ALS) (uh-my-oh-TROH-fik LAT-ur-ul skluh-ROE-sis)	amyotrophy means muscular atrophy, derived from *a-* (without), *mus* (muscle), and *trophē* (nourishment); *later-* (side); sclerosis means body tissue hardening, derived from *sklērōsis* (harden)	progressive nervous system disease affecting neurons in the brain and spinal cord leading to loss of muscle control and muscle atrophy (wasting)

Term and Pronunciation	Analysis	Meaning
Disorders		
aneurysm (AN-yur-izm)	from the Greek *ana* (up) and *eurys* (broad)	localized dilation of an artery due to vessel wall weakness
anxiety disorder (ANG-zigh-ih-tee DIS-or-der)	from the Latin word *anxius* (to choke)	a feeling of apprehension or uneasiness that results from anticipation of danger
aphasia (uh-FAY-jhah)	*a-* (absence of); from the Greek word *phases* (speech)	loss of speech
astrocytoma (a-stroh-sigh-TOH-muh)	from the Greek word *astron* (star); *cyt/o* (cell); *-oma* (tumor)	star-shaped tumor that usually develops in the cerebrum; frequently in people younger than 20 years old
ataxia (ah-TAK-see-uh)	*a-* (without); from the Greek word *taxis* (order)	lack of muscular coordination
bipolar disorder (bye-POLE-ur DIS-or-der)	*bi-* (twice, double); from the Latin word *polus* (the end of an axis)	disorder characterized by manic episodes alternating with depressive episodes
cerebral palsy (CP) (seh-REE-brul PAL-zee)	cerebral refers to the brain and palsy means weakness or paralysis	motor impairment affecting muscle coordination, movement, balance, and posture typically caused by brain damage before birth or at birth
cerebral thrombosis (seh-REE-brul throm-BOH-sis)	*cerebr/o* (brain); *-al* (adjective suffix); *thromb/o* (of or relating to a blood clot); *-sis* (abnormal condition)	blood clot in the brain
cerebrovascular accident (CVA) (seh-REE-bro-VAS-kyu-lur AKS-ih-dent)	*cerebr/o* (brain); *vascul/o* (blood vessel); *-ar* (adjective suffix)	a synonym for *cerebral stroke*, an acute clinical event, related to impairment of cerebral circulation, lasting more than 24 hours
cerebrovascular disease (seh-REE-bro-VAS-kyu-lur de-ZEEZ)	*cerebr/o* (brain); *vascul/o* (blood vessel); *-ar* (adjective suffix)	brain disorder involving a blood vessel
concussion (kun-KUSH-un)	from the Latin word *concussionem* (a shaking)	brain injury resulting from a hit to the head or violent shaking
delirium (duh-LEER-ee-um)	from the Latin word *deliro* (to be crazy)	altered state of consciousness
delusion (deh-LOO-zhun)	from the Latin word *ludere* (to play)	false belief or wrong judgment despite evidence to the contrary
dementia (duh-MEN-shuh)	from Latin *de* (apart, away); *mens* (mind)	impaired intellectual function
demyelination (dee-my-uh-lin-AY-shun)	from the Greek word *myelos* (marrow, inner part of the brain)	loss of myelin
depression (dih-PRESH-un)	from the Latin word *depressio*	prolonged period where there is a loss of interest or pleasure in almost all activities
dopamine (DA) (DOH- puh-meen)	from the acronym for the amino acid dioxyphenylalanine (DOPA)	neurotransmitter in the CNS and PNS; depletion of dopamine causes Parkinson's disease
dysphasia (DIS-fay-jhuh)	*dys-* (bad, difficult); from the Greek word *phases* (speaking)	impaired speech
encephalitis (en-seff-uh-LYE-tis)	*encephal/o* (of or pertaining to the brain); *-itis* (inflammation)	inflammation of the brain

(continues)

Study Table The Nervous System		*(continued)*
Term and Pronunciation	**Analysis**	**Meaning**
Disorders		
epidural hematoma (EH-pih-dur-ul hee-muh-TOH-muh)	*epi-* (above); dural (relating to the dura mater); *hemat/o* (blood); *-oma* (tumor)	a collection of blood in the space between the skull and dura mater
epilepsy (EPP-ih-lepp-see)	from the Greek *epilepsia* (seizure)	central nervous system (CNS) disorder often characterized by seizures
glioblastoma (GLY-oh- blass-TOH-muh)	*glio* (glue); from the Greek word *blastos* (germ); *-oma* (tumor)	a cerebral tumor occurring most frequently in adults
glioma (gly-OH-muh)	*glio-* (glue); *-oma* (tumor)	tumor of glial tissue
grand mal seizure (GRAND-MAHL SEE-zhur)	French words meaning "big sickness"	type of severe seizure with tonic–clonic convulsion; also called tonic–clonic seizure
hallucination (huh-LOO-sih-nay-shun)	from the Latin word *alucinor* (to wander in mind)	subjective perception of an object or voice when no such stimulus exists
hemiparesis (hem-ee-puh-REE-sus)	*hemi-* (one-half); *-paresis* (slight paralysis)	partial paralysis of one side of the body
hemiplegia (hem-ee-PLEE-jee-uh)	*hemi-* (one-half); *-plegia* (paralysis)	paralysis of one side of the body
Huntington's disease (HUN-ting-tunz de-ZEEZ)	named after American physician George Huntington who described the disorder in 1872	hereditary disorder of the CNS
hydrocephalus (hy-dro-SEFF-uh-lus)	*hydro-* (water); *cephal/o* (of or pertaining to the head)	excessive cerebrospinal fluid (CSF) in the brain
hyperesthesia (hy-per-ess-THEE-zyuh)	*hyper-* (extreme or beyond normal); *esthesi/o* (sensation)	abnormal sensitivity to touch
kleptomania (klep-toh-MAY-knee-uh)	from the Greek word *klepto-* (to steal); from the Latin *-mania* (insanity)	uncontrollable impulse to steal
lesion (LEE-zhun)	from the Latin, *laedo* (to injure)	wound or injury; pathologic tissue change
meningioma (meh-nin-jee-OH-muh)	*mening/o* (membrane); *-oma* (tumor)	benign tumor of the meninges
meningitis (meh-nin-JYE-tis)	*mening/o* (membrane); *-itis* (inflammation)	inflamed meninges
mood disorder (MOOD DIS-or-der)	variant of *mode*, meaning mood	a group of mental disorders involving a disturbance of mood not due to any other mental disorder
multiple sclerosis (MS) (MUL-ti-pul skleh-ROH-sis)	multiple (from the English word meaning "many"); *scler/o* (hardness); *-osis* (abnormal condition)	disease of the CNS characterized by demyelination and the formation of plaques in the brain and spinal cord
myasthenia gravis (MG) (MY-us-THEE-nee-uh GRAV-is)	*my/o* (muscle); *astheneia* (weakness)	muscle weakness, lack of strength

Term and Pronunciation	Analysis	Meaning
Disorders		
myelitis (my-eh-LYE-tis)	*myel/o* (bone marrow or spine); *-itis* (inflammation)	inflammation of the spinal cord
myelomeningocele (MY-loh-mih-NIN-gee-oh-seel)	*myel/o* (bone marrow or spine); *meningi/o* (membrane); *-cele* (hernia)	incomplete closure of the vertebra enabling protrusion of the meninges and spinal cord through the opening
neuralgia (nur-ALL-juh)	*neur/o* (nerve); *-algia* (pain)	pain in a nerve
neuropathy (nur-OP-uh-thee)	*neur/o* (nerve); *-pathy* (disease)	disease or dysfunction of peripheral nerves causing numbness or weakness
obsessive–compulsive disorder (OCD) (ub-SESS-iv kum-PULS-iv DIS-or-der)	from medieval Latin, *compulsivus* meaning driven or forced	type of anxiety disorder characterized by persistent thoughts and impulses with repetitive responses that interfere with daily activities
paralysis (puh-RALL-ih-sis)	*para-* (abnormal, alongside); *-lysis* (destruction)	loss of one or more muscle functions
paranoia (pair-uh-NOY-yuh)	*para-* (abnormal, alongside); from Greek word *noeo* (to think)	a serious mental disorder characterized by unreasonable suspicion or jealousy, along with a tendency to interpret everything others do as hostile
paraplegia (pair-uh-PLEE-jee-uh)	*para-* (abnormal, alongside); *-plegia* (paralysis)	paralysis of the lower extremities and, often, the lower trunk of the body
paresthesia (pair-ess-THEE-zyuh)	*para-* (abnormal); *esthesi/o* (sensation)	numbness
Parkinson's disease (PD) (PAR-kin-suns de-ZEEZ)	named for English physician James Parkinson, who described it in 1817	disease of the nerves in the brain due to an imbalance of dopamine; also called parkinsonism
phobia (FOH-bee-uh)	*phob/o* (exaggerated fear); *-ia* (noun suffix)	a fear of something that is not a hazard from a statistical point of view
plegia (PLEE-jee-uh)	*-plegia* (paralysis)	paralysis
poliomyelitis (poh-lee-oh-MY-eh-LYE-tis)	*polio-* (denoting gray color); *myel/o* (bone marrow or spine); *-itis* (inflammation)	inflamed gray matter of the spinal cord
posttraumatic stress disorder (PTSD) (post-truh-MAT-ik stres dis-OR-der)	*post-* (after); *trauma* (Greek for wound); *-ic* (forming adjective)	development of characteristic long-term symptoms following a psychologically traumatic event that is generally outside the range of usual human experience
psychosis (sigh-KOH-sis)	*psych/o* (mind); *-sis* (condition of)	a serious disorder involving a marked distortion of, or sharp break from, reality; general term covering severe mental or emotional disorders
psychotic disorder (sigh-KOT-ik dis-OR-der)	*psych/o* (mind); *-ic* (adjective)	a mental and behavioral disorder causing gross distortion or disorganization of a person's mental capacity, affective response, and capacity to recognize reality

(continues)

Study Table The Nervous System		*(continued)*
Term and Pronunciation	**Analysis**	**Meaning**
Disorders		
quadriplegia (kwad-rih-PLEE-jee-uh)	*quadr/i* (four); *-plegia* (paralysis)	paralysis of all four limbs
schizophrenia (skits-oh-FREN-ee-uh)	*schiz/o* (denoting split or double sided); from the Greek word *phren* (mind)	a severe mental illness characterized by auditory hallucinations, paranoia, and an inability to distinguish reality from fiction
seizure (SEE-zhur)	from the French word *seisir* (to grasp)	sudden disturbance in brain function sometimes producing a convulsion
somnambulism (sahm-NOM-bu-liz-um)	from Latin words *somnus* (sleep) and *ambulo* (walk); *-ism* (a medical condition)	sleep walking
spina bifida (SPY-nuh BIF-ih-duh)	from Latin words *spina* (backbone) and *bifidus* (doubly split)	congenital defect in which the spinal cord protrudes through a gap in the backbone (vertebra), often causing lower limb paralysis
subdural hematoma (SUB-dur-uhl hee-muh-TOH-muh)	*sub-* (beneath); *dura* (hard); *-al* (adjective suffix); *hemat/o* (blood); *-oma* (tumor)	a collection of blood trapped in the space beneath the dura mater, between the dura and arachnoid layers of the meninges
syncope (SIN-kuh-pee)	from the Greek word *syncope* (a cutting short, a swoon)	fainting
torticollis (tor-tih-KOH-lis)	also called wryneck; from the Latin words *tortus* (crooked, twisted) and *collum* (neck)	neurological condition causing the head to persistently turn to one side, often with accompanying painful muscle spasms
transient ischemic attack (TIA) (TRANS-ee-ent IH-skee-mik uh-TACK)	from Greek *isch,* (to restrict), and the suffix *-emia* (blood)	temporary interruption in the blood supply to the brain
vertigo (VUR-tih-goh)	from the Latin word *verto* (turn)	dizziness
Diagnostic Tests, Treatments, and Surgical Procedures		
antianxiety agent (an-tee-ang-ZYE-ih-tee A-jent)	*anti-* (against); from the Greek word *angho* (to squeeze, embrace, throttle)	drug used to suppress anxiousness and relax muscles
anticonvulsant agent (an-tee-con-VUL-sunt A-jent)	*anti-* (against); from the Latin *con* (with) and *vulsus* (to tear up)	drug used to decrease seizure activity
antipsychotic agent (an-tee-sigh-KOT-ik A-jent)	*anti-* (against); *psych/o* (mind); *-tic* (adjective suffix)	drug given to patients to affect behavior and treat psychiatric disorders
computed tomography (CT) (com-PUTE-ed tuh-MOG-ruh-fee)	*tomos* (Greek "to slice"); *-graph* (instrument for recording)	X-ray imaging using cross-sectional planes of the body
craniectomy (KRAY-nee-ek-tuh-mee)	*crani/o* (cranium); *-ec-tomy* (excision)	excision of part of the skull
craniotomy (KRAY-nee-ot-uh-mee)	*crani/o* (cranium); *-tomy* (cutting operation)	incision into the skull
electroconvulsive therapy (ECT) (eh-LEK-troh-kun-VULS-iv THER-uh-pee)	*electr/o* (electric); from the Latin words *con* (with) and *vulsus* (to tear up); also called electroshock therapy (EST)	a controlled convulsion produced by passing an electric current through the brain

Term and Pronunciation	Analysis	Meaning
Diagnostic Tests, Treatments, and Surgical Procedures		
electroencephalography (EEG) (ee-LEK-troh-en-sef-uh-LOG-ruh-fee)	*electr/o* (electric); *encephal/o* (brain); *-graphy* (process of recording)	record of the electrical activity of the brain
electromyography (EMG) (ee-lek-troh-my-OG-ruh-fee)	*electro-* (electric); *myo* (muscle); *-graphy* (writing, recording)	test used to measure electrical activity of muscles by inserting a needle electrode through the skin into various muscles as they contract and relax; test can diagnose or rule out amyotrophic lateral sclerosis (ALS)
electroshock therapy (EST) (eh-LEK-troh-SHOCK THER-uh-pee)	*electr/o* (electric); from the Latin words *con* (with) and *vulsus* (to tear up); also called electroconvulsive therapy (ECT)	a controlled convulsion produced by passing an electric current through the brain
lobotomy (loh-BOT-uh-mee)	*lob/o* (lobe); *-tomy* (cutting operation)	incision into a lobe
lumbar puncture (LP) (LUM-bar PUNK-cher)	from the Latin word *lum- bus* (loin)	insertion of a needle into the subarachnoid space between the third and fourth or fourth and fifth lumbar vertebrae to withdraw fluid for diagnosis
magnetic resonance imaging (MRI) (mag-NET-ik REZ-uh-nunce im-ih-JING)	from the Latin, *imago* (to imitate) and *resonantia* (echo)	uses radio waves and a very strong magnetic field to produce images of the soft tissue
myelography (my-eh-LOG-ruh-fee)	*myel/o* (bone marrow or spine); *-graphy* (process of recording)	radiography of the spinal cord and nerve roots
nerve conduction study (NCS) (NURV kun-DUCK-shun stud-EE)	from the Latin, *conduction* (channel or conduit); also called a nerve conduction velocity test	medical test used to evaluate nerve function by measuring electrical conduction in a nerve and is used to determine nerve function or nerve disease
neuroplasty (NUR-oh-plass-tee)	*neur/o* (nerve); *-plasty* (repair)	surgery to repair a nerve
sedatives (SED-uh-tivz)	from the Latin *sedeo* (sit); from the Greek word *hypnotikos* (causing one to sleep)	drugs used to induce calming effect or sleep
Practice and Practitioners		
neurologist (nur-OL-oh-jihst)	*neur/o* (nerve); *-logist* (practitioner)	a medical specialist who treats nervous system disorders
neurology (nur-OL-oh-jee)	*neur/o* (nerve); *-logy* (the study of)	medical specialty dealing with the nervous system
neurosurgeon (NOO-roh-sur-jun)	*neur/o* (nerve); from the Greek word *kheirourgos* (working or done by hand)	surgeon who specializes in operations on the nervous system
psychiatrist (sigh-KYE-uh-trist)	*psych/o* (mind); *iatr/o* (of or pertaining to medicine or a physician); *-ist* (one who specializes in)	a medical doctor who specializes in the diagnosis and treatment of psychological disorders
psychologist (sigh-KOL-oh-jist)	*psych/o* (mind); *-logist* (one who studies a certain field)	a (nonmedical) doctor of psychology who specializes in the diagnosis and treatment of psychological disorders

CASE STUDY WRAP-UP

By the time Pierce got into the clinic, 2 months had passed and his speech was slurring, his hand weakness had progressed, muscle twitching in his left arm was prevalent, and he had great difficulty buttoning his shirt. Pierce told his doctor that he felt like he couldn't control his body and playing the guitar was really hard. The clinic physician sent Pierce to a neurologist, who saw him that same day. Given the rapid change in his signs and symptoms, the neurologist ordered several diagnostic tests including an electromyogram (EMG), nerve conduction study, and routine blood and urine tests. The results of these tests indicated possible amyotrophic lateral sclerosis (ALS) with both upper motor neuron (brain) and lower motor neuron (spinal cord) involvement.

Case Study Application Questions

1. Describe amyotrophic lateral sclerosis (ALS).
2. Upper motor neurons originate in the _____, while lower motor neurons originate in the _____.
3. What signs indicate that Pierce has motor neuron issues?
4. What test evaluates the electrical activity of muscles during contraction and relaxation?
5. Why was a nerve conduction study ordered?

END-OF-CHAPTER EXERCISES

Exercise 7.1 Labeling

Label the parts of the neuron. Select from the following list of terms.

axon   dendrites   nucleus

cell body   myelin

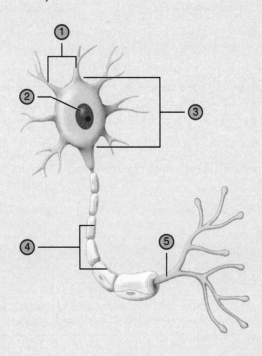

1. _____   4. _____

2. _____   5. _____

3. _____

Exercise 7.2 Word Parts

Break each of the following terms into its word parts: root, prefix, or suffix. Give the meaning of each word part and then define each term.

1. *psychosis*

    root: _____

    suffix: _____

    definition: _____

2. *electroencephalography*

    root: _____

    root: _____

    suffix: _____

    definition: _____

3. *astrocytoma*

    root: _____

    root: _____

    suffix: _____

    definition: _____

4. *cerebrovascular*

    root: _____

    root: _____

    suffix: _____

    definition: _____

5. *encephalitis*

    root: _____

    suffix: _____

    definition: _____

6. *epidural*

    prefix: _____

    root: _____

    suffix: _____

    definition: _____

7. *psychiatrist*

    root: _____

    root: _____

    suffix: _____

    definition: _____

8. *meningioma*

     root: _____

     suffix: _____

     definition: _____

Exercise 7.3 Word Building

Use the listed word parts to build the defined terms.

neur/o	-oma	sympathetic	-noia
-paresis	para-	-plasty	esthesia
gli/a	-itis	-tomy	hemi-
di-	-on	lob/o	encephala/o

1. _____ inflammation of the brain

2. _____ tumor of glial tissue

3. _____ partial paralysis of one side of the body

4. _____ incision into a lobe

5. _____ cells that are a part of nerve tissue and are external to neurons

6. _____ division of the ANS responsible for rest and digestive responses

7. _____ a mental disorder characterized by unreasonable suspicion or jealousy

8. _____ surgery to repair a nerve

9. _____ the part of the brain containing both the thalamus and the hypothalamus

10. _____ numbness

Exercise 7.4 Matching

Match the term in the first column with its definition in the second column.

1. _____ cerebrum   a. accumulation of fluid on the brain

2. _____ cerebral cortex   b. nerve pain

3. _____ brainstem   c. contains the mesencephalon (midbrain), pons, and medulla oblongata

4. _____ somatic nerves   d. dizziness

5. _____ pons   e. hernia of the meninges and the spinal cord

6. _____ autonomic nerves   f. outer layer of the cerebrum

7. _____ meningomyelocele   g. fainting

8. _____ neuralgia   h. smallest part of brain

9. _____ convulsion   i. contact point between two nerves

10. _____ syncope   j. involuntary nerves

11. _____ vertigo   k. largest part of the brain

12. _____ hydrocephalus

13. _____ neuritis

14. _____ synapse

l. inflammation of a nerve

m. seizure

n. voluntary nerves

Exercise 7.5 Multiple Choice

Choose the correct answer for the following multiple-choice questions.

1. Which term means paralysis on one side of the body?
   a. diplegia
   b. paraplegia
   c. monoplegia
   d. hemiplegia

2. Which of the following terms means a disease of the CNS characterized by the formation of plaques in the brain and spinal cord?
   a. amyotrophic lateral sclerosis (ALS)
   b. Parkinson's disease (PD)
   c. multiple sclerosis (MS)
   d. poliomyelitis

3. The term *cerebrocranial* refers to the
   a. brain and cranium.
   b. cerebellum and cranium.
   c. cerebrum and brain.
   d. cerebrum and cerebellum.

4. The axon is a process that extends from a neuron cell body. What is another process from the neuron cell body?
   a. effector
   b. dendrite
   c. neurotransmitter
   d. ganglia

5. Which of the following means *accumulation of blood under the outermost meningeal layer*?
   a. epidural hematoma
   b. intracerebral hematoma
   c. subdural hematoma
   d. cerebral concussion

6. Which of the following means *hardening of the brain*?
   a. multiple sclerosis (MS)
   b. encephalosclerosis
   c. encephalomyelopathy
   d. depilepsy

7. What is cerebral meningitis?
   a. inflammation of the cerebellum
   b. inflammation of the medulla
   c. inflammation of the meninges of the brain
   d. inflammation of the meninges of the spinal cord

8. Which part of the nervous system conducts impulses to skeletal muscle and is under *conscious* control?
   a. autonomic
   b. central
   c. somatic
   d. afferent

9. Parkinson's disease (PD) is a disease of the nerves in the brain due to an imbalance of what?
   a. glucose
   b. serotonin
   c. oxygen
   d. dopamine (DA)

10. A craniectomy is an _____.
    a. incision into a lobe
    b. incision into the skull
    c. excision of part of the skull
    d. surgery to repair a nerve

11. This is given to reduce seizure activity.
    a. antianxiety agent
    b. anticonvulsant agent
    c. antipsychotic agent
    d. sedative

12. Of the following choices, which is the best place to perform an LP?
    a. between T2 and T3
    b. between T12 and L1
    c. between L5 and S1
    d. between L3 and L4

13. What is another name for an absence seizure?
    a. grand mal seizure
    b. petit mal seizure
    c. somnambulism
    d. syncope

14. A TIA involves primarily the nervous system and which other body system?
    a. respiratory
    b. cardiovascular
    c. muscular
    d. digestive

15. Delirium is _____.
    a. a false belief or wrong judgment despite evidence to the contrary
    b. a subjective perception of an object or voice when no such stimulus exists
    c. impaired intellectual function
    d. altered state of consciousness

Exercise 7.6 Fill in the Blank

Fill in the blank with the correct answer.

1. Abnormal sensitivity to touch is called _____.
2. The name for "inflamed" gray matter of the spinal cord is_____.
3. Impaired intellectual function is called _____.
4. The demyelinization of the spinal cord nerves is called _____.
5. The protrusion of the meninges and spinal cord tissue through an opening in the vertebra is called a(n) _____.
6. The term for a blood clot in the brain is _____.
7. _____ is characterized by a lack of muscular coordination.
8. CNS disorder often characterized by seizures is termed _____.
9. _____ is synonymous with fainting.
10. Pain in a nerve is _____.

Exercise 7.7 Abbreviations

Write out the term for the following abbreviations.

1. _____ ICP
2. _____ CSF
3. _____ LP
4. _____ EEG
5. _____ MS

6. _____ OCD
7. _____ PD
8. _____ PNS
9. _____ CVA
10. _____ DA

Write the abbreviation for the following terms.

11. _____ posttraumatic stress disorder
12. _____ peripheral nervous system

13. _____ cerebrovascular accident
14. _____ magnetic resonance imaging
15. _____ transient ischemic attack

Exercise 7.8 Spelling

Select the correct spelling of the medical term.

1. _____ is the loss, due to brain damage, of the ability to speak or write or to comprehend the written or spoken word.
   a. Aphasia
   b. Afasia
   c. Aphazia
   d. Aphesia
2. _____ is a type of psychosis that may manifest itself as paranoia, withdrawal, or psychotic symptoms.
   a. Skitzophrenia
   b. Schizofrenia
   c. Schizophrenia
   d. Skizophrenia

3. _____ are the potent chemicals in the synapse between neurons.
   a. Nuerotransmiters
   b. Neurotransmiters
   c. Neurotransmitters
   d. Neuritransmitters
4. _____ is a collection of blood in the subdural space.
   a. Subdaral hemitoma
   b. Subdural hemitonia
   c. Subdural henitoma
   d. Subdural hematoma

5. A _____ is a protrusion of the membranes of the brain or spinal cord through a defect in the vertebral column.
   a. myelomeningocele
   b. myelomenengocele
   c. myelomenegocell
   d. meylomeningocele

6. The membranes that surround the brain and spinal cord are called _____.
   a. menenges
   b. meninges
   c. meninnges
   d. meningis

7. The plural of nucleus is _____.
   a. nuclie
   b. neuclei
   c. nuclius
   d. nuclei

8. TIA stands for transient _____ attack.
   a. ichemic
   b. ischemic
   c. ischimic
   d. ischeimic

9. A sudden disturbance in brain function which sometimes produces a convulsion is called a _____.
   a. seisure
   b. siezure
   c. seizure
   d. seizur

10. An _____ is a localized dilation of an artery due to vessel wall weakness.
    a. aneurysm
    b. aneurism
    c. anurism
    d. anurysm

Exercise 7.9 Medical Report

Read the following excerpt from an emergency room record and answer the questions.

CHIEF COMPLAINT: Mental status changes and aphasia.

BRIEF HISTORY: B.B. is an 85-year-old female who presents to the emergency department with difficulty talking. Her daughter states that B.B. has had garbled speech for the past few days, repeatedly says, "How do you do?" and answers the same to any questions asked. This has happened in the past, but the daughter says her mother has always "gotten better." This morning B.B. woke up and has weakness on the right side of her body. There are no other modifying factors or associated signs or symptoms.

ASSESSMENT: Probable history of TIA; now CVA with resulting dysphasia and right hemiparesis.

1. What is a TIA? _____
2. What does the abbreviation CVA represent? _____
3. Break up the medical term *dysphasia* and define its word parts. _____
4. What does the root word *paresis* mean? _____
5. What is the difference between *hemiparesis* and *hemiplegia*? _____
6. Break up the term *hemiplegia* and define the word parts. _____

Exercise 7.10 Reflection

1. What terms from this chapter were you already familiar with?
2. Of the disorders described in this chapter, which two do you think present the greatest challenges for people living with the conditions? Explain your answers.

CHAPTER 8

The Special Senses of Sight and Hearing

LEARNING OUTCOMES

Upon completion of this chapter, you should be able to:

- Name the structures of the eyes and ears.
- Label diagrams showing major components of the eyes and ears.
- Pronounce, spell, and define medical terms related to the eyes and ears and its disorders.
- Interpret abbreviations associated with the eyes and ears.
- Apply knowledge gained to case study questions.

CASE STUDY

Purple Rain

Thad was attending a professional conference about 2 hours from home. During the last session, he noticed spots appearing in his right eye. He didn't think much of it because he was tired, the last presentation was long, and he habitually rubbed his eyes. These spots floated across his field of vision, darting sporadically like rain streaks. Thad wasn't too concerned because he'd experienced these "floaters" in the past after rubbing his eyes or after a camera flash. Driving home that night, he lost vision in his right eye. It felt like a purplish-black sheet was drawn across his eyeball. He kept opening and closing his eye trying to clear whatever was there. However, after 10 minutes or so, his vision was still blurry in some parts and totally gone in others. Thad finished driving home and immediately called his friend to take him to the emergency room at the hospital.

Introduction

The English word *sense* is derived from the Latin verb *sentire*, which means "to feel." Thus, *special senses* refer to the five senses of sight, hearing, smell, taste, and touch. This chapter describes the structures and functions involved with special senses. Sight and hearing are discussed in a single chapter because unlike smell, taste, and touch, which rely on chemical responses, sight and hearing include terminology associated with body organs that process electromagnetic energy (sight) and mechanical energy (hearing).

Sight and hearing are discussed in two separate sections within this chapter.

Word Parts Related to the Eye

Several word roots are related to the word *eye*. The word root ocul/o comes from the Latin word *oculus* (eye). The word root ophthalm/o comes from the Greek word *ophthalmos*, which also means eye. Words such as *optic* and *optical* are derived from the Latin word *opticus*, which means "of sight or seeing." The suffixes -opia and -opsia both mean "vision." Many word parts refer to specific structures within the eye. **Table 8.1** lists word parts related to the eye.

Table 8.1 Word Parts Related to the Eye

Word Part	Meaning
blephar/o	eyelid
conjunctiv/o	conjunctiva (*conjunctivae*, plural)
corne/o	horny
dacry/o	tears, lacrimal sac, or lacrimal duct
dipl/o	two, double
irid/o	iris
kerat/o	hard, cornea
lacrim/o	tear, lacrimal apparatus
ocul/o	eye
ophthalm/o	eye
-opia	vision
opt/o	light, eye, vision
phac/o	lens
presby/o	old age
pupil/o	pupil
retin/o	retina
scler/o	relating to the sclera, hard
uve/o	denoting the pigmented middle eye layer

After studying Table 8.1, write the meaning of each of the word parts.

Word Part	Meaning
1. retin/o	1. _____
2. kerat/o	2. _____
3. lacrim/o	3. _____
4. opt/o	4. _____
5. ocul/o	5. _____
6. uve/o	6. _____
7. dipl/o	7. _____
8. dacry/o	8. _____
9. irid/o	9. _____
10. ophthalm/o	10. _____
11. phac/o	11. _____
12. presby/o	12. _____
13. blephar/o	13. _____
14. conjunctiv/o	14. _____
15. pupil/o	15. _____
16. corne/o	16. _____
17. scler/o	17. _____

Structure and Function of the Eye

Light waves are part of the electromagnetic spectrum, and the eyes work like a motion picture camera, taking continuous pictures and transmitting them instantaneously to the brain, which converts them to images in motion. Although light energy and brain waves are both part of the electromagnetic spectrum, brain waves have much lower frequencies and, therefore, much longer wavelengths than those of light. Thus, the eyes must also convert detected light frequencies, so that the brain can enable people to "see" objects and their motions.

The eye, also called the eyeball, is the organ of vision that is found within the **orbit**, a bony cavity (socket) formed by seven skull bones. Accessory structures of each eyeball include the *extraocular muscles, eyebrows, eyelids, eyelashes, conjunctivae,* and *lacrimal apparatus.* **Extraocular muscles** are those muscles within the orbit but outside the eyeball that move the eyes. They are not visible from the exterior.

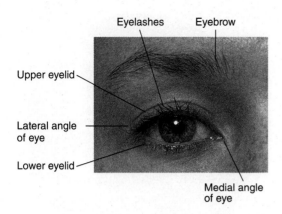

Figure 8.1 Protective structures of the eyeball.

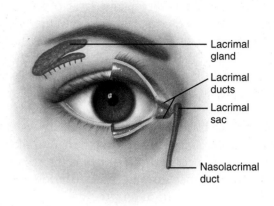

Figure 8.2 Structures of the right lacrimal apparatus.

Eyebrows are the crescent-shaped line of hairs on the superior edge of the orbit. The movable upper and lower folds that cover the surface of the eyeballs when they close are called **eyelids** (*palpebrae*), and the stiff hairs projecting from the eyelid margins are the **eyelashes**. The angle formed by the junction of the lateral parts of the upper and lower eyelids is known as the *lateral angle of eye* (*lateral canthus*), and the medial angle formed by their union is the *medial angle of eye* (*medial canthus*) (see **Figure 8.1**). The **conjunctiva** is the mucous membrane that lines the anterior surface of the eyeball and the underside of the eyelid. This membrane covers and protects the exposed surface of the eyeball (see **Figure 8.3**).

Several structures associated with tear production and flow make up the **lacrimal apparatus**. These structures are the lacrimal gland, lacrimal ducts, lacrimal sac, and nasolacrimal duct. Located superior to the outer corner of each eye is the **lacrimal gland**, which secretes tears to cleanse and moisten the eyeball surface. The **lacrimal sac** stores tears. **Lacrimal ducts** are channels that carry tears to the eyes, whereas the **nasolacrimal duct** carries tears from the lacrimal gland to the nose (see **Figure 8.2**).

The eyeball is made up of three layers, listed from the outermost to the innermost layer: *fibrous layer*, *vascular layer*, and *inner layer*. The fibrous layer consists of the *sclera* and *cornea*; the vascular layer (also called the *uvea*) is made up of the *choroid*, *ciliary body*, and *iris*; the inner layer has the *retina* and *optic nerve*. The **sclera**, also known as the white of the eye, helps maintain the eyeball shape and extends from the cornea to the optic nerve. The **cornea** is the transparent portion that provides most of the optical power by bending light rays to focus on the retinal surface (see Figure 8.3).

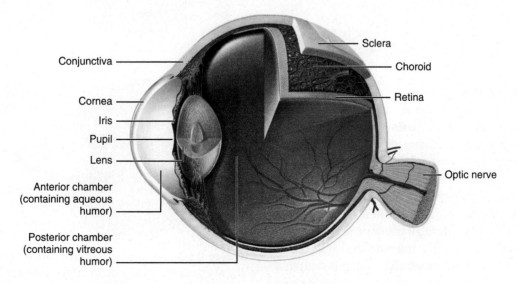

Figure 8.3 Structures of the eyeball.

The **choroid** is the opaque layer of the eyeball that contains vessels supplying blood to the eye. The **ciliary body** is a thickened portion between the choroid and iris. Ciliary body muscles suspend the lens and adjust it to direct the light entering the eye. The **lens** is a transparent structure posterior to the pupil that bends and focuses light rays on the retina. It is held in place by the ligaments of the ciliary body. The *ciliary muscles* control the shape of the lens to allow for far vision and near vision. The **iris** is the pigmented muscular ring that surrounds and controls the size of the **pupil**, the opening in the middle of the iris through which light enters the eye.

The innermost layer of the eye that contains visual receptors (rod and cones) is the **retina**. The first cranial nerve, called the **optic nerve**, carries nerve impulses from the retina to the brain to give the sense of sight (see Figure 8.3). It exits the eyeball through the optic foramen (opening) in the orbit.

The interior spaces (chambers) of the eyeball contain fluid. The *anterior chamber* is the space between the cornea and the lens, and it is filled with a watery fluid called the **aqueous humor**. The *posterior chamber* is the large open space between the lens and retina that contains a semi-gelatinous liquid, the **vitreous humor** (see Figure 8.3).

QUICK CHECK

Fill in the blanks.

1. The three layers of the eyeball are the
   _____ layer,
   the _____ layer, and
   the _____ layer.
2. The _____ contains
   vessels for supplying blood to the eye.
3. The opening in the middle of the iris is the
   _____ .

Photoreceptors are the specialized visual receptor cells in the retina. There are two types of photoreceptors: rods and cones. **Rods** are black and white receptors that respond to dim light, and **cones** are color receptors that provide color vision and sharp vision (visual acuity). These photosensitive cells receive the light waves that come in through the cornea and convert them into nerve impulses. These nerve impulses are carried to the brain through the optic nerve. An oval area of the retina is called the **macula**, and at its center is a pit called the **fovea centralis**, which is saturated with cones and thus permits the best possible color vision. The **optic disc** is the location where nerve fibers from the retina converge to form the optic nerve.

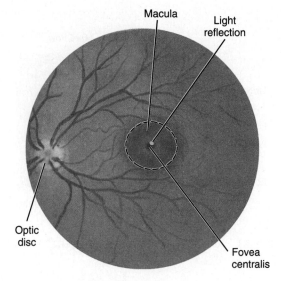

Figure 8.4 Structures of the internal right eye.

Because it has no photoreceptors, it is referred to as the *blind spot* (see **Figure 8.4**).

Refraction, the bending of light rays, is the ability of the eye to change the direction of light to focus it on the retina. Light rays are refracted by the cornea and lens to focus an image on the retina. People see because of **accommodation**, the automatic adjustment of focusing the eye by flattening or thickening the lens (see **Figure 8.5**).

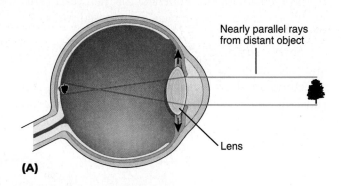

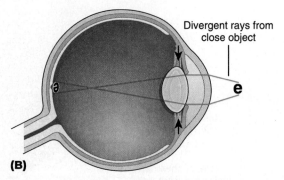

Figure 8.5 Accommodation. The ciliary muscles control the shape of the lens to allow for far and near vision. **(A)** The figure has an elongated lens allowing the eye to focus on distant objects. **(B)** The figure has a shortened lens, allowing the eye to focus on close objects.

Disorders Related to the Eye

Refractive errors, infections, and disorders of the eyelids are common. Refractive errors can be corrected with glasses, contact lenses, or operations that include the reshaping of the cornea. Other eye conditions may be treated with medications or surgery.

Refractive Errors

Hyperopia is the medical term for *farsightedness*, a condition in which the image falls behind the retina. With hyperopia, people cannot see nearby objects clearly, but they can see distant objects. **Myopia** is the medial term for *nearsightedness*, a condition in which the image falls in front of the retina. People with myopia cannot see objects clearly unless they are close to the eyes (see **Figure 8.6**). **Presbyopia** is farsightedness caused by aging. Another refractive error is called **astigmatism**, which means the light coming into the eye does not focus on a single point; this condition is caused by an irregularity of the curve of the cornea or lens that distorts light entering the eye. Corrective lenses can usually compensate for any refractive error.

Infections

Conjunctivitis, commonly known as *pinkeye*, is an inflammation of the conjunctiva and is commonly caused by a viral infection. The inflammation causes small blood vessels in the conjunctiva to become more prominent, giving the sclera a pink or red color. **Keratitis** is an inflammation of the cornea that occurs when the cornea has been scratched or otherwise damaged. Infective keratitis is typically caused by a viral, bacterial, or fungal infection. An inflamed lacrimal sac is called **dacryocystitis**.

Disorders of the Eyelids

Blepharoptosis is drooping of the upper eyelid. **Ectropion** is a condition in which the eyelid is turned outward away from the eyeball. **Entropion** is a condition that causes the eyelid to roll inward against the eyeball. A **hordeolum**, commonly called a **sty**, is an infection of the oil gland of an eyelash.

Other Disorders of the Eye

Xerophthalmia, also known as dry eyes, occurs when the surface of the eye becomes dry, often from wearing contact lenses or from diminished flow of tears.

Glaucoma is a disease characterized by increased intraocular pressure (IOP) that causes damage to the optic nerve. If left untreated, it can result in permanent blindness. Symptoms frequently go unnoticed by the patient until the optic nerve has been damaged.

A cloudiness, or opacity, of the lens is called a **cataract** (see **Figure 8.7**). Disease, injury, chemicals, or exposure to various physical elements may cause

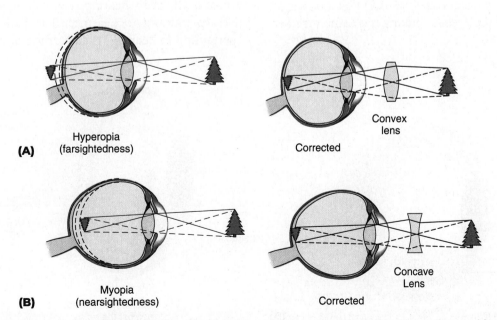

(A) Hyperopia (farsightedness)

(B) Myopia (nearsightedness)

Convex lens
Corrected

Concave Lens
Corrected

Figure 8.6 Refractive errors. **(A)** Hyperopia or farsightedness. The image falls behind the retina, making it difficult to see up close. The corrective lens places the image properly on the retina. **(B)** Myopia or nearsightedness. The image falls in front of the retina, making it difficult to see faraway. The corrective lens places the image properly on the retina.

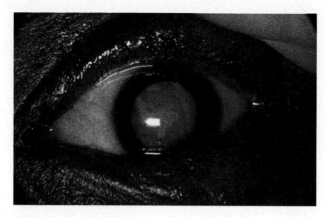

Figure 8.7 Cataract.

cataracts. Surgery to replace the clouded lens with an artificial intraocular lens is a common treatment for cataracts.

Diagnostic Tests, Treatments, and Surgical Procedures of the Eye

An **ophthalmoscope** is an instrument used by practitioners to examine the eye's interior by looking through the pupil.

A procedure to correct vision problems, such as myopia, hyperopia, and astigmatism, is **laser-assisted in situ keratomileusis (LASIK)**. This procedure uses a laser to create a corneal flap and reshape the cornea. Treatment for a detached retina or retinal tear may include scleral buckling. A **scleral buckle** is a permanent silicone band that attaches to the outside of the eyeball, pulling the retina together (see **Figure 8.8**).

Practice and Practitioners of the Eye

An **ophthalmologist** provides eye care ranging from examining eyes and prescribing corrective lenses to performing surgery. Such a wide range of activities and responsibilities requires ophthalmologists to have completed an undergraduate college degree, a doctorate in medicine, a 1-year internship, and 3 or more additional years of specialized clinical training in the field of **ophthalmology** (medical specialty concerned with the eye). **Optometry** is the profession concerned with examination of the eyes and related structures. An **optometrist** is a doctor of optometry (O.D.) who examines eyes and prescribes corrective lenses. In the United States, optometrists complete a preprofessional undergraduate education plus 4 years of professional education at an accredited college of optometry. The technicians who fill eyeglass prescriptions and dispense eyewear are called **opticians**. This occupation requires a high school diploma and successful completion of an accredited optician program, which consists of about 1 year of study.

Word Parts Related to the Ear

The three root words that mean ear are aur/o, auricul/o, and ot/o. These refer to the structure of the ear, but more commonly words related to the function of the ear are used. Acous/o, acus/o, and accost/o all mean hearing, from the Greek *akoustikos* (pertaining to hearing). The Latin word for "pertaining to hearing" is *auditorius*, which gives us

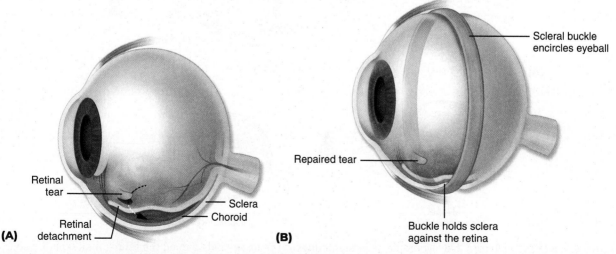

Figure 8.8 Scleral buckle. **(A)** Detached retina. The arrow shows the movement of fluid. **(B)** Repair of retinal tear by attaching a buckle (band) around the sclera to keep the retina from pulling away.

the word part audi/o and makes up words like *auditory* and *audible*. **Table 8.2** lists word parts related to the ear.

Table 8.2 Word Parts Related to the Ear

Word Part	Meaning
acous/o, acus/o, acoust/o	hearing
audi/o	sound
aur/o	ear
auricul/o	ear
myring/o	tympanic membrane (eardrum)
ot/o	ear
staped/o	stapes (smallest ear bone)
tympan/o	eardrum

Word Parts Exercise

After studying Table 8.2, write the meaning of each of the word parts.

Word Part	Meaning
1. audi/o	1. _____
2. ot/o	2. _____
3. acous/o, acus/o, acoust/o	3. _____
4. myring/o	4. _____
5. tympan/o	5. _____
6. aur/o	6. _____
7. staped/o	7. _____
8. auricul/o	8. _____

Structure and Function of the Ear

The ear is an organ of hearing and equilibrium (balance). The ear is divided into three sections: the external ear, middle ear, and internal ear. The **external ear** consists of the auricle (outer ear), external acoustic meatus (passageway), and tympanic membrane (eardrum). It directs sound waves into the ear. Numerous ceruminous glands line the external acoustic meatus and secrete **cerumen**, better known as *earwax*. Cerumen protects the ear by preventing

dust, insects, and some bacteria from entering the middle ear; cerumen also keeps the eardrum soft and pliable. The **middle ear** consists of the tympanic cavity with its auditory ossicles (bones), associated muscles, and the auditory tube. The **internal ear** contains the vestibule, which includes the bony labyrinth of semicircular canals and the cochlea (see **Figure 8.9**).

Sound waves entering the ear vibrate the **tympanic membrane** (eardrum). Just beyond the tympanic membrane is the middle ear. A tiny *tympanic cavity* in the skull houses the **auditory ossicles**, three small bones called the **malleus**, **incus**, and **stapes** (see **Figure 8.10**). These are also sometimes referred to as the hammer, anvil, and stirrup because of their shapes. Sound waves affect these tiny bones and cause them to transmit sound vibrations to the internal ear. Also found inside the middle ear is the **auditory tube**, which reaches from the tympanic cavity to the nasopharynx to help equalize pressure in the ear with outside atmospheric pressure (see Figure 8.9).

The internal ear has a **bony labyrinth** (maze) that contains the sensory receptors for hearing and balance. Major structures of the bony labyrinth include the **semicircular canals** (organ of balance) and **cochlea** (organ of hearing). Receptors in the cochlea change sound waves into nerve impulses that the brain can process.

Disorders Related to the Ear

Ear disorders can occur in any part of the ear. **Impacted cerumen**, an accumulation of earwax in the external acoustic meatus, may cause hearing loss. An earache, termed **otalgia** or **otodynia**, may be caused by trauma or infection. **Otitis** is any inflammation of the ear but can be divided into otitis externa (inflammation of the outer ear), otitis media (OM) (inflammation of the middle ear), or otitis interna (inflammation of the inner ear), with otitis media being the most common type.

Hearing loss may range from a partial loss of hearing that includes only a certain range of frequencies to full loss, which leaves a person completely **deaf** (unable to hear). **Conductive hearing loss** occurs when sound waves are not conducted through the external ear to the ossicles of the middle ear. **Sensorineural hearing loss** occurs when there is damage to the cochlea of the internal ear or to the nerve pathways to the brain. **Presbycusis** is progressive hearing loss that occurs with aging. **Anacusis** is total deafness.

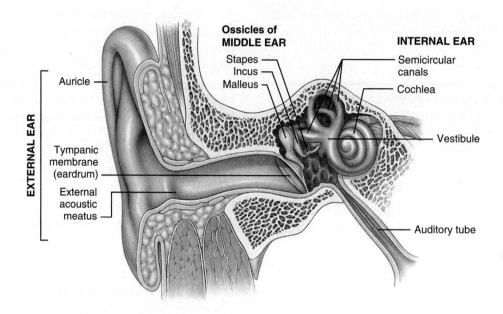

Figure 8.9 Structures of the external, middle, and internal ear.

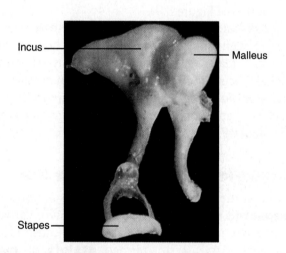

Figure 8.10 The auditory ossicles.

QUICK CHECK

Fill in the blanks.

1. What are the medical terms for the ossicles, sometimes referred to as the hammer, anvil, and stirrup? _____

2. Identify the types of hearing loss.

   _____

3. Identify the structure in the labyrinth that changes sound waves into nerve impulses.

   _____

Other inflammatory ear conditions are **myringitis**, inflammation of the tympanic membrane; **mastoiditis**, inflammation of the mastoid air cells, which are intercommunicating cavities in the mastoid process of the temporal bone; and **labyrinthitis**, inflammation of the labyrinth.

Two other disorders of the ear include **otosclerosis** (hardening of the stapes, resulting in sound waves being unable to travel from the outer ear to the internal ear) and **Ménière's syndrome**, a chronic disease of the internal ear characterized by vertigo, tinnitus, and periodic hearing loss. **Vertigo** is dizziness and/or a loss of balance. **Tinnitus** is ringing, buzzing, or roaring sounds in the ears.

Diagnostic Tests, Treatments, and Surgical Procedures of the Ear

Some ear disorders are treated by surgery. These procedures include the following:

- **Otoplasty**: surgical repair of the auricle of the ear
- **Mastoidectomy**: surgical removal of the mastoid process of the temporal bone
- **Myringectomy** or **tympanectomy**: surgical removal of all or part of the tympanic membrane
- **Myringotomy**: surgical incision of the eardrum to create an opening for placement of drainage tubes
- **Tympanoplasty**: surgical correction of a damaged tympanic membrane
- **Stapedectomy**: surgical removal of the stapes
- **Labyrinthotomy**: a surgical incision into the labyrinth

Practice and Practitioners of the Ear

Audiology is the specialty dealing with hearing and hearing disorders. An **audiologist** is the specialist who measures hearing and treats hearing impairments. An **otoscope** is an instrument with light and lenses used to visually examine the external ear and eardrum. **Otology** is the study of the ear and its related structures. An **otologist** is the specialist who diagnoses and treats diseases of the ear and its related structures. An **otorhinolaryngologist** is a physician who specializes in the diagnosis and treatment of diseases that involve not only the ear but also the nose and throat.

Abbreviations

The following table lists common abbreviations relating to the eyes and ears. The Latin words *dexter* and *sinister* mean, respectively, "right" and "left." These two Latin words give us many English words, such as ambidextrous (able to use either hand equally well), dexterous (good with one's hands), and sinister (odd or spooky—probably because most of the population is right-handed). The first letter of each of these two words, namely D and S, have also found their way into abbreviations for the eyes and ears. AD means right ear because *A* refers to auris/audio meaning "ear," and *D* refers to *dexter* "right side." Likewise, AS refers to the left ear. The root ocul/o refers to the eye, abbreviated with O; thus, OD is the right eye, and OS is the left eye.

The abbreviation OU means both eyes and is derived from the Latin term *oculus uterque*, meaning "both eyes."

Are abbreviations good or bad? The good thing about abbreviations is that they save time. The bad thing about them is that time saved often equals lost accuracy. Looking up the abbreviation AS gives many answers, one of which is "left ear" and another of which is "aortic stenosis." Heart surgery is not going to help someone who is suffering hearing loss in the left ear.

Abbreviation Table Sight and Hearing

Abbreviation	Meaning
AD	right ear
AS	left ear
AU	both ears
EOM	extraocular movement
IOP	intraocular pressure
LASIK	laser-assisted in situ keratomileusis
OD	right eye
O.D.	doctor of optometry
OM	otitis media
OS	left eye
OU	both eyes

Study Table Sight and Hearing

Term and Pronunciation	Analysis	Meaning
Structure and Function: Eye		
accommodation (ah-KOM-moh-DAY-shun)	from the Latin word *accommodare* (fit one thing to another)	the process that allows the shape of the lens to change for near and far vision
aqueous humor (ah-kwee-us HUE-mor)	from the Latin word *aqua* (water) + humor, from the Latin word *umor* (body fluid)	watery substance filling the space between the lens and the cornea
canthus (KAN-thus)	from the Greek word *kanthus* (corner of the eye)	angle where the upper and lower eyelids meet
choroid (KOH-royd)	derived from the Greek words *chorion* (skin, leather; a spot or plot of ground) and *eidos* (form, likeness, appearance, resemblance)	opaque middle layer of the eyeball
ciliary body (SIL-ee-air-ee)	from the Latin word *ciliaris* (pertaining to eyelashes) + body	set of muscles and suspensory ligaments that adjust the shape of lens

(continues)

Study Table Sight and Hearing		*(continued)*
Term and Pronunciation	**Analysis**	**Meaning**
Structure and Function: Eye		
cones (KONZ)	from the Greek word *konos* (cone)	color receptors of the retina that have high visual acuity
conjunctiva (kon-JUNK-tih- vuh); plural: conjunctivae (kon-JUNK-tih-vay)	from the Latin words *con* (with) and *jungere* (to join)	the mucous membrane covering the anterior of the eyeball and inner eyelid
cornea (KOR-nee-uh)	from the Latin word *cornus* (horn)	transparent shield of tissue forming the outer wall of the eyeball
dacryocyst (DACK-ree-oh-sist)	from the Greek words *dakryon* (tear) and *kytis* (bag)	dilated upper portion of nasolacrimal duct; tear sac, lacrimal sac
extraocular muscles (EX-truh-AWK-yu-lur MUS-ulz)	*extra-* (outside); *ocul/o* (eye); *-ar* (adjective suffix)	muscles within the eye orbit but outside the eyeball
eyebrows (EYE-browz)	related to German word *Auge* (eye) and possibly from Norwegian *bru* (bridge)	arched line of hairs on the superior edge of the orbit
eyelashes (EYE-LASH-ez)	common English word	stiff hairs projecting from the margins of the eyelids
eyelids (EYE-lidz)	related to German word *Auge* (eye) and Dutch *lid* (cover)	movable folds that cover the front of the eyes when they close; also called *palpebrae*
fovea centralis (FOH-vee-uh sen-TRAH-lis)	*fovea*, a Latin word meaning "small pit" + *centralis*, a Latin word meaning "central"	a depression in the middle of the retina that is the area of sharpest vision
iris (EYE-ris) plural: irides (IHR-ih-deez)	a Greek word meaning "lily," "iris of the eye," originally "messenger of the gods," personified as the rainbow	the anterior part of the vascular tunic; it is the colored part of the eye
lacrimal apparatus (LAK-rih-mul app-uh-RAT-us)	from the Latin words *lacrima* (tear) + *ad* (toward) and *parare* (to make ready)	collectively: the lacrimal gland, lacrimal ducts, lacrimal sac, and nasolacrimal duct
lacrimal ducts (LAK-rih-mul DUKTZ)	from the Latin words *lacrima* (tear)	channels that carry tears to the eyes
lacrimal glands (LAK-rih-mul GLANDZ)	from the Latin words *lacrima* (tear)	glands that secrete tears
lacrimal fluid (LAK-rih-mul FLOO-id)	from the Latin words *lacrima* (tear) and *fluidus* (fluid)	a watery, physiologic saline; tears
lacrimal sac (LAK-rih-mul SAK)	from the Latin words *lacrima* (tear)	dilated upper part of the nasolacrimal duct
lateral angle of eye (LAT-er-ul AN-gul UV EYE)	from the Latin words *lateralis* (side) and *angulus* (corner)	angle formed by the union of the lateral (side) parts of the upper eyelid and lower eyelid; also called *lateral canthus*
lens (LENZ)	from Latin word *lentil* (because of its similar shape)	the refractive structure of the eye, lying between the iris and the vitreous humor

Term and Pronunciation	Analysis	Meaning
Structure and Function: Eye		
medial angle of eye (ME-dee-ul AN-gul UV EYE)	from the Latin word *medialis* (middle)	angle formed by the union of the upper eyelid and lower eyelid; also called *medial canthus*
nasolacrimal ducts (NAY-zo LACK-rih-mul DUKTZ)	naso- (nose); from the Latin word *lacrima* (tear)	ducts that carry tears from the lacrimal glands to the nose
ocular (OCK-yoo-lur)	*ocul/o* (eye); -ar (adjective suffix)	adjective referring to the eye
optic disc (OP-tik DISK)	*opt/o* (light, eye, vision); -ic (adjective suffix)	oval area in eye without light receptors; *blind spot*
optic nerve (OP-tik nurv)	*opt/o* (light, eye, vision); -ic (adjective suffix) + nerve	the cranial nerve responsible for vision
orbit (OR-bit)	from the Latin word *orbita* (wheel track, course, orbit)	bony depression in the skull that houses the eyeball
palpebra (pal-PEH-bruh)	From the Latin word *palpebra* (eyelid)	eyelid
photoreceptors (FOH-toh-ree-SEPP-turz)	from the Greek word *phos* (light) and the Latin word *recipere* (to receive)	retinal cones and rods
pupil (PYOO-pul)	from the Latin word *pupilla* (doll); named for the tiny image one sees of oneself reflected in the eye of another	the dark part in the center of the iris through which light enters the eye
retina (RETT-ih-nuh)	from Medieval Latin *retina* probably from the Latin word *rete* (net)	light-sensitive membrane forming the innermost layer of the eyeball
rods (RODZ)	probably from Old Norse word *rudda* (club); rods are shaped like little clubs	black and white receptors on the innermost layer of the eyeball
sclera (SKLER-uh) plural: sclerae (SKLER-ay)	from the Greek word *skleros* (hard)	the outer surface of the eye; part of the fibrous tunic; white part of eye
uvea (YOO-vee-uh)	from the Latin word *uva* (grape)	vascular layer of the eye
vitreous body (VIH-tree-us BOD-ee)	from the Latin word *vitreus* (glass) + body	a transparent jellylike substance filling the interior of the eyeball
vitreous humor (VIH-tree-us HYU-mur)	from the Latin words *vitreus* (glass) and *humere* (body fluid)	the fluid component of the vitreous body
Disorders: Eye		
amblyopia (am-blee-OH-pee-uh)	from the Greek word *ambly* (dim); -opia (eye, vision)	condition that occurs when visual acuity is not the same in both eyes; also called lazy eye
astigmatism (uh-STIG-muh-tizm)	From a- (without) and from the Greek word *stigma* (point) + -ism (suffix forming a noun denoting a condition)	fuzzy vision caused by the irregular shape of one or both eyeballs
blepharitis (bleff-uh-RYE-tis)	*blephar/o* (eyelid); -itis (inflammation)	inflammation of the eyelid

(continues)

Study Table Sight and Hearing		*(continued)*
Term and Pronunciation	**Analysis**	**Meaning**
Disorders: Eye		
blepharoconjunctivitis (BLEFF-uh-roh-kon-junk-tih-VYE-tis)	*blephar/o* (eyelid); *conjunctiv/o* (mucous membrane covering the anterior surface of the eyeball and inner eyelid); *-itis* (inflammation)	inflammation of the palpebral conjunctiva; inflammation of the inner lining of the eyelids
blepharoplegia (BLEFF-uh-roh-pleej-ee-uh)	*blephar/o* (eyelid); *-plegia* (paralysis)	paralysis of an eyelid
blepharoptosis (BLEFF-ar-opp-TOH-sis)	*blephar/o* (eyelid); *-ptosis* (falling, downward placement, prolapse)	drooping eyelid
blepharospasm (BLEFF-ar-oh-SPAZ-um)	*blephar/o* (eyelid); from the Greek *spasmos* (spasm, convulsion)	involuntary contraction of the eyelid
cataract (KAT-uh-rakt)	from the Latin word *cataracta* (waterfall)	complete or partial opacity of the ocular lens
conjunctivitis (kon-junk-tih-VYE-tis)	*conjunctiv/o* (mucous membrane covering the anterior surface of the eyeball); *-itis* (inflammation)	inflammation of the conjunctiva; pinkeye
dacryocele (DAK-ree-oh-seel)	*dacry/o* (tears); *-cele* (hernia)	enlargement of the lacrimal sac with fluid
dacryocystitis (DAK-ree-oh-SIST-eye-tis)	*dacryocyst/o* (tear sac); *-it is* (inflammation)	inflammation of the tear sac
dacryolith (DAK-ree-oh-lith)	*dacry/o* (tears); *-lith* (stone)	a "stone" in the lacrimal apparatus; also called ophthalmolith
dacryorrhea (DAK-ree-uh-REE-uh)	*dacry/o* (tears); *-rrhea* (discharge)	excessive discharge of tears
diplopia (dih-PLOH-pee-uh)	*diplo-* (from the Greek *diploos* meaning "double") *and -opia* (eye, vision)	condition in which a single object is perceived as two objects; double vision
ectropion (ek-TROH-pee-un)	*ex-* (out); *trope* (Greek "that which turns")	eversion (turning out) of the eyelid
entropion (en-TROH-pee-un)	*en-* (in); *trope* (Greek "that which turns")	inversion (turning in) of the eyelid
floaters (FLOAT-urz)	from Old English verb *flotian* (fleet—move quickly) and Middle English from Old French word *floter*	Flashes of light (like a camera flash), spots, specks, or "cobwebs" seen in the field of vision
glaucoma (glaw-KOH-muh)	from the Greek word *glaucoma* (cataract, opacity of the lens) (note: cataracts and glaucoma not distinguished until around 1705)	disease of the eye characterized by increased intraocular pressure and atrophy of the optic nerve
hordeolum (hor-DEE-oh-lum)	from the Latin word *hordeum* (barley)	an infection of a gland in the eye; also called *sty*
hyperopia (hy-pur-OH-pee-uh)	*hyper-* (above normal); *-opia* (eye, vision)	farsightedness
iridomalacia (IHR-ih-doh-muh-LAY-shee-uh)	*irid/o* (iris); *-malacia* (softening)	softening of the iris

Term and Pronunciation	Analysis	Meaning
Disorders: Eye		
iritis (eye-RYE-tiss)	*ir/o* (iris); *-itis* (inflammation)	inflammation of the iris
keratitis (ker-uh-TYE-tis)	*kerat/o* (hard, cornea); *-itis* (inflammation)	inflammation of the cornea
lacrimal (LAK-rih-mul)	*lacrim/o* (tear, lacrimal apparatus); *-al* (adjective suffix)	referring to or related to tears or the tear ducts and glands
lacrimation (LAK-rih-MAY-shun)	*lacrim/o* (tear, lacrimal apparatus); *-ation* (noun suffix)	secretion of tears, especially in excess
myopia (my-OH-pee-uh)	from the Greek word *myops* (nearsighted)	nearsightedness
oculodynia (OCK-yu-loh-DIN-ee-ah)	*ocul/o* (eye); *-dynia* (pain)	pain in the eyeball; also called ophthalmalgia
oculopathy (OCK-yu-loh-path-ee)	*ocul/o* (eye); *-pathy* (disease)	any disease of the eyes; also called ophthalmopathy
ophthalmolith (op-THAL-moh-lith)	*ophthalm/o* (eye); *-lith* (stone)	a stone in the lacrimal apparatus; also called dacryolith
ophthalmomalacia (op-THAL-moh-muh-LAY-shee-uh)	*ophthalm/o* (eye); *-malacia* (softening)	softening of the eyeball
ophthalmopathy (op-THAL-moh-path-ee)	*ophthalm/o* (eye); *-pathy* (disease)	any disease of the eyes; also called oculopathy
presbyopia (prez-bee-OH-pee-uh)	from the Greek word *presbys* (old man); *-opia* (eye, vision)	farsightedness resulting from loss of elasticity of the lens due to aging
retinal detachment (RET-ih-nul dee-TACH-ment)	from the Latin word *rete* (net) and the French word *detacher* (to detach)	condition in which the retina pulls away from the nourishing blood vessels at the back of the eyeball
retinitis (rett-ih-NYE-tis)	*retin/o* (retina); *-itis* (inflammation)	inflammation of the retina
retinopathy (rett-ihn-OP-uh-thee)	*retin/o* (retina); *-pathy* (disease)	disease of the retina
scleroiritis (skler-oh-EYE-RYE-tis)	*sclera/o* (sclera); *ir/o* (iris); *-itis* (inflammation)	inflammation of the sclera and iris
strabismus (struh-BIZ-mus)	from the Greek word *strabismos*, from *strabos* (squinting, squint-eyed)	lack of parallelism in the visual axes; also called crossed eyes
xerophthalmia (zee-roh-OP-thal-mee-uh)	from the Greek word *xeros* (dry); *ophthalm/o* (eye); *-ia* (condition)	dry eyes
Diagnostic Tests, Treatments, and Surgical Procedures: Eye		
blepharectomy (bleff-uh-REK-tuh-mee)	*blephar/o* (eyelid); *-ectomy* (excision)	surgical removal of part of or all an eyelid
blepharoplasty (BLEFF-uh-roh-plass-tee)	*blephar/o* (eyelid); *-plasty* (surgical repair)	surgery to correct a defective eyelid
blepharotomy (BLEFF-uh-rot-uh-mee)	*blephar/o* (eyelid); *-tomy* (incision into)	surgical incision of an eyelid

(continues)

Study Table Sight and Hearing		*(continued)*
Term and Pronunciation	**Analysis**	**Meaning**
Diagnostic Tests, Treatments, and Surgical Procedures: Eye		-
conjunctivoplasty (kon-JUNK-tih-voh-plass-tee)	*conjunctiv/o* (conjunctiva *-plasty* (surgical repair)	surgery on the conjunctiva
dacryocystectomy (dak-ree-oh-sist-EK-toh-mee)	*dacryocyst/o* (tear sac); *-ectomy* (excision)	surgical removal of the lacrimal sac
dacryocystotomy (dak-ree-oh-sist-OT-toh-mee)	*dacryocyst/o* (tear sac); *-tomy* (incision into)	incision into the lacrimal sac
lacrimotomy (lakk-rih-MOT-uh-mee)	*lacrim/o* (tear, lacrimal apparatus); *-tomy* (incision into)	incision into the lacrimal sac or lacrimal duct
ophthalmoscope (OP-THAL-moh-skope)	*ophthalm/o* (eye); *-scope* (instrument for viewing)	device for examining the interior of the eyeball by looking through the pupil
ophthalmoscopy (OP-thal-MOS-kuh-pee)	*ophthalm/o* (eye); *-scopy* (use of instrument for viewing)	examination of the eye with an ophthalmoscope
phacolysis (fay-KOL-ih-sis)	*phac/o* (lens); *-lysis* (destruction)	operative removal of the lens in pieces
refraction (ree-FRAK-shun)	from late Latin *refractio*, from *refringere* (to break up)	deflection of a ray of light into the eye for accommodation or correction of vision as it passes from one medium to another of different densities
retinectomy (ret-in-EK-tuh-mee)	*retin/o* (retina); *-ectomy* (excision)	surgical removal of part of the retina
retinopexy (RET-in-oh-pexx-ee)	*retin/o* (retina); *-pexy* (surgical fixation)	surgical fixation of a detached retina
retinotomy (ret-in-OT-uh-mee)	*retin/o* (retina); *-tomy* (incision into)	incision through the retina
scleral buckle (SKLEER-ul BUCK-ul)	*scler/o* (hard) and Latin word *buccula* (cheek strap)	an operation to place a silicone band on the scleral periphery to tighten the retina
vitrectomy (vih-TREK-toh-mee)	from the Latin word *vitrum* (glass) and *-ectomy* (surgical removal of a specific structure)	surgical operation to remove the vitreous humor of the eyeball and replace it with a gel-like substance that simulates vitreous humor
Practice and Practitioners: Eye		
ophthalmologist (op-thul-MAWL-uh-jist)	*ophthalm/o* (eye); *-logist* (one who studies a specific field)	physician whose specialty is the diagnosis and treatment of eye disorders
ophthalmology (op-thul-MAWL-uh-jee)	*ophthalm/o* (eye); *-logy* (study of)	medical specialty dealing with the eye
optician (op-TISH-ihn)	*opt/o* (light, eye, vision)	person who fills prescriptions for ophthalmic lenses, dispenses glasses, and makes and fits contact lenses
optometrist (op-TOM-uh-trist)	*opt/o* (light, eye, vision); *-metrist* (one who measures)	one trained in examining the eyes and prescribing corrective lenses

Term and Pronunciation	Analysis	Meaning
Practice and Practitioners: Eye		
optometry (op-TOM-uh-tree)	*opt/o* (light, eye, vision); *-metry* (measurement)	science of examining eyes
Structure and Function: Ear		
auditory tube (AW-dih-tor-ee TOOB)	from the Latin word *auditorius* (pertaining to hearing)	for impaired vision and other disorders
auditory tube (AW-dih-tor-ee TOOB)	from the Latin word *auditorius* (pertaining to hearing)	canal that connects the middle ear to the pharynx (throat); also called pharyngotympanic tube and eustachian tube
auricle (AW-rih-kul)	*auri-* (ear)	external portion of the ear that directs sound waves; also called pinna
cerumen (se-ROO-men)	from the Latin word *cera* (wax)	waxy substance produced by glands of the external acoustic meatus
external acoustic meatus (EKS-tur-nul uh-KOOS-tick mee-AY-tus)	from the Latin, *externus* (outside) + from the Greek, *akoustikos* (pertaining to sound) + from the Latin, *meatus* (passage)	passage leading inward from the auricle to the tympanic membrane (eardrum); also called external auditory canal
eustachian tube (yu-STAY-shun)	named after Bartolomeo Eustachi (died 1574), who discovered the passages from the ears to the throat	canal that connects the middle ear to the pharynx (throat); also called the auditory tube and pharyngotympanic tube
incus (INK-us)	a Latin word meaning "anvil"	one of the auditory ossicles (the anvil)
labyrinth (LAB-uh-rinth)	from the Greek word *labyrinthos* (maze, large building with intricate passages)	canals of the inner ear
malleus (MAL-ee-us)	a Latin word meaning "hammer"	one of the auditory ossicles (the hammer)
ossicles (OSS-ih-kulz)	from the Latin word *ossiculum* (a small bone)	three small bones in the middle ear: the malleus (hammer), the incus (anvil), and the stapes (stirrup)
pinna (PIN-uh)	from the Latin word *pinna* (feather, wing, fin)	external portion of the ear that directs sound waves; also called auricle
stapes (STAY-peez)	from the Latin word *stapes* (stirrup)	one of the auditory ossicles (the stirrup)
tympanic cavity (tim-PAN-ik)	*tympan/o* (eardrum); *-ic* (adjective suffix) + cavity	air chamber between the external acoustic meatus and the internal ear that contains the ossicles
tympanic membrane (tim-PAN-ik MEM-brain)	*tympan/o* (eardrum); *-ic* (adjective suffix)	eardrum
Disorders: Ear		
anacusis (an-uh-KYU-sis)	*a-* (without); cusis, from the Greek word *akousis* (hearing)	total deafness
conductive hearing loss (kon-DUK-tiv HEAR-ing LOSS)	common English words	hearing loss caused by interference with sound transmission in the external acoustic meatus, middle ear, or ossicles

(continues)

Study Table Sight and Hearing		*(continued)*
Term and Pronunciation	**Analysis**	**Meaning**
Disorders: Ear		
deaf (DEF)	related to Dutch word *doof* and German word *taub*	unable to hear
labyrinthitis (lab-ih-rin-THIGH-tis)	*labyrinth/o* (internal ear); *-itis* (inflammation)	inflammation of the labyrinth
mastoiditis (mas-toid-EYE-tis)	mastoid (mastoid process); and *-itis* (inflammation)	inflammation of any part of the mastoid air cells of the mastoid process of the temporal bone
Ménière's syndrome (men-YEHRS SIN-drome)	named for Prosper Ménière, the French physician who first described the illness in 1861	chronic disease of the internal ear characterized by vertigo, tinnitus, and periodic hearing loss
myringitis (mir-in-JIGH-tis)	*myring/o* (tympanic membrane); *-itis* (inflammation)	inflammation of the tympanic membrane
otalgia (oh-TAHL-jee-ah)	*ot/o* (ear); *-algia* (pain)	pain in the ear
otitis (oh-TYE-tis)	*ot/o* (ear); *-itis* (inflammation)	inflammation of the ear (otitis externa = the outer ear; otitis media = the middle ear; otitis interna = the inner ear)
otodynia (oh-toh-DIN-ee-uh)	*ot/o* (ear); *-dynia* (pain)	earache
otopathy (oh-TOP-uh-thee)	*ot/o* (ear); *-pathy* (disease)	any disease of the ear
otoplasty (OH-toh-plas-tee)	*ot/o* (ear); *-plasty* (surgical repair)	surgical repair of the auricle of the ear
otorrhea (oh-toh-REE-uh)	*ot/o* (ear); *-rrhea* (discharge)	fluid discharge from the ear
otosclerosis (OH-toh-skler-OH-sis)	*ot/o* (ear); *scler/o* (hardening); *-osis* (abnormal condition)	formation of spongy bone in the internal ear producing hearing loss
presbycusis (PREZ-be-KYU-sis)	*presby-* (old); cusis, from the Greek word *akousis* (hearing)	hearing loss that occurs with aging
sensorineural hearing loss (SENTZ-oh-rih-NOO-rul LOSS)	*sensor-* (sensory); *neur/o* (nervous system); *-al* (adjective suffix)	hearing loss caused by a neural condition
tinnitus (TIN-ih-tus; tin-EYE-tus)	from the Latin word *tinnire* (to ring)	sensation of noises (such as ringing) in the ears
vertigo (VUR-tih-go)	a Latin word meaning "dizziness"	sensation of spinning or whirling; dizziness; can be caused by infection or other disorder in the inner ear
Diagnostic Tests, Treatments, and Surgical Procedures: Ear		
audiogram (AW-dee-oh-gram)	*audi/o* (sound, hearing); *-gram* (record or picture)	a graphic record produced by the results of hearing tests with an audiometer
audiometer (aw-dee-OM-ih-ter)	*audi/o* (sound, hearing); *-meter* (measurement)	electrical device for measuring hearing

Term and Pronunciation	Analysis	Meaning
Diagnostic Tests, Treatments, and Surgical Procedures: Ear		
audiometry (aw-dee-OM-ih-tree)	*audi/o* (sound, hearing); *-metry* (process of measuring)	measuring hearing with an audiometer
cochlear implant (KOK-lee-ur IM-plant)	from the Latin word *cochlea* (snail shell); *-ar* (adjective suffix) + implant	surgically implanted hearing aid in the cochlea
labyrinthotomy (lab-ih-rin-THOT-uh-mee)	*labyrinth/o* (internal ear); *-tomy* (incision into)	a surgical incision into the labyrinth
mastoidectomy (mas-toid-ECK-toh-mee)	mastoid (mastoid process) + *-ectomy* (excision)	surgical removal of the mastoid process
myringectomy (mir-in-JECK-toh-mee)	*myring/o* (tympanic mem- brane); *-ectomy* (excision)	surgical removal of all or part of the tympanic membrane; also called tympanectomy
myringoplasty (mir-ING-oh-PLASS-tee)	*myring/o* (tympanic mem- brane); *-plasty* (surgical repair)	surgical repair of the tympanic membrane (eardrum)
myringotomy (mir-ing-OT-uh-mee)	*myring/o* (tympanic mem- brane); *-tomy* (incision into)	incision or surgical puncture of the eardrum; also called tympanotomy
otoplasty (OH-toh-plass-tee)	*ot/o* (ear); *-plasty* (surgical repair)	surgical repair of the auricle of the ear
otoscope (OH-toh-skope)	*ot/o* (ear); *-scope* (instrument for viewing)	device for looking into the ear
otoscopy (oh-TOSS-kuh-pee)	*ot/o* (ear); *-scopy* (use of an instrument for viewing)	looking into the ear with an otoscope
Rinne test (RIN-eh TEST)	named after Heinrich A. Rinne, German otologist (1819–1868)	hearing test using a tuning fork; checks for differences in bone conduction and air conduction
stapedectomy (stay-peh-DECK-toh-mee)	*staped/o* (stapes); *-ectomy* (excision)	surgical removal of the stapes
tuning fork (TOON-ing FORK)	common English words	an instrument that vibrates when struck and is used to test hearing and vibratory sensations
tympanectomy (TIM-puh-NEK-tuh-mee)	*tympan/o* (eardrum); *-tomy* (incision into)	surgical removal of the eardrum; also called myringectomy
tympanocentesis (TIM-puh-noh-senn-TEE-sis)	*tympan/o* (eardrum); *-centesis* (surgical puncture for aspiration)	puncture of the tympanic membrane with a needle to aspirate middle ear fluid
tympanoplasty (TIM-puh-noh-plass-tee)	*tympan/o* (eardrum); *-plasty* (surgical repair)	surgery performed on the eardrum
tympanotomy (TIM-puh-NOT-oh-mee)	*tympan/o* (eardrum); *-tomy* (incision)	incision or surgical puncture of the eardrum; also called myringotomy
Weber test (VAY-behr TEST)	named after Wilhelm Edward Weber, German physicist (1804–1891)	hearing test using a tuning fork; distinguishes between conductive and sensorineural hearing loss
Practice and Practitioners: Ear		
audiologist (aw-dee-OL-oh-jist)	*audi/o* (sound, hearing); *-logist* (one who studies a certain field)	specialist who measures hearing efficiency and treats hearing impairment

(continues)

Study Table Sight and Hearing   (continued)

Term and Pronunciation	Analysis	Meaning
Practice and Practitioners: Ear		
audiology (aw-dee-OL-oh-jee)	*audi/o* (sound, hearing); *-logy* (the study of a certain field)	specialty dealing with hearing and hearing disorders
otologist (oh-TOL-oh-jist)	*ot/o* (ear); *-logist* (one who studies a certain field)	specialist in otology, the branch of medical science concerned with the study, diagnosis, and treatment of diseases of the ear and its related structures
otology (oh-TOL-oh-jee)	*ot/o* (ear); *-logy* (the study of a certain field)	branch of medical science concerned with the study, diagnosis, and treatment of diseases of the ear and its related structures
otorhinolaryngologist (oh-TOH-RYE-no-lair-in-GOL-oh-jist)	*ot/o* (ear); *rhin/o* (nose); *g/o* (throat); *-logist* (one who studies a certain field)	physician who specializes in the diagnosis and treatment of ear, nose, and throat disorders

CASE STUDY WRAP-UP

The emergency room was crowded, but the check-in clerk took Thad back to the non-COVID exam area. Using an ophthalmoscope, the physician peered into Thad's eyes and told him he needed to see an ophthalmologist soon. The next morning, Thad saw his ophthalmologist, Dr. Dogra, who had performed cataract surgery on Thad 6 months ago. Dr. Dogra examined Thad and told him he had retinal detachment with vitreous hemorrhage and required a vitrectomy.

Case Study Application Questions

1. Describe floaters.
2. Why did Thad see an ophthalmologist instead of a family physician?
3. What was Thad's diagnosis?
4. Identify the medical procedure that Thad needed.

END-OF-CHAPTER EXERCISES

Exercise 8.1 Labeling: The Eye
Using the following list, choose the terms to label the diagram correctly.

anterior chamber (containing aqueous humor)

choroid

conjunctiva

cornea

fovea centralis

iris

lens

optic nerve

posterior chamber (containing vitreous humor)

pupil

retina

sclera

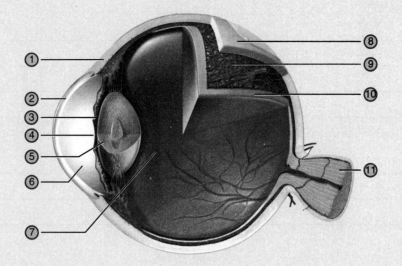

1. _____
2. _____
3. _____
4. _____
5. _____
6. _____

7. _____
8. _____
9. _____
10. _____
11. _____

Exercise 8.2 Word Parts

Break each of the following terms into its word parts: prefix, root, or suffix. Give the meaning of each word part and then define the term.

1. *extraocular*

   prefix: _____

   root: _____

   suffix: _____

   definition: _____

2. *xerophthalmia*

   root: _____

   root: _____

   suffix: _____

   definition: _____

3. *scleroiritis*

   root: _____

   root: _____

   suffix: _____

   definition: _____

4. *blepharoconjunctivitis*

    root: _____

    root: _____

    suffix: _____

    definition: _____

5. *audiometry*

    root: _____

    suffix: _____

    definition: _____

6. *otosclerosis*

    root: _____

    root: _____

    suffix: _____

    definition: _____

7. *mastoidectomy*

    root: _____

    suffix: _____

    definition: _____

8. *otorhinolaryngologist*

    root: _____

    root: _____

    root: _____

    suffix: _____

    definition: _____

Exercise 8.3 Word Building

Use the word parts listed to build the terms defined.

-lith	-centesis	irid/o	-rrhea	-malacia
tympano	myringo	-pexy	-tomy	-lysis
phac/o	ot/o	-dynia	retin/o	-itis
cyst/o	dacryo			

1. _____ a "stone" in the lacrimal apparatus

2. _____ operative removal of the lens in pieces

3. _____ surgical removal of the lacrimal sac

4. _____ surgical fixation of a detached retina

5. _____ softening of the iris

6. _____ puncture of the tympanic membrane with a needle to aspirate middle ear fluid

7. _____ earache

8. _____ incision or surgical puncture of the eardrum

9. _____ fluid discharge from the ear

10. _____ inflammation of the ear

Exercise 8.4 Matching: The Eye

Match the term with its definition.

1. _____ ophthalmology   a. transparent shield of tissue covering the iris

2. _____ vitreous humor   b. adjective associated with tears

3. _____ pupil   c. sensitive inner nerve layer of the eye that contains the rods and cones

4. _____ iris   d. the "colored" part of the eye

5. _____ sclera   e. the dark part in the very center of the eye

6. _____ cornea   f. mucous membrane that covers the anterior surface of the eyeball and lines the underside of each eyelid

7. _____ conjunctiva   g. gelatinous liquid between the lens and retina

8. _____ ophthalmoscope   h. part of the outermost layer of the eye, which is white in color

9. _____ retina   i. a device for examining the interior of the eyeball by looking through the pupil

10. _____ lacrimal   j. name of the medical specialty dealing with the eye

Exercise 8.5 Matching: The Ear

Match the term with its definition.

1. _____ audiologist   a. the eardrum

2. _____ cerumen   b. maze-like portion of the inner ear

3. _____ otoscope   c. specialist treating abnormal hearing

4. _____ tympanoplasty   d. device for looking into the ear

5. _____ labyrinth   e. inflammation of the middle ear

6. _____ auditory ossicles   f. part of the bony labyrinth (internal ear)

7. _____ otitis media   g. wax-like secretion in the external auditory canal

8. _____ tympanic membrane   h. passageway that connects the middle ear to the nasopharynx

9. _____ auditory tube   i. surgical repair on the tympanic membrane

10. _____ cochlea   j. three small bones in the middle ear: the malleus, incus, and stapes

Exercise 8.6 Multiple Choice

Choose the correct answer for the following multiple-choice questions.

1. The medical specialist who treats ear disorders is called a(n) _____.
   a. ophthalmologist
   b. otologist
   c. audiologist
   d. optometrist

2. A term for eardrum is _____.
   a. tympanic membrane
   b. malleus
   c. oval window
   d. none of the above

3. The function(s) of the ear include _____.
   a. equilibrium
   b. hearing
   c. sound vibrations
   d. both a and b

4. The ability of the eye to adjust to variations in distance is _____.
   a. eversion
   b. strabismus
   c. accommodation
   d. presbycusis

5. An inflammation of the tear sac is called _____.
   a. dacryocystitis
   b. scleroiritis
   c. blepharitis
   d. keratitis

6. The layer of the eye that contains the rods and cones is the _____.
   a. sclera
   b. choroid
   c. uvea
   d. retina

7. Hearing loss that is due to nerve damage is _____.
   a. conductive hearing loss
   b. sensorineural hearing loss
   c. tympanitis
   d. tinnitus

8. The cornea is the transparent part of the eye and is an extension of the _____.
   a. choroid
   b. iris
   c. sclera
   d. both a and c

9. The ciliary body is _____.
   a. a group of muscles that suspends the lens
   b. the curved portion of the eye that refracts light
   c. the area between the lens and retina
   d. the protective layer of the eye

10. Farsightedness is called _____.
    a. myopia
    b. hyperopia
    c. presbyopia
    d. both b and c

Exercise 8.7 Fill in the Blank

Fill in the blank with the correct answer.

1. A cloudiness or opacity of the lens is called a(n) _____.
2. Difficulty hearing due to the aging process is termed _____.
3. The medical term for double vision is _____.
4. Another name for dizziness due to an internal ear disturbance is _____.
5. _____ is a ringing or buzzing of the ears.
6. _____ The external ear component is called the pinna or _____.
7. Another name for a sty is _____.
8. _____ means pain in the ear or an earache.
9. An irregularity of the curve of the cornea that distorts the light entering the eye is called _____.
10. An inflammation of the cornea is called _____.
11. The _____ contains the sensory receptors for hearing.
12. The internal ear contains the _____ canals and cochlea.
13. The passageway that goes from the middle ear to the nasopharynx is the _____.
14. _____ is the medical term for a drooping eyelid.
15. A(n) _____ hearing loss is one in which the external or middle ear cannot conduct the sound vibrations to the internal ear.

Exercise 8.8 Abbreviations

Write out the term for the following abbreviations.

1. _____ AD
2. _____ OM
3. _____ OD
4. _____ AS
5. _____ OU
6. _____ OS
7. _____ LASIK

Write the abbreviation for the following terms.

8. _____ both ears
9. _____ extraocular movement
10. _____ right ear
11. _____ intraocular pressure
12. _____ left eye
13. _____ doctor of optometry

Exercise 8.9 Spelling

Select the correct spelling of the medical term.

1. _____ is the medical condition known as double vision.
   a. Diplopia
   b. Diploplia
   c. Dioplia
   d. Diplopea

2. The mucous membrane covering the anterior of the eyeball and the inner eyelid is the

   _____.
   a. conjuctivah
   b. conjunktiva
   c. conjunctiva
   d. conjuncteva

3. The adjective _____ is used to describe tears.
   a. lacrimul
   b. lacrimal
   c. lacrimle
   d. lacramal

4. An eye disease characterized by an increase in intraocular pressure is _____.
   a. glacoma
   b. glaucoma
   c. gluacoma
   d. glocoma

5. An _____ is a healthcare professional who examines eyes and prescribes corrective lenses.
   a. optomatrist
   b. optomotrist
   c. optomitrist
   d. optometrist

6. The purpose of the _____ is to funnel sound waves into the auditory canal.
   a. aricle
   b. oricle
   c. auricel
   d. auricle

7. A synonym for otodynia is _____.
   a. otalgia
   b. otoalgia
   c. otalga
   d. otoalga

8. The three auditory ossicles are the incus, the stapes, and the _____.
   a. maleus
   b. malleus
   c. mallius
   d. malleous

9. A _____ is a puncture of the tympanic membrane with a needle to aspirate middle ear fluid.
   a. timpanacentesis
   b. timpanocentesis
   c. tympanocentesis
   d. tympanocentisis

10. An _____ is a specialist who measures hearing efficiency and treats hearing impairments.
    a. audiologist
    b. adiologist
    c. audilogist
    d. auddiologist

Exercise 8.10 Medical Report

Read the following report and define the italicized medical terms.

PREOPERATIVE DIAGNOSIS: Chronic (1) *otitis media*

OPERATIVE PROCEDURE: Bilateral (2) *myringotomy* and placement of tubes

INDICATIONS: Recurrent ear infections with persistent fluid buildup despite prolonged medical treatment

PROCEDURE: The patient was brought to the operating suite and placed under general mask anesthesia. The ear canals were cleaned of dry (3) *cerumen* and crust. Myringotomies were done bilaterally. Cultures were taken of the fluid present in the middle ear spaces. Ear tubes were placed in the myringotomy sites bilaterally. Antibiotic drops and cotton balls were placed in the (4) *external acoustic meatus.*

   The patient tolerated the procedure well and was taken to the recovery room.

1. _____
2. _____
3. _____
4. _____

Exercise 8.11 Reflection

1. What terms were already familiar to you?
2. What terms were the most difficult to learn?
3. What one thing did you learn that you think you will never forget?

CHAPTER 9

The Endocrine System

LEARNING OUTCOMES

Upon completion of this chapter, you should be able to:

- Name the major endocrine glands and the hormones each gland secretes.
- Pronounce, spell, and define medical terms related to the endocrine system and its disorders.
- Interpret abbreviations associated with the endocrine system.
- Apply knowledge gained to case study questions.

CASE STUDY

Felicity's Fatigue

Felicity is a 45-year-old employed female who is a mother to three teenage daughters. She reports that she is always on the go because in addition to working a full-time day job, she is taking night classes at the local community college to become a registered nurse. Felicity has always wanted to work in health care, but life events focused her attention elsewhere, and she took a job as a bookkeeper directly out of high school. She enjoys her work and her new college courses, but she's very tired and constantly hungry and thirsty. Felicity didn't think much about her fatigue and eating, but she noticed that she was frequently getting up from her desk to urinate. When her vision started to blur, she made an appointment with her nurse practitioner. She hoped all her signs and symptoms could be attributed to stress and lack of sleep.

Introduction

The **endocrine system** consists of ductless *glands* and organs that secrete *hormones* directly into the bloodstream. **Glands** are cell groupings that function as secretory organs. In the case of the endocrine system, the secretion is called a **hormone**. Hormones are transported in the bloodstream to stimulate specific cells or tissues. Working together with the nervous system, the endocrine system helps to maintain **homeostasis** (chemical balance) throughout the body. The nervous system also contributes to this process by either stimulating or delaying hormone release by feedback mechanisms.

Word Parts Related to the Endocrine System

The term endocrine comes from the prefix *endo-* (within) and the Greek word *krinein* (to separate) and refers to secreting internally. This can be contrasted with **exocrine glands**, which secrete hormones through ducts instead of directly into the bloodstream, as endocrine glands do. An example of an exocrine gland is a sweat gland, which secretes onto the skin surface through a duct. *Aden/o* is the root for gland and comes from the Greek word for gland, *aden*. Be careful not to confuse aden/o with adren/o. Adren/o refers specifically to the adrenal glands, which are structures capping the kidneys; the term adrenal comes from the Latin *ad-* (near) and *ren/o* (kidney). **Table 9.1** lists word parts that make up endocrine system terms.

Table 9.1 Word Parts Related to the Endocrine System

Word Part	Meaning
acr/o	extremities
aden/o	gland
adren/o	adrenal glands
adrenal/o	adrenal glands
calc/i	calcium
crin/o	to separate or secrete
endocrin/o	secreting internally
gluc/o	sugar, glucose, glycogen
glyc/o	sugar, glucose, glycogen
hypophys/o	pituitary gland
-ine	suffix used in the formation of names of chemical substances
-megaly	enlargement
-oma	tumor
pancreat/o	pancreas
parathyr/o	parathyroid gland
parathyroid/o	parathyroid gland
thyr/o	thyroid gland
thyroid/o	thyroid gland
-tropin	suffix meaning nourishment or stimulation

Word Parts Exercise

After studying Table 9.1, write the meaning of each of the word parts.

Word Part	Meaning
1. endocrin/o	1._____
2. hypophys/o	2._____
3. adren/o, adrenal/o	3._____
4. -ine	4._____
5. -tropin	5._____
6. -oma	6._____
7. pancreat/o	7._____
8. acr/o	8._____
9. aden/o	9._____
10. thyr/o, thyroid/o	10._____
11. -megaly	11._____
12. gluc/o, glyc/o	12._____
13. crin/o	13._____
14. parathyr/o, parathyroid/o	14._____
15. calc/i	15._____

Structure and Function

Several glands make up the endocrine system. These glands include the **pineal**, **pituitary** (made up of three lobes: anterior, intermediate, and posterior), **thyroid**, **parathyroid** (two paired glands, superior and inferior), **thymus**, **adrenal** (cortex and medulla), **pancreas** (pancreatic islets), **testes** (in males), and **ovaries** (in females) (see **Figure 9.1**). The hormones and primary functions of each of these hormones are noted in **Table 9.2**.

What do the words *endocrine* and *hormone* mean? Endocrine glands are so-called because they secrete hormones directly into the bodily fluids that surround them, and those hormones eventually find their way into the bloodstream. In other words, endocrine gland secretions do not travel through ducts. Glands that direct their secretions through ducts are called exocrine glands. The word *hormone* comes from Greek and means "to urge on or set in motion." So, a hormone is a chemical "messenger" transported through blood to other parts of the body. When the hormone reaches its target destination, the "message" has been delivered and can be acted upon.

Pituitary Gland

Located in the brain, the **pituitary gland**, or *hypophysis*, is suspended from the base of the hypothalamus. (The *hypothalamus* coordinates the autonomic nervous system and the activities of the pituitary gland.) The pituitary gland controls other endocrine glands by releasing special hormones that regulate glandular functions. The pituitary gland is divided into an **anterior lobe**, or *adenohypophysis*, and a **posterior lobe**, or *neurohypophysis*.

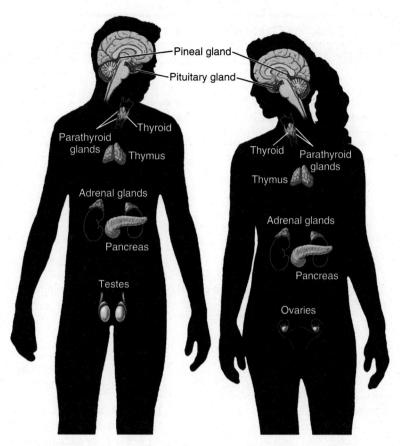

Figure 9.1 The endocrine system.

Table 9.2 Summary of the Endocrine Glands, Hormones, and Hormone Functions

Gland	Hormone	Hormone Function
pineal gland	melatonin	affects sleep–wake cycles and reproduction
pituitary gland		regulates activities of other glands; referred to as the "master gland"
anterior lobe of pituitary gland		
	growth hormone (GH)	growth and development of bones, muscles, and other organs
	thyroid-stimulating hormone (TSH)	growth and development of thyroid gland
	adrenocorticotropic hormone (ACTH)	growth and development of adrenal cortex
	follicle-stimulating hormone (FSH)	stimulates production of sperm in males and growth of ovarian follicles in females
	luteinizing hormone (LH)	stimulates the production of testosterone in males and secretion of estrogen and progesterone in females
	prolactin (PRL) also called lactotropin	stimulates milk secretion in the mammary glands
intermediate lobe of pituitary gland		
	melanocyte-stimulating hormone (MSH)	regulates skin pigmentation

(continues)

Table 9.2 Summary of the Endocrine Glands, Hormones, and Hormone Functions   *(continued)*

Gland	Hormone	Hormone Function
posterior lobe of pituitary gland		
	antidiuretic hormone (ADH); also called vasopressin	stimulates the reabsorption of water by the kidneys
	oxytocin	stimulates the uterus to contract during labor and delivery
thyroid gland	thyroxine (T_4); also called tetraiodothyronine (T_4)	influences growth and development, both physical and mental
	triiodothyronine (T_3)	maintenance and regulation of metabolism
	calcitonin (CT)	decreases the blood level of calcium
parathyroid gland	parathyroid hormone (PTH); also called parathormone	increases the blood level of calcium
thymus	thymosin	aids T-cell development; T cells play a role in immunity
adrenal gland		consists of outer region (cortex) and inner region (medulla)
cortex	cortisol	regulates carbohydrate, protein, and fat metabolism; anti-inflammatory effect; helps the body cope during stress
	aldosterone	regulates water and electrolyte balance
	androgen (sex hormone)	develops male secondary sex characteristics
medulla	epinephrine; also called adrenaline	acts as a vasoconstrictor, cardiac stimulant (increases heart rate and cardiac output), and antispasmodic; releases glucose into the bloodstream (giving the body a spurt of energy)
	norepinephrine; also called noradrenaline	acts as a vasoconstrictor; increases blood pressure and heart rate
pancreas		
pancreatic islets; also called islets of Langerhans	insulin	transports glucose into the cells; decreases blood glucose levels
	glucagon	promotes release of glucose by liver; increases blood glucose levels
ovaries		
	estrogen	promotes growth, development, and maintenance of female sex organs
	progesterone	prepares uterus for pregnancy; promotes development of mammary glands
testes	testosterone	promotes growth, development, and maintenance of male sex organs

The anterior lobe secretes several hormones essential for the development of sex glands, muscles, bones, thyroid gland, and other organs. The posterior lobe secretes two hormones that are produced in the hypothalamus: **antidiuretic hormone** (ADH) and **oxytocin** (OXT). Antidiuretic hormone, also called *vasopressin*, helps regulate fluid balance by reducing urination. Oxytocin enhances labor contractions during childbirth and promotes milk release during lactation (milk secretion). During ejaculation in males, a spurt of OXT stimulates reproductive tract contractions to aid sperm release. In humans, it also appears to play a role in social bonding.

Thyroid Gland and Parathyroid Gland

The **thyroid gland** is a butterfly-shaped gland lying in front and to the sides of the upper part of the trachea (windpipe) and lower part of the larynx (voice box) (see **Figure 9.2**). It secretes hormones needed for cell growth, metabolism, and calcium regulation. Thyroid hormones include *triiodothyronine* (T_3), *thyroxine* (T_4), and *calcitonin* (CT). **Triiodothyronine** (T_3) and **thyroxine** (T_4) play roles in many body functions, including growth and development, metabolic rate, body temperature, and heart rate. **Calcitonin** helps control blood calcium levels by decreasing the level of calcium in the bloodstream.

There are four **parathyroid glands** consisting of a superior pair and an inferior pair. They are located on the posterior surface of the thyroid gland (see **Figure 9.3**). The hormone **parathyroid hormone** (PTH), also called *parathormone*, helps maintain correct calcium levels in the blood by increasing the blood level of calcium.

Adrenal Glands

The **adrenal glands**, also called *suprarenal glands*, consist of two triangular-shaped glands, each located on the superior border of the kidneys. Each adrenal gland is divided into an outer part called the **adrenal cortex** and an inner part called the **adrenal**

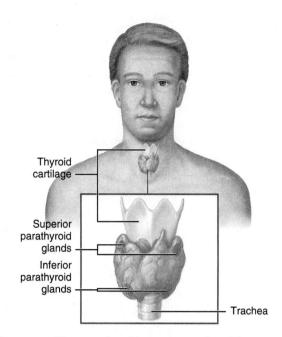

Figure 9.3 The parathyroid glands consist of four glands, a superior pair and an inferior pair. They are found on the posterior surface of the thyroid gland but are highlighted in this anterior view.

medulla (see **Figure 9.4**). The adrenal cortex secretes the steroid hormones, **cortisol**, which helps the body cope with stress, and **aldosterone**, which helps with sodium regulation. It also produces **androgens**, which contribute to the development of male sex characteristics.

The adrenal medulla secretes **epinephrine** (*adrenaline*), which stimulates the sympathetic nervous system. It also secretes **norepinephrine** (*noradrenaline*), a hormone structurally like epinephrine that also stimulates the sympathetic nervous system.

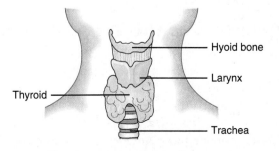

Figure 9.2 The thyroid gland and adjacent structures.

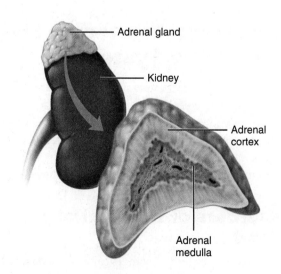

Figure 9.4 The adrenal glands are positioned above each kidney and have an outer adrenal cortex and an inner adrenal medulla.

Pancreas

The pancreas is a feather-shaped organ located posterior to the stomach. It contains clusters of specialized cells called the **pancreatic islets** (*islets of Langerhans*), which produce *insulin* and *glucagon*. These chemicals control blood glucose (sugar) levels and glucose metabolism throughout the body. **Insulin**, produced by the beta cells (β cells) of the pancreas, decreases blood glucose. **Glucagon**, produced by the alpha cells (α cells) of the pancreas, increases blood glucose.

Gonads

Reproductive organs that produce sex cells are called **gonads**. The female gonads are the **ovaries**, and the male gonads are the **testes**. The ovaries secrete estrogen and progesterone. **Estrogen** affects the development of female organs, regulates the menstrual cycle, and plays a role in pregnancy. **Progesterone** stimulates the uterus in preparation for and maintenance of pregnancy. The testes secrete **testosterone**, a hormone that affects development of sexual organs in males and secondary sexual characteristics.

QUICK CHECK

Fill in the blanks.

1. Another name for the pituitary gland is the
   _____.
2. Another name for the adrenal gland is the
   _____ because it is
   located on the superior border of the kidney.
3. _____ glands secrete
   hormones directly into the bloodstream.

Disorders Related to the Endocrine System

Disorders of the endocrine system are almost always the result of an excess or a deficit in hormone production. In other words, either too much or too little of a hormone causes a problem. If there is too much, surgery or radiation may be needed. If there is too little, hormone replacement therapy is the usual treatment.

Disorders of the Pituitary Gland

One cause of pituitary disorders can be an **adenoma**, a benign tumor that causes excessive hormone secretion. This condition may also destroy pituitary cells and cause too little hormone secretion.

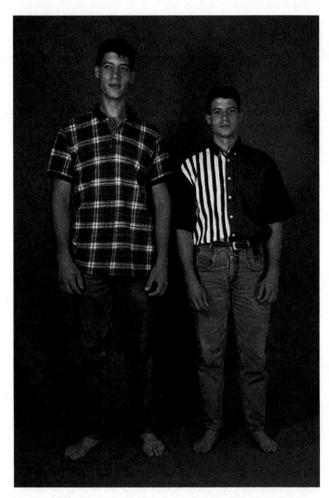

Figure 9.5 A 22-year-old male with gigantism is shown next to his identical twin, who does not have the condition.

Diabetes insipidus is a disorder in which the posterior lobe of the pituitary gland no longer releases enough antidiuretic hormone or because the response to antidiuretic hormone is impaired. This results in **polydipsia** (excessive thirst) and **polyuria** (excessive urination).

Gigantism, or *giantism*, is a disorder caused by excessive secretion of growth hormone (GH) before puberty, resulting in abnormally long bones (see **Figure 9.5**). When excessive growth hormone secretion occurs in adulthood, this results in **acromegaly**, which is characterized by abnormally thick bones in the extremities, especially the hands and feet.

Disorders of the Thyroid Gland

As with other endocrine disorders, excessive or deficient thyroid hormone results in homeostatic imbalance. **Hypothyroidism**, deficient hormone production by the thyroid gland, is characterized by decreased metabolic rate, weight gain, and tiredness. Excessive thyroid hormone production leads to **hyperthyroidism**, characterized by increased metabolic rate, weight

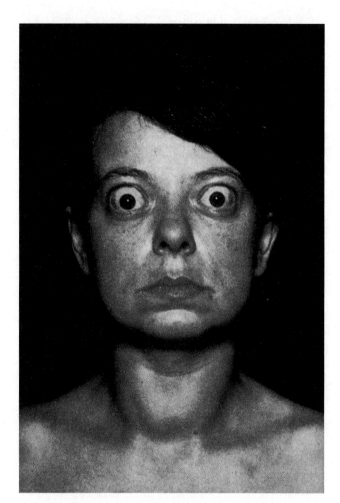

Figure 9.6 A young female exhibiting the signs of Graves' disease, including goiter and exophthalmos.

loss, and rapid heartbeat. A form of hyperthyroidism is **Graves' disease**, which is an autoimmune disorder (condition in which the body's antibodies are directed against itself) resulting in **goiter** (neck swelling caused by an enlarged thyroid gland) and **exophthalmos** (eye protrusion) (see **Figure 9.6**). Graves' disease is named for Irish physician, Robert J. Graves (1796–1853), who first identified the condition.

What causes thyroid enlargement? Enlargement of the thyroid gland is caused by a dietary deficiency of iodine. Iodine is necessary to make thyroid hormones. Recall that these hormones have the word part *iodo* in their names. Although this condition is no longer common in the United States, it still affects people in less developed parts of the world. The reason for its rarity in the United States is that in 1924, members of the Michigan State Medical Society championed the fight against goiter by convincing salt producers to include small amounts of iodine in their product. The discovery that goiter was a result of too little iodine in the diet had previously been noted by French physician J. B. Boussingault nearly a century earlier.

Disorders of the Adrenal Gland

Inflammatory conditions and viral infections involving the adrenal glands can cause a decrease in hormone production. Benign tumors are often the cause of increased hormone production from the adrenal glands.

Addison's disease is a progressive disorder caused by inadequate secretion of hormones from the adrenal cortex. These hormones are cortisol and aldosterone. Insufficient cortisol and aldosterone production in the adrenal gland may result from failure of the pituitary gland to produce a stimulating hormone that targets the adrenal gland. It is characterized by skin discoloration (known as bronzing), weakness, progressive anemia, low blood pressure, and loss of appetite (see **Figure 9.7**).

Cushing's syndrome is caused by an excessive amount of cortisol production by the adrenal glands. It is characterized by fat pads in the chest and abdomen and a "moon face" appearance.

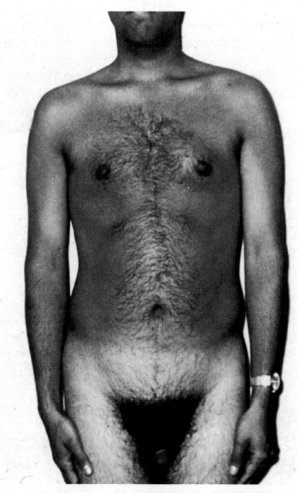

Figure 9.7 Darkening (bronzing) of the skin caused by Addison's disease.

The naming of disorders for persons who first identified them is a well-established practice. Using the possessive form of the founder's name in the names of the disorders has been questioned, and one may, therefore, see and hear both *Addison's disease* and *Addison disease*. The problem is one of tradition versus logic. Those who eschew tradition in favor of logic say that Addison's disease is not something that 19th-century British physician Thomas Addison contracted but rather a disorder he identified. Likewise, Harvey Cushing identified and did not contract Cushing's syndrome. In this book, the traditional naming is used because when you search these terms on the Internet, the apostrophe appears more often. Medical dictionaries, however, often do not include the apostrophe.

There is an exception: Graves' disease, although a traditional spelling, is not a true possessive. The rule for forming possessives specifies that this should be Graves's disease. Robert Graves was an Irish physician who described exophthalmic goiter in 1835. In this one case, therefore, tradition defies not only logic but also the rules of grammar and punctuation.

Disorders of the Pancreas

Diabetes mellitus (DM) is a disorder caused by insulin deficiency or insulin resistance. This results in poor carbohydrate metabolism and high blood glucose (sugar) level. There are several types: **Type 1 diabetes** is a metabolic disorder caused by insufficient insulin production that usually develops in childhood. Symptoms in the early stages include **glycosuria** (excess glucose in the urine) and **hyperglycemia** (excess glucose in the blood). **Type 2 diabetes** is caused by either a lack of insulin or the body's inability to use insulin efficiently. It usually develops in middle-aged or older adults, but it can develop during childhood. **Prediabetes** is a condition in which blood glucose levels are higher than normal, but not high enough to be classified as type 2 diabetes. **Gestational diabetes**, characterized by elevated blood glucose, occurs in females during pregnancy. It usually goes away after pregnancy but places the person at greater risk for developing type 2 diabetes later in life. Diabetes is often described by the three "polys"—**polydipsia** (excessive thirst), **polyphagia** (excessive hunger), and **polyuria** (excessive urination).

Diagnostic Tests, Treatments, and Surgical Procedures

Hormone replacement therapy (HRT) is often used to correct endocrine conditions, where the problem is a low hormone level. Examples of conditions treatable by hormone replacement are hypothyroidism and diabetes mellitus. In hypothyroidism, patients are given a medication called levothyroxine to replace low thyroxine levels. In diabetes, patients are given medications to treat high glucose levels. Most commonly, people with type 1 diabetes are given insulin. People with type 2 diabetes are often prescribed dietary modifications and exercise to control glucose levels. If they do need medications, these patients are more likely to receive oral medications to help decrease blood glucose. In Addison's disease, cortisol is the deficient hormone, so **corticosteroids** may be administered. Corticosteroids are immunosuppressant and anti-inflammatory drugs.

Practice and Practitioners

Endocrinology is the medical practice of treating endocrine and hormonal disorders. The practitioner, an **endocrinologist**, specializes in caring for patients with endocrine diseases and hormonal dysfunctions that may involve sexual development, body growth, or other bodily functions.

Abbreviation Table The Endocrine System	
Abbreviation	**Meaning**
ACTH	adrenocorticotropic hormone
ADH	antidiuretic hormone
CT	calcitonin
DM	diabetes mellitus
FBS	fasting blood sugar
FSH	follicle-stimulating hormone
GH	growth hormone
GTT	glucose tolerance test
HbA1c	hemoglobin A1c (glycosylated hemoglobin)
HRT	hormone replacement therapy
LH	luteinizing hormone
MSH	melanocyte-stimulating hormone
OXT	oxytocin
PRL	prolactin
PTH	parathyroid hormone
TSH	thyroid-stimulating hormone
T_3	triiodothyronine
T_4	thyroxine, tetraiodothyronine

Term and Pronunciation	Analysis	Meaning
Study Table The Endocrine System		
Structure and Function		
adenogenous (ad-eh-NAW-jeh-nus)	*aden/o* (gland); *-genous* (originating)	originating in a gland
adenohypophysis (AD-eh-noh-hy-POFF-ih-sis)	*aden/o* (gland); *hypophys/o* (pituitary gland)	the anterior lobe of the pituitary gland
adrenal cortex (uh-DREE-nul KOR-teks)	*adren/o* (adrenal glands); *cortex* (a Latin word meaning "bark")	the outer region of the adrenal gland
adrenal glands (uh-DREE-nul GLANDZ)	*adren/o* (adrenal glands)	triangular-shaped glands located above each kidney that secrete hormones that aid in metabolism, electrolyte balance, and stress reactions; each gland has an outer cortex and an inner medulla; also called *suprarenal glands*
adrenal medulla (uh-DREE-nul muh-DOOL-uh)	*adren/o* (adrenal glands); *medulla* (a Latin word meaning "marrow, innermost part")	the inner region of the adrenal gland
adrenaline (uh-DREN-uh-lin)	*adren/o* (adrenal glands); *-ine* (a suffix used to form names of chemical substances)	chemical secreted by the adrenal medulla that increases heart rate, breathing rate, and carbohydrate metabolism; also called *epinephrine*
adrenocorticotropic hormone (ACTH) (uh-DREE-oh-KOR-tih-koh-TROH-pik HOR-mone)	*cortic/o* (from *cortex* meaning bark); from the Greek word *trophe* (nourishment); *-in* (a suffix used to form names of biochemical substances)	pituitary secretion that stimulates the adrenal glands
androgen (AN-droh-jen)	*andro-* (masculine); *-gen* (suffix meaning "source of")	male hormone secreted by the adrenal cortex
aldosterone (al-DOS-teh-rone)	ald (ehyd) + ster(ol) + *-one* (chemical suffix)	a corticosteroid; hormone produced by the adrenal glands
antidiuretic hormone (ADH) (AN-tee-dye-uh-RET-ik HOR-mone)	*anti-* (against); from the Greek *dia* (through); *-uresis* (urina- tion); from the Greek word *hormon* (to set in motion)	hormone secreted by the posterior pituitary gland to prevent the kidneys from expelling too much water
calcitonin (CT) (kal-sih-TOH- nin)	*calci-* (calcium); from the Greek *tonos* (to stretch); *-in* (suffix used to form names of biochemical substances)	hormone secreted by the thyroid that lowers blood calcium level
corticosteroids (KOR-tih-koh-STAIR-oydz)	*cortic/o* (from Latin word *cortex* meaning bark); from steros (solid); *-oid* (resemblance to)	steroids produced by the cortices of the adrenal glands; synthetic drugs that replace natural adrenal cortex hormones
cortisol (KOR-tih-sul)	from the Latin word *corticus* (cortex)	main glucocorticoid produced in the adrenal cortex; inhibits inflammation and immune response; also called *hydrocortisone*
endocrine (EN-doh-krin)	*endo-* (within, inner); from the Greek word *krino* (to separate)	adjective describing a gland that delivers its secretions directly into bloodstream
epinephrine (EP-ih-NEFF-rin)	*epi-* (upon); *nephr/o* (kidney); *-ine* (suffix used to form the names of chemical substances)	chemical secreted by the adrenal medulla that increases heart rate, breathing rate, and carbohydrate metabolism; also called *adrenaline*

(continues)

Study Table The Endocrine System		*(continued)*
Term and Pronunciation	**Analysis**	**Meaning**
Structure and Function		
estrogen (ES-troh-jen)	from the Greek word *oistrus* (estrus); *-gen* (producing)	hormone secreted by the female ovaries
exocrine gland (EX-oh-krin GLAND)	*exo-* (outside of); from the Greek word *krino* (to separate)	gland that delivers its secretions through a duct onto the skin or other epithelial surface
follicle-stimulating hormone (FSH) (FOL-ih-kul STIM-yoo-leyt-ing HOR-mone)	from the Latin words *folliculus* (little bag) and *stimulatus* (rouse to action); from the Greek word *hormon* (to set in motion)	hormone promoting gonadal growth
glands (GLANDZ)	From the Latin, *glans* (acorn)	organized group of cells that function as a secretory or excretory organ
glucagon (GLOO-kuh-gon)	*gluc/o* (glucose); from the Greek word *ago* (to lead)	hormone secreted by the pancreas that increases blood glucose level
homeostasis (hoh-mee-oh-STAY-sis)	from two Greek words *homos* (same) and *stasis* (existence)	tendency toward equilibrium; remaining normal
hormone (HOR-mone)	from the Greek word *hormon* (to set in motion)	chemical messenger that is secreted by an endocrine gland directly into the bloodstream
hydrocortisone (hy-droh-KOR-tih-zone)	*hydro-* (water); *cortic/o* (from the Greek word *cortex* meaning "bark"); *-one* (chemical suffix)	an adrenal gland hormone secretion
hypophysis (hy-POFF-ih-sis)	*hypophys/o* (pituitary gland)	major endocrine gland in the brain that controls growth, development, and functioning of other endocrine glands; *pituitary gland*
hypothalamus (high-poh-THAL-uh-mus)	*hypo-* (below); from the Greek word, *thalamus* (bed, bedroom)	part of the brain located near the pituitary gland that secretes releasing hormones that control the release of other hormones by the pituitary gland
insulin (IN-suh-lin)	from the Latin word *insula* (island)	hormone produced in the pancreas that decreases blood glucose level
islets of Langerhans (EYE-lets UV LAN-gur-hans)	after German pathologist Paul Langerhans, who described it in 1869; islets are the regions of the pancreas that contain its hormone-producing cells	clusters of specialized cells in the pancreas that secrete insulin (β cells) and glucagon (α cells)
luteinizing hormone (LH) (LOO-tee-uh-nize-ing HOR-mone)	from the Latin word *luteus* (yellow); from the Greek word *hormon* (to set in motion)	hormone that stimulates final ripening of follicles, oocyte release, and conversion of the ruptured follicle into the corpus luteum
melanocyte-stimulating hormone (MSH) (MUH-lan-oh-site STIM-yoo-late-ing HOHR-mone)	*melan/o* (black); *-cyte* (cell); from the Latin word *stimulatus* (rouse to action); from the Greek word *hormon* (to set in motion)	hormone secreted from the anterior lobe of the pituitary gland that is involved with skin pigmentation changes
melatonin (mel-uh-TONE-in)	melanophore + Greek *tonos* (to stretch); *-in* (suffix used to form names of biochemical substances)	hormone secreted by the pineal gland that is involved with sleep–wake cycles and reproduction

Term and Pronunciation	Analysis	Meaning
Structure and Function		
neurohypophysis (NUR-oh-hy-POFF-ih-sis)	*neur/o* (nerve); *hypophys/o* (pituitary gland)	posterior lobe of the pituitary gland that stores and releases oxytocin and antidiuretic hormone, which are produced in the hypothalamus
noradrenaline (nor-uh-DREN-uh-lin)	*nor-* (chemical prefix); *adrenal/o* (adrenal glands); *-ine* (a suffix used to denote chemical substances)	chemical secreted by the adrenal medulla that aids the body during stress and increases blood pressure; also called *norepinephrine*
norepinephrine (NOR-ep-ih-NEFF-rin)	*nor-* (chemical prefix); *epi-* (upon); from the Greek word *nephros* (kidney); *-ine* (a suffix used to denote chemical substances)	chemical secreted by the adrenal medulla that aids the body during stress and increases blood pressure; also called *noradrenaline*
ovaries (OH-vuh-reez)	from the Latin word *ovum* (egg)	female gonads; two oval-shaped glands located in the pelvic cavity that secrete the hormones estrogen and progesterone
oxytocin (OXT) (ox-ih-TOH-sin)	from the Greek word *oxytokos* (swift birth); *-in* (suffix used to form names of biochemical substances)	hormone secreted by the posterior pituitary gland that stimulates uterine contractions and mammary gland milk ejection
pancreas (PAN-kree-us)	from the Greek word *pancreas* (sweet bread)	feather-shaped organ that lies posterior to the stomach that contains islets of Langerhans (α cells and β cells that secrete glucagon and insulin, respectively)
parathyroid gland (pair-uh-THIGH-royd GLAND)	*para-* (prefix denoting involvement of two like parts; also denoting adjacent, alongside, near); *thyr/o* (thyroid gland)	gland that secretes parathyroid hormone
parathyroid hormone (PTH) (pair-uh-THIGH-royd HOR-mone)	*para-* (prefix denoting involvement of two like parts; also denoting adjacent, alongside, near); *thyr/o* (thyroid gland); from the Greek word *hormon* (to set in motion)	a hormone secreted by the parathyroid gland that regulates calcium and phosphorus levels in the blood and bones; also called *parathormone*
parathormone (pair-uh-THOR-mone)	*para-* (prefix denoting involvement of two like parts; also denoting adjacent, alongside, near); *thyr/o* (thyroid gland); from the Greek word *hormon* (to set in motion)	a hormone secreted by the parathyroid gland that regulates calcium and phosphorus levels in the blood and bones; also called *parathyroid hormone*
pineal gland (PIE-nee-uhl GLAND)	from the Latin word *pinus* (pine); *-al* (adjective ending)	small, cone-shaped gland that secretes melatonin, which affects sleep–wake cycles and reproduction
pituitary gland (pih-TOO-ih-tair-ee GLAND)	from the Latin word *pituita* (phlegm)	major endocrine gland in the brain that controls growth, development, and functioning of other endocrine glands; also called *hypophysis*
progesterone (proh-JES-ter-ohn)	from the Latin *pro* (for); from the Latin *gestare* (to carry); *-one* (chemical suffix)	female hormone secreted by the ovary that stimulates uterus in preparation for and maintenance of pregnancy
prolactin (PRL) (pro-LAK-tin)	from the Latin *pro* (for); from the Latin *lacteus* (milky)	a secretion of the anterior lobe of the pituitary gland that stimulates milk production

(continues)

Study Table The Endocrine System		*(continued)*
Term and Pronunciation	**Analysis**	**Meaning**
Structure and Function		
suprarenal glands (SOO-pruh-REEN-ul GLANDZ)	*supra-* (above); *ren-* (kidney); *-al* (pertaining to)	triangular-shaped glands located above each kidney that secrete hormones that aid in metabolism, electrolyte balance, and stress reactions; each has an outer cortex and an inner medulla; also called *adrenal glands*
testes (TES-teez)	from the plural form of the Latin *testis* (testicle)	male gonads; two oval organs that lie in the scrotum that secrete testosterone
testosterone (tes-TOS-tuh-rone)	from the Latin *testis* (testicle); ster(ol); *-one* (chemical suffix)	male hormone secreted by the testes that affects development of sexual organs in males and secondary sexual characteristics
thymus (THIGH-mus)	from the Greek word *thymos* (a warty outgrowth)	gland located in the upper chest behind the sternum (breastbone) that plays a role in immunity by "training" specialized white blood cells called T cells
thyroid gland (THIGH-royd GLAND)	*thyr/o* (thyroid gland)	bilobed gland located in the neck that secretes thyroid hormone that is needed for cell growth and metabolism
thyroid-stimulating hormone (TSH) (THIGH-royd STIM-yoo-late-ing HOR-mone)	*thyr/o* (thyroid gland)	hormone produced in the anterior lobe of the pituitary gland that stimulates the growth and function of the thyroid gland; also called *thyrotropin*
thyrotropin (thigh-ROH-troh-pin)	*thyr/o* (thyroid gland); from the Greek *trophe* (nourishment); *-in* (suffix used to form names of biochemical substances)	hormone produced in the anterior lobe of the pituitary gland that stimulates the growth and function of the thyroid gland; also called *thyroid-stimulating hormone*
thyroxine (T_4) (thigh-ROK-sin)	*thyr/o* (thyroid gland); *-ine* (suffix used to form names of biochemical substances)	a secretion of the thyroid gland
triiodothyronine (T_3) (try-EYE-oh-doh-THIGH-roh-neen)	*tri-* (three); *iodo* (iodine); *thyr/o* (thyroid gland); *-ine* (a suffix used to form names of chemical substances)	a secretion of the thyroid gland that is often synthesized from thyroxine (T_4) by bodily organs
Disorders		
acromegaly (AK-roh-meg-uh-lee)	from the Greek *akron* (extremity); *-megaly* (enlargement)	enlargement of the extremities (mostly hands and feet) caused by excessive secretion of growth hormone *after* puberty
Addison's disease (AD-uh- sens dih-ZEEZ)	named after the British physician, Thomas Addison, who first described the condition in 1855	disorder in which the adrenal glands do not produce sufficient cortisol; characterized by skin darkening (bronzing), weakness, and loss of appetite
adenitis (ad-en-EYE-tis)	*aden/o* (gland); *-itis* (inflammation)	inflammation of a gland
adenohypophysitis (AD-en-oh-hy-poff-ih-SIGH-tis)	*aden/o* (gland); *hypophys/o* (pituitary gland); *-itis* (inflammation)	inflammation of the anterior pituitary, often related to pregnancy

Term and Pronunciation	Analysis	Meaning
Disorders		
adenoma (ad-en-OH-muh)	*benignus* (Latin for *aden/o* (gland) *-oma* (tumor)	benign (nonmalignant) neoplasm in which the tumor cells form glands or gland-like structures
adrenalitis (uh-dren-ul-EYE-tis)	*adrenal/o* (adrenal glands); *-itis* (inflammation)	inflammation of an adrenal gland
adrenalopathy (uh-dren-ul-OP-uh-thee)	*adrenal/o* (adrenal glands); *-pathy* (disease)	any disease of the adrenal glands; also called *adrenopathy*
adrenomegaly (uh-dren-oh-MEG-uh-lee)	*adren/o* (adrenal gland); *-megaly* (enlargement)	enlargement of the adrenal glands
adrenopathy (uh-dren-OP-uh-thee)	*adrenal-* (adrenal glands); *-pathy* (disease)	any disease of the adrenal glands; also called *adrenalopathy*
Cushing's syndrome (KOOSH-ingz SIN-drum)	named after Harvey Cushing, American physician, who described the disorder in 1932	a hormonal disorder caused by too much cortisol; characterized by fat pads in the chest and abdomen and a "moon face" appearance
diabetes insipidus (DYE-uh-BEED-eez in-SIP-ih-dis)	from the Greek word *diabetes* meaning *siphon*; *insipidus* (lacking flavor)	condition brought about by the posterior pituitary's failure to produce enough antidiuretic hormone
diabetes mellitus (DM) (DYE-uh-BEED-eez muh-LYE-tis)	from the Greek word *diabetes* meaning *siphon*; *mellitus*, a Latin word meaning "sweet"	condition brought about by insufficient production of insulin in the pancreas or the failure of the body's cells to absorb glucose
exophthalmos (eks-off-THAL-mus)	*ex* (out) + *ophthalmos* (eye)	protruding or bulging eyes from their sockets
gestational diabetes (juh-STAY-shen-ul DYE-uh-BEED-eez)	from the Latin *gestation* meaning *carry in the womb* and from the Greek word *diabetes* meaning *siphon*	condition of increased blood glucose level in female during pregnancy that typically resolves after childbirth
giantism (JYE-en-tiz-um)	from the Latin, *gigant-* meaning giant or large	excessive growth due to hypersecretion of growth hormone before puberty; also called *gigantism*
gigantism (JYE-gan-tiz-um)	*giant* (common English word); *-ism* (condition)	excessive growth due to hypersecretion of growth hormone before puberty; also called *giantism*
glycosuria (GLYE-kose-YOUR-ee-uh)	*glyc/o/s* (sugar); *-uria* (urine)	sugar (glucose) in the urine
goiter (GOY-tur)	from the Latin word *gutter* (throat)	neck swelling caused by thyroid gland enlargement
Graves' disease (GRAVZ dih-ZEEZ)	named after Robert James Graves (1796–1853), an Irish physician who first described exophthalmic goiter in 1835	a common form of hyperthyroidism resulting from overproduction of thyroxine caused by a false immune system response
Hashimoto's thyroiditis (hah-shee-MOE-tohz thigh-roid-EYE-tis)	Hashimoto (Japanese surgeon, 1881–1934); *thyr/o* (thyroid gland); *-itis* (inflammation)	an autoimmune disorder that attacks the thyroid gland causing hypothyroidism
hyperglycemia (high-pur-gly-SEE-mee-uh)	*hyper-* (above normal); *glyc/o* (sugar); *-ia* (condition)	excessive sugar (glucose) in the blood
hyperpituitarism (high-pur-pih-TOO-ih-tair-iz-um)	*hyper-* (above normal); from the Latin word *pituita* (phlegm)	excessive hormone secretion by the pituitary gland

(continues)

Study Table The Endocrine System		*(continued)*
Term and Pronunciation	**Analysis**	**Meaning**
Disorders		
hyperthyroidism (HIGH-pur-THIGH-royd-iz-um)	*hyper-* (above normal); *thyr/o* (thyroid); *-ism* (condition)	excessive production of thyroid hormone by the thyroid gland; overactive thyroid
hypophysitis (high-poh-fih-SIGH-tis)	*hypophys/o* (pituitary gland); *-itis* (inflammation)	inflammation of the pituitary gland
hypopituitarism (hogh-poh-pih-TOO-ih-tair-iz-um)	*hypo-* (below normal); from the Latin word *pituita* (phlegm); *-ism* (condition)	condition of diminished hormone secretion from the anterior pituitary gland
hypothyroidism (high-poh-THIGH-roid-iz-um)	*hypo-* (below normal); thyroid refers to the thyroid gland; *-ism* (state of)	decrease in thyroid hormone production
pituitarism (pih-TOO-ih-tair-iz-um)	from the Latin word *pituita* (phlegm); *-ism* (condition)	pituitary dysfunction
polydipsia (pol-ee-DIP-see-uh)	from the Greek words *polus* (much) and *dipsa* (thirst)	excessive thirst that is usually indicative of diabetes
polyphagia (pol-ee-FAJE-ee-uh)	from the Greed words *polus* (much) and *phagein* (eating)	
polyuria (pol-ee-YOUR-ee-uh)	from the Greek words *polus* (much) and *ouron* (urine)	excessive urination
prediabetes (pree-DYE-uh-BEED-eez)	*pre-* (prefix meaning before); from the Greek word *diabetes* meaning *siphon*	condition of elevated blood glucose level without diagnosed diabetes and is indicative that a person is progressing toward developing type 2 diabetes
thyroaplasia (THIGH-roh-uh-PLAY-zee-uh)	*thyr/o* (thyroid gland); aplasia from the Greek *a plassein* (not to form)	congenital condition characterized by low thyroid output
thyroiditis (thigh-roid-EYE-tis)	*thyr/o* (thyroid gland); *-itis* (inflammation)	inflammation of the thyroid gland
thyromegaly (thigh-roh-MEG-uh-lee)	*thyr/o* (thyroid gland); *-megaly* (enlargement)	enlargement of the thyroid gland
toxic goiter (TOK-sik GOY-tur)	from two Latin words *toxicus* (poisoned); *gutter* (throat)	a goiter that forms excessive secretions causing signs and symptoms of hyperthyroidism
type 1 diabetes (TYPE 1 DYE-uh-BEED-eez)	from the Greek word *diabetes* meaning *siphon*	condition brought about by insufficient production of insulin in the pancreas and generally appearing in childhood
type 2 diabetes mellitus (TYPE 2 DYE-uh-BEED-eez)	from the Greek word *diabetes* meaning *siphon*	condition brought about by insufficient production of insulin in the pancreas or the failure of the body's cells to absorb glucose generally appearing in adulthood
Diagnostic Tests, Treatments, and Surgical Procedures		
adenectomy (ad-uh-NEK-toh-mee)	*aden/o* (gland); *-ectomy* (excision)	excision of a gland
adenotomy (ad-en-OT-oh-mee)	*aden/o* (gland); *-tomy* (cutting operation)	incision of a gland
adrenalectomy (uh-dree-nul-EK-toh-mee)	*adrenal/o* (adrenal glands); *-ectomy* (excision)	surgical removal of one adrenal gland or both adrenal glands

Term and Pronunciation	Analysis	Meaning
Diagnostic Tests, Treatments, and Surgical Procedures		
fasting blood sugar (FSB) test (FAST-ing BLUD SHOOG-ur TEST)	*fasting* (to not eat)	test for diabetes; after drinking a glucose solution, the patient fasts and then their blood is tested for glucose; also called *glucose tolerance test* (GTT)
glucose tolerance test (GTT) (GLUE-kose TAL-ur-ence TEST)	from the Greek *gleukos* (sweet wine) and the Latin *tolerantia* (ability to endure continued subjection to something)	test for diabetes; after drinking a glucose solution, the patient fasts and then their blood is tested for glucose; also called *fasting blood sugar*
glycosylated hemoglobin (HbA1c) (glye-KOS-ih-late-ed HE-muh-gloh-bin)	*glyco-* (glucose, sugar); *hem-* (blood)	blood test that indicates the amount of glucose in the blood over the previous 3 months; used to indicate how well diabetes mellitus is being controlled; also called a *glycated hemoglobin* (A1C) *test*
hypoglycemic (HIGH-poh-gly-SEE-mik)	*hypo-* (below normal); *glyc/o* (sugar); *-ic* (pertaining to)	drug used to lower blood glucose
hypophysectomy (HIGH-poh-fih-SEK-toh-mee)	*hypophys/o* (pituitary gland); *-ectomy* (excision)	surgical removal of the hypophysis (pituitary gland)
parathyroidectomy (PAIR-uh-thigh-royd-EK-toh-mee)	*parathyr/o* (parathyroid gland); *-ectomy* (excision)	surgical excision of the parathyroid gland
thyroidectomy (THIGH-royd-EK-toh-mee)	*thyr/o* (thyroid gland); *-ectomy* (excision)	removal of the thyroid gland
thyroparathyroidectomy (THIGH-roh-pair-uh-THIGH-royd-EK-toh-mee)	*thyr/o* (thyroid gland); *parathyr/o* (parathyroid gland); *-ectomy* (excision)	removal of the thyroid and parathyroid glands
thyrotomy (thigh-ROT-oh-mee)	*thyr/o* (thyroid gland); *-tomy* (cutting operation)	surgery performed on the thyroid gland
urinalysis (your-in-AL-ih-sis)	From the Latin word *urina* (urine)	physical, chemical, and microscopic examination of urine
Practice and Practitioners		
endocrinologist (en-doe-krin-OL-oh-jist)	*endocrin/o* (endocrine); *-logist* (one who specializes)	medical specialist in endocrinology
Endocrinology (en-doe-krin-OL-oh-jee)	*endocrin/o* (endocrine); *-logy* (study of)	medical specialty of the endocrine system

CASE STUDY WRAP-UP

Felicity's nurse practitioner performed a complete history and physical examination. Because Felicity reported polyphagia, polydipsia, polyuria, and fatigue, the nurse practitioner ordered a urinalysis, a fasting blood sugar test, and a glycosylated hemoglobin (HbA1c) test. Felicity returned a week later for her follow-up visit. She was diagnosed with type 2 diabetes and was scheduled for a consult with a registered dietician.

Case Study Application Questions

1. What signs and symptoms exhibited by Felicity correlate with polyphagia, polydipsia, and polyuria?
2. Describe a fasting blood sugar test.
3. Why was an HbA1c test ordered?

END-OF-CHAPTER EXERCISES

Exercise 9.1 Labeling

Using the following list, choose the terms to label the diagram correctly.

adrenal glands   parathyroid glands   testes

ovaries   pineal gland   thymus

pancreas   pituitary gland   thyroid

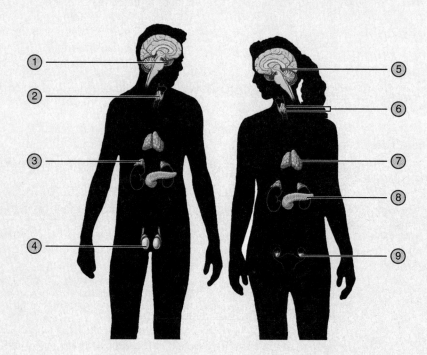

1. _____   4. _____   7. _____

2. _____   5. _____   8. _____

3. _____   6. _____   9. _____

Exercise 9.2 Word Parts

Break each of the following terms into its word parts: prefix, root, or suffix. Give the meaning of each word part and then define the term.

1. *adenogenous*

    root: _____

    suffix: _____

    definition: _____

2. *epinephrine*

    prefix: _____

    root: _____

    suffix: _____

    definition: _____

3. *suprarenal*

    prefix: _____

    root: _____

    suffix: _____

    definition: _____

4. *adrenomegaly*

    root: _____

    suffix: _____

    definition: _____

5. *hyperglycemia*

    prefix: _____

    root: _____

    suffix: _____

    definition: _____

6. *adenotomy*

    root: _____

    suffix: _____

    definition: _____

7. *thyroparathyroidectomy*

    root: _____

    root: _____

    suffix: _____

    definition: _____

8. *endocrinology*

    root: _____

    suffix: _____

    definition: _____

Exercise 9.3 Word Building

Use *adren/o* to build the medical words meaning:

1. enlargement of the adrenal gland _____
2. surgical removal of an adrenal gland _____
3. disease of the adrenal glands _____

Use *thyr/o or thyroid/o* to build the medical words meaning:

4. condition of minimal functioning of the thyroid gland _____
5. inflammation of the thyroid gland _____
6. incision of the thyroid gland _____
7. enlargement of the thyroid gland _____

Use *pancreat/o* to build the medical words meaning:

8. tumor of the pancreas _____
9. inflammation of the pancreas _____
10. originating in the pancreas _____

Exercise 9.4 Matching

Match the term with its definition.

1. _____ adrenalopathy
2. _____ hyperpituitarism
3. _____ adenogenous
4. _____ antidiuretic hormone
5. _____ adrenaline
6. _____ master gland, hypophysis
7. _____ calcitonin
8. _____ goiter
9. _____ parathyroid gland
10. _____ thyrotropin
11. _____ thyromegaly
12. _____ adenohypophysitis
13. _____ thyroparathyroidectomy

a. synonym for epinephrine
b. thyroid-stimulating hormone, secreted by the anterior lobe of the pituitary gland
c. enlargement of the thyroid gland
d. disease of the adrenal glands
e. synonym for pituitary gland
f. hormone secreted by the thyroid to decrease blood calcium level
g. originating in a gland
h. removal of the thyroid and parathyroid glands
i. hormone released by the posterior lobe of the pituitary gland
j. secretes PTH (parathyroid hormone)
k. excessive pituitary secretion
l. inflammation of the anterior pituitary gland
m. chronic enlargement of the thyroid

Exercise 9.5 Multiple Choice

Choose the correct answer for the following multiple-choice questions.

1. The master gland is known as the_____.
   a. pituitary gland
   b. thymus gland
   c. thyroid gland
   d. pineal gland
2. The ovaries produce which two hormones?
   a. insulin and glucagon
   b. estrogen and progesterone
   c. testosterone and thymosin
   d. T_3 and T_4
3. Endocrine means_____.
   a. to cringe from within
   b. to secrete within
   c. to cry inside
   d. disease of the gland

4. Over secretion of GH in an adult produces a condition called_____.
   a. hyperthyroidism
   b. adenitis
   c. acromegaly
   d. tetany
5. _____ is an enlargement of the thyroid gland.
   a. Hypothyroidism
   b. Goiter
   c. Thyroidectomy
   d. Addison's disease
6. A chemical secreted from an endocrine gland is called_____.
   a. a hormone
   b. a lymph
   c. a neurotransmitter
   d. insulin

7. Hypersecretion of GH may cause_____.
   a. insulin
   b. diabetes
   c. hypothyroidism
   d. gigantism

8. _____is associated with excessive hormone secretion from the adrenal cortex.
   a. Cushing's syndrome
   b. Exophthalmos
   c. Goiter
   d. Gigantism

9. The two-lobed gland in the neck is called the_____.
   a. Adam's apple
   b. thymus
   c. pituitary gland
   d. thyroid gland

Exercise 9.6 Fill in the Blank

Fill in the blank with the correct answer.

1. Another term for enlargement of the thyroid gland besides goiter is _____.
2. Insufficient insulin production or insulin resistance results in the condition called _____.
3. An abnormally high level of glucose in the blood is termed _____.
4. Excessive urination is called _____.
5. The term _____ means sugar (glucose) in the urine.
6. The hormone _____ increases blood glucose level.
7. The enlargement of extremities caused by the overproduction of GH in adults is _____.
8. _____ is the tendency toward equilibrium.

Exercise 9.7 Abbreviations

Write out the term for the following abbreviations.

1. _____ GTT
2. _____ PTH
3. _____ T_4
4. _____ FBS
5. _____ ADH
6. _____ HbA1c
7. _____ GH
8. _____ PTH
9. _____ adrenocorticotropic hormone

Write the abbreviation for the following terms.

10. _____ follicle-stimulating hormone
11. _____ diabetes mellitus
12. _____ calcitonin
13. _____ melanocyte-stimulating hormone
14. _____ triiodothyronine
15. _____ prolactin
16. _____ thyroid-stimulating hormone
17. _____ luteinizing hormone

Exercise 9.8 Spelling

Select the correct spelling of the medical term.

1. An _____ is a physician who specializes in caring for patients with endocrine diseases and hormonal dysfunctions.
   a. enocreenologist
   b. endokrineologist
   c. endocrineologist
   d. endocrinologist

2. A medication that can be taken orally to lower the circulating level of blood glucose is called a _____ .
   a. hypogysemic
   b. hyperglycemic
   c. hypoglycemic
   d. hyperglysemik

3. _____ is one of the hormones produced in the pancreas that regulates blood sugar.
   a. Insullin
   b. Insulin
   c. Insalin
   d. Insulen

4. One of the main disorders of the pancreas is called _____.
   a. diabetes mellitus
   b. diabetis mellitus
   c. diabetis melletes
   d. diabetes melletes

5. The _____ is located posterior to the stomach.
   a. pancreas
   b. pancrease
   c. pankreas
   d. pankrease

6. In addition to insulin, the pancreas also produces _____, which increases blood sugar.
   a. glukagon
   b. glucagun
   c. glucagon
   d. glucagone

7. The _____ gland controls the activities of the other endocrine glands.
   a. pituatary
   b. pitooatary
   c. patuitary
   d. pituitary

8. A _____ is a chronic enlargement of the thyroid gland.
   a. goyter
   b. goiter
   c. goitar
   d. goytar

9. Enlargement of the extremities, especially the hands and feet, that is caused by excessive GH after puberty is called _____.
   a. acromeguly
   b. acromegaly
   c. acrohmegaly
   d. akromegaly

10. The male sex hormone secreted by the adrenal cortex is _____.
    a. andragen
    b. androhgen
    c. androjen
    d. androgen

Exercise 9.9 Medical Report

ENDOCRINOLOGY OFFICE CONSULTATION

After reading the case study, answer the following questions.

OFFICE NOTE: This 59-year-old female has previously been in good health. On a routine physical examination, she was noted to have a thyroid nodule on the right lobe of the thyroid gland. She complained of hoarseness, dysphasia, local tenderness, and a slight enlargement on the right side of her neck. She also stated that she feels anxious and cannot sleep throughout the night.

On physical examination, the right side of the neck was visibly enlarged, and a nodule was felt; it was noted that the patient's eyes were bulging outward. A blood test to check her thyroid hormone levels indicated a high value of TSH. No other modifying factors or associated signs or symptoms were present.

1. What does dysphasia mean? _____
2. What is a medical term for an "enlargement of the thyroid gland"? _____
3. What does TSH stand for? _____

Exercise 9.10 Reflection

1. When you first read the opening Case Study, what did you think was wrong with Felicity?
2. After reading this chapter, what stood out as the most interesting information?
3. Were you aware of the differences between endocrine glands and exocrine glands?

CHAPTER 10

The Cardiovascular System

LEARNING OUTCOMES

Upon completion of this chapter, you should be able to:

- Understand blood flow through the heart and through the body.
- Name the elements that form blood.
- Pronounce, spell, and define medical terms related to the cardiovascular system and its disorders.
- Interpret abbreviations associated with the cardiovascular system.
- Apply knowledge gained to case study questions.

CASE STUDY

Brian's Blood Bruise

Brian is a 50-year-old male with a history of hypertension who smokes tobacco products and is not physically fit. One day while cleaning windows, he stepped off the ladder and experienced excruciating pain in his left calf. For several days following the incident, he had significant pain and tenderness in his lower leg, which was red, slightly swollen, and warm to the touch. He wasn't sure what to do since he didn't remember injuring himself and he hadn't done any physical exertion beyond washing windows. By day 5, he went to the urgent clinic, where the physician assistant (PA) completed a history and physical examination and ordered an ultrasound. When the PA returned with the test results, she ordered him to the emergency room of the local hospital for a direct admit.

Introduction

The **cardiovascular system** is made up of the heart and blood vessels, which transport blood. The blood vessels include all the **arteries** (carrying blood *away* from the heart), **veins** (carrying blood *toward* the heart), and **capillaries** (vessels between the arteries and veins). Together they form a transportation system that delivers oxygen and nutrients to the body's cells, returns carbon dioxide and wastes to be eliminated, and helps regulate body temperature. The heart pumps the blood within the blood vessels to all parts of the body. When discussing the cardiovascular system, it is typically divided into the *pulmonary circuit* and the *systemic circuit*. The **pulmonary circuit** passes blood from the heart's right ventricle, through the lung's pulmonary arteries, and then back through the pulmonary veins to the heart's left atrium. The **systemic circuit** passes blood the through the arteries, capillaries, and veins of the general circulation (see **Figure 10.1**).

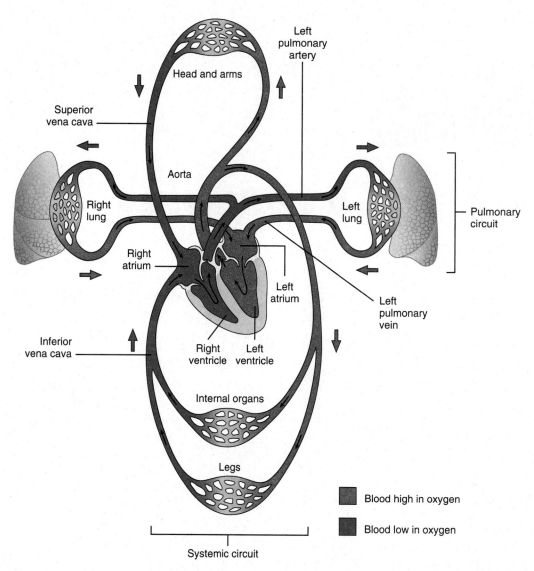

Figure 10.1 The cardiovascular system. The cardiovascular system allows blood flow in a closed system of vessels. The pulmonary circuit carries blood to and from the lungs, and the systemic circuit carries blood to and from all other parts of the body. Blood that is low in oxygen leaves the right side of the heart and enters the lungs, whereas blood that is rich in oxygen leaves the lungs and is returned to the left side of the heart to be pumped out to the systemic circuit. The vessels depicted in red signify blood that is high in oxygen; the vessels depicted in blue signify blood that is low in oxygen.

Word Parts Related to the Cardiovascular System

The term *cardiovascular* introduces two different word parts: cardi/o, which comes from the Greek *kardia* (heart), and vas/o, which comes from the Latin *vas* (vessel). The third component to this system besides the heart and vessels is blood. The root words hem/o and hemat/o both mean blood, as does the suffix -emia. **Table 10.1** lists word parts related to the cardiovascular system terms.

Table 10.1 Word Parts Related to the Cardiovascular System

Word Part	Meaning
angi/o	vessel
aort/o	aorta
arteri/o	artery
ather/o	fatty
atri/o	atrium
brady-	slow

Table 10.1 Word Parts Related to the Cardiovascular System   *(continued)*

Word Part	Meaning
cardi/o	heart
coron/o	crown; encircling, such as in the coronary blood vessels encircling the heart
-ectasis	dilation, expansion
electr/o	electricity
-emia	blood
endo-	within, inner
-gram	written record
hem/o	blood
hemat/o	blood
isch	restricting, thinning
my/o	muscle
peri-	around, surrounding
phleb/o	vein
-stenosis	a narrowing
tachy-	fast
thromb/o	clot
valv/o	valve
valvul/o	valve
varic/o	dilated
vas/o	vessel
ven/o	vein
ventricul/o	ventricle

Meaning	Word Part
7. prefix meaning around, surrounding	7. _____
8. root meaning fatty	8. _____
9. root meaning atrium	9. _____
10. suffix meaning written record	10. _____
11. suffix meaning blood	11. _____
12. root meaning muscle	12. _____
13. suffix meaning a narrowing	13. _____
14. root meaning blood	14. _____
15. root meaning artery	15. _____
16. root meaning vein	16. _____
17. root meaning valve	17. _____
18. root meaning aorta	18. _____
19. prefix meaning slow	19. _____
20. root meaning dilated	20. _____
21. root meaning crown	21. _____
22. suffix meaning dilation or expansion	22. _____
23. root meaning vessel	23. _____
24. root meaning electricity	24. _____
25. root meaning ventricle	25. _____
26. root meaning restricting, thinning	26. _____

Word Parts Exercise

After studying Table 10.1, write the correct word part for the meaning given.

Meaning	Word Part
1. root meaning vein	1. _____
2. root meaning heart	2. _____
3. root meaning vessel	3. _____
4. root meaning within, inner	4. _____
5. prefix meaning fast	5. _____
6. root meaning clot	6. _____

Structure and Function

The Heart

The heart is a four-chambered hollow organ with three layers. Its lowermost tip is called the **apex**. The innermost layer is called the **endocardium**. The middle layer, which is the actual heart muscle and the thickest of the three layers, is called the **myocardium**. The outer layer of the heart is called the **epicardium**, which is surrounded by the **pericardium**, a sac that surrounds the heart (see **Figure 10.2**).

The heart is a double pump whose chambers are separated by a wall called the **septum**. Remember anatomic position when thinking about blood flow and how it relates to the figures. The right side of the

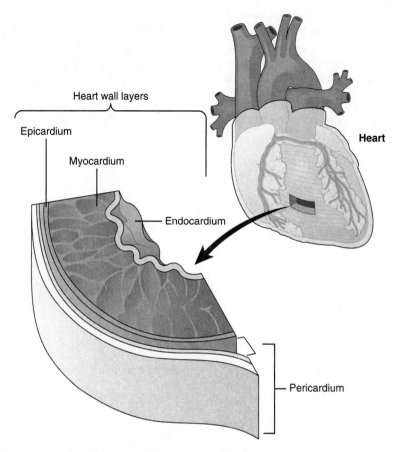

Heart wall layers

Epicardium

Myocardium

Endocardium

Heart

Pericardium

Figure 10.2 Layers of the heart and pericardium. The heart wall is composed of three layers: the epicardium, myocardium, and endocardium. Note the thickness of the myocardium or "muscle" layer. The pericardium is composed of two layers and has fluid in the space between the layers. This fluid helps to reduce friction when the heart beats.

heart is the right side of the patient, and in figures on book pages facing you, it is on the left-hand side of the image. The right side of the heart pumps deoxygenated blood to the **lungs** where the blood picks up oxygen. Because the right side is pumping blood a shorter distance, the muscle in this side of the heart is thinner. The left side of the heart receives blood that has been oxygenated in the lungs, and it pumps the oxygenated blood through the entire body. In the heart, blood travels through four distinct chambers. The atria are the superior (top) chambers, and the ventricles are the inferior (bottom) chambers. The four chambers are as follows:

- **Right atrium**: upper right chamber that receives blood from the systemic circuit via the superior vena cava, inferior vena cava, and coronary sinus; the **interatrial septum** separates the right and left **atria** (plural of *atrium*).
- **Right ventricle**: lower right chamber that receives blood from the right atrium and pumps it to the lungs; the **interventricular septum** separates the right and left ventricles.
- **Left atrium**: upper left chamber that receives oxygen-rich blood as it returns from the lungs.

- **Left ventricle**: lower left chamber that pumps blood out the aorta (large artery) to all parts of the body.

Blood Flow Through the Heart

Blood first enters the heart from the **superior vena cava**, **inferior vena cava**, and **coronary sinus**. The venae cavae are large veins that drain into the right atrium. The **coronary sinus** is a wide channel receiving blood from the heart's coronary veins that empties into the right atrium. Blood leaves the heart at the left ventricle by way of a large artery called the **aorta**. Blood flow through the heart is directed by one-way valves located at the entrance and exit to each of the ventricles. The **atrioventricular (AV) valves** are found at the entrance to the ventricles and are so named because they are between the atria and ventricles. The **right atrioventricular valve** is also known as the **tricuspid valve** because it has three cusps (flaps) that open and close. It controls the opening between the right atrium and right ventricle. The **left atrioventricular valve** is located between the left atrium and left ventricle and is called the bicuspid valve or mitral valve. It has two cusps that control blood flow.

> Why is the left AV valve also named the mitral valve? This name comes from the valve's visual similarity to a miter, which is a tall ceremonial hat that is tapered to a point and worn by some clergymen as a symbol of their office.

The exit valves separate the ventricles from the lungs on the right side and the rest of the body on the left side. These valves are named **semilunar** because the flaps resemble half-moons. The exit point at the right ventricle is called the **pulmonary valve** (*pulmonary semilunar valve*), and it is located between the right ventricle and the **pulmonary arteries**, the vessels that lead to the lungs. The **aortic valve** (*aortic semilunar valve*) is located between the left ventricle and the aorta, the vessel that leads to the rest of the body. The pathway of blood through the heart is illustrated in **Figure 10.3**.

> Use the adjective "ventricular" only when you are sure of the meaning you want. The reason for caution is that the brain, as well as the heart, contains ventricles.

The Heartbeat

To pump blood effectively throughout the body, the heart must contract and relax in a rhythmic cycle known as a **heartbeat**. The **conducting system of the heart** generates and transmits signals that stimulate the myocardium of the heart to contract and relax in sequence (see **Figure 10.4**). The conducting system of the heart includes the following:

- **Sinoatrial node** (SA node): located in the upper posterior wall of the right atrium; action potential (impulse) is generated here and distributed to other cells of the conducting system; conducting cells form **intermodal pathways** that distribute

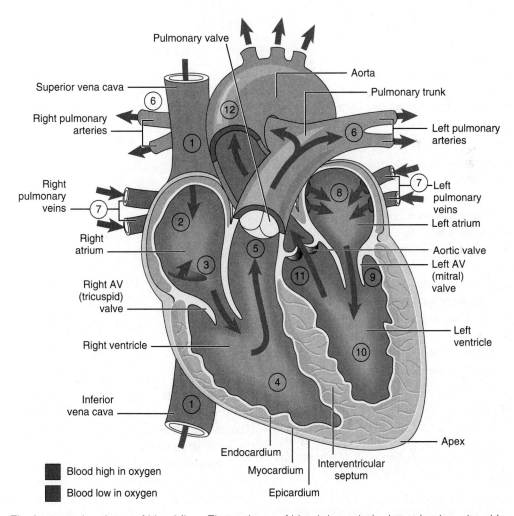

Figure 10.3 The heart and pathway of blood flow. The pathway of blood through the heart begins when blood is returned to the venae cavae ① and coronary sinus ③ and exits the heart through the aorta ⑫ to the rest of the body. The blue coloration indicates blood low in oxygen, and the red coloration indicates blood high in oxygen.

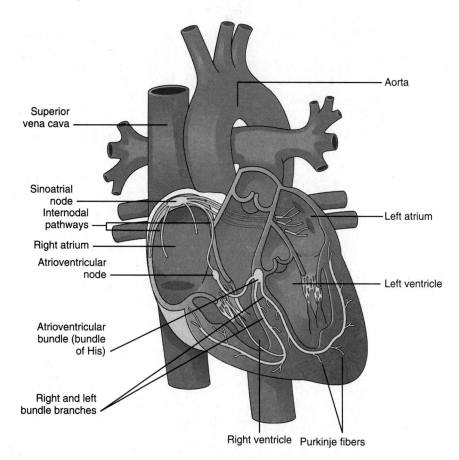

Figure 10.4 Conducting system of the heart. The electrical stimulus begins in the sinoatrial node. The electrical stimulus moves from the sinoatrial node, through the internodal pathways, to the atrioventricular node, through the atrioventricular bundle, through the right and left bundle branches, and terminates in the Purkinje fibers where excitation of the ventricles occurs.

the impulse across the atria as it travels toward the ventricles; also called the pacemaker of the heart.

- **Atrioventricular node** (AV node): located at the junction between the atria and ventricles; continues to generate impulses toward the atrioventricular bundle.

- **Atrioventricular bundle** (AV bundle or bundle of His) and **right and left bundle branches**: atrioventricular bundle is located at the top of the interventricular septum; right and left bundle branches travel down each side of the septum toward the apex; transmit impulses to the Purkinje fibers.

- **Purkinje fibers**: peripheral fibers extending from the bundle branches that end in the right and left ventricles; stimulation from the atrioventricular bundle causes excitation of the ventricular muscles, resulting in contraction.

The electrical activity of the heart can be recorded on an **electrocardiogram** (ECG, EKG). The machine that does the recording is called an **electrocardiograph**.

Why bundle of His? Why not "bundle of His or Hers"? In 1893, German physician Wilhelm His figured out that a heartbeat starts in a particular group of AV fibers, which were, subsequently, named for him. A Czech anatomist/physiologist, Jan Evangelista Purkyně, likewise discovered the Purkinje (or Purkyně) fibers. Born in 1787, Purkyně contributed many other scientific discoveries to the world. For example, he was the first to show that fingerprints could be used to establish identity, and his studies of the human eye foreshadowed motion pictures.

Each heart contraction, called **systole**, is followed by a relaxation called **diastole**. These complete rounds of cardiac systole and diastole make up the **cardiac cycle** and are illustrated in **Figure 10.5**.

Heart rate (HR) is the number of times the heart beats per minute. The blood that is forced through the vessels by contraction creates an increased arterial pressure that can be felt as a pulse. The radial artery on the thumb side of the anterior wrist is a common location for feeling an arterial pulse.

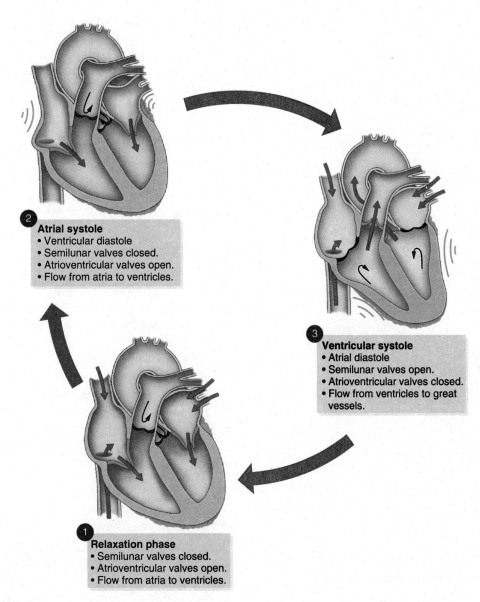

Figure 10.5 The three phases of the cardiac cycle.

(2) **Atrial systole**
- Ventricular diastole
- Semilunar valves closed.
- Atrioventricular valves open.
- Flow from atria to ventricles.

(3) **Ventricular systole**
- Atrial diastole
- Semilunar valves open.
- Atrioventricular valves closed.
- Flow from ventricles to great vessels.

(1) **Relaxation phase**
- Semilunar valves closed.
- Atrioventricular valves open.
- Flow from atria to ventricles.

Blood Vessels

Blood vessels are tubular structures that convey blood. The types of blood vessels include arteries, arterioles, capillaries, venules, and veins (see **Figure 10.6**).

- **Arteries**: thick-walled, muscular, elastic blood vessels that carry blood away from the heart. Except for pulmonary and umbilical arteries, which carry deoxygenated blood, arteries carry oxygenated blood.
- **Arterioles**: branches of the arteries that carry blood to the capillaries.
- **Capillaries**: blood vessels that connect the arterial and venous systems; they are only one cell thick and allow for the exchange of nutrients, gases, and wastes.
- **Venules**: vessels that are continuous with capillaries and transport blood to the veins.
- **Veins**: blood vessels that carry blood toward the heart. Except for pulmonary and umbilical veins, which carry oxygenated blood, veins carry deoxygenated blood.

The **lumen** of a blood vessel is the tubular interior space through which blood flows. The nervous system can stimulate the lumen to be opened, known as **vasodilation**, or closed, which is called **vasoconstriction**. Vasodilation and vasoconstriction each can influence blood pressure (BP).

Blood pressure is a measurement of the amount of pressure exerted against the walls of blood vessels. Blood pressure is recorded as a fractional

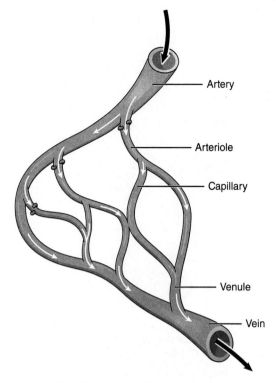

Figure 10.6 The five types of blood vessels.

number, **systolic** over **diastolic**. For example, 120/80 means that the systolic pressure is 120 and the diastolic pressure is 80. Systolic pressure occurs when the highest pressure is exerted against the vessel walls, and diastolic pressure occurs when the lowest pressure is exerted against the vessel walls. Blood pressure is measured with an instrument called a **sphygmomanometer**, commonly called a BP cuff.

Blood

Blood is a fluid connective tissue made up of plasma (55%) and formed elements (45%). **Plasma** is a clear, straw-colored fluid that is composed mostly of water (92%), along with proteins and other solutes (organic nutrients, electrolytes, and organic wastes) in solution. The formed elements in blood consist of red blood cells (RBCs), also called **erythrocytes**; white blood cells (WBCs), also called **leukocytes**; and platelets, also called **thrombocytes**. Each element has an important role, ranging from oxygen transport in erythrocytes, to defense against harmful organisms by leukocytes, to blood clotting via platelets. The following list identifies the structure and function of each formed element:

Red blood cells: The main function of red blood cells is to transport oxygen. The oxygen binds to **hemoglobin (Hb)**, a protein within red blood cells.

White blood cells: White blood cells are the body's main defense against harmful organisms; there are five types of white blood cells: **neutrophils**, **eosinophils**, **basophils**, **lymphocytes**, and **monocytes**. White blood cells play important roles in the body's defense, so they will be discussed again in Chapter 11, which covers the lymphatic system and immunity.

Platelets: These cell fragments play an important role in the blood-clotting process. They are the smallest of the formed elements, about half the size of erythrocytes.

Blood Groups

The four major blood groups (types) are **A**, **B**, **AB**, and **O**. Blood type compatibility is an important consideration when blood is transfused from one person to another. **Table 10.2** lists the blood type compatibilities for donors and recipients.

The presence or absence of a protein on the surface of a red blood cell is responsible for what is known as the **Rh factor**. The Rh factor is named for the first two letters in the word *rhesus*, a reference to the rhesus monkey, whose blood was used in early experiments. A person whose blood contains the Rh factor is **Rh positive** (Rh+). People with blood that does not contain the Rh factor are **Rh negative** (Rh-).

QUICK CHECK

Fill in the blanks.

1. Arteries transfer blood to _____.
2. _____ are blood vessels that return blood to the heart.
3. Erythrocyte is another term for _____.

Table 10.2 Blood Types as Donors and Recipients

Blood Type	Can Donate To	Can Receive From
A	A or AB only	A or O only
B	B or AB only	B or O only
AB (universal recipient)	AB only	A, B, AB, O
O (universal donor)	A, B, AB, O	O only

Disorders Related to the Cardiovascular System

Heart disease includes numerous problems and is a leading cause of death. This section discusses disorders related to the cardiovascular system.

Coronary Artery Disease

Coronary artery disease (CAD) is narrowing of the lumen of one or more of the coronary arteries, usually due to atherosclerosis. Normal blood vessels have a smooth lumen. When there is a progressive buildup of plaque or fatty deposits on inner arterial walls, the lumen narrows, creating **atherosclerosis**. One cause of plaque buildup in the coronary arteries is a condition of increased blood fat (lipid) called **hyperlipidemia**. Common types of lipids are high-density lipoproteins (HDLs) and low-density lipoproteins (LDLs). When there is a hardening and loss of elasticity in the artery, impeding blood flow to the heart muscle, the condition is called **arteriosclerosis** (see **Figure 10.7**). An inadequate supply of blood and oxygen to tissues is called **ischemia**. In the heart, the myocardium is affected the most when blood flow and oxygen are deficient.

Blood Clots

A **thrombus** is a blood clot in a blood vessel, which can impede blood flow to the myocardium and cause ischemia. **Thrombosis** is the formation of a thrombus. An **embolus** is a blood clot that moves throughout the bloodstream.

Myocardial Infarction and Congestive Heart Failure

Myocardial infarction (MI), commonly called a *heart attack*, results from a lack of oxygen supply to the myocardium. Various diagnostic tests are used to identify abnormal cardiac function. Among these are an electrocardiogram (ECG); **echocardiography** (ultrasonic examination of the heart); **cardiac catheterization** (insertion of a catheter and contrast dye into the coronary arteries to detect blockage); and a stress test.

A simple blood test to discover the presence of *troponin* may confirm a diagnosis of myocardial infarction. **Troponin** is a muscle protein released into the bloodstream when a myocardial infarction occurs.

Congestive heart failure (CHF) occurs when the heart cannot pump enough blood to meet the body's needs for oxygen and nutrients. This leads to edema (swelling) in the legs and fluid buildup in the lungs.

> The acronym MONA was formerly used to refer to standard emergency treatment for a suspected heart attack. M stands for morphine, O for oxygen, N for nitroglycerin, and A for aspirin. Practitioners have moved away from MONA as new evidence suggests a different treatment with the mnemonic THROMBINS$_2$: T stands for thienopyridines, H for heparin, R for renin–angiotensin system blockers, O for oxygen, M for morphine, B for beta blocker, I for intervention, N for nitroglycerin, and S$_2$ for statin and salicylate (aspirin).

Arrhythmias

A normal heart rhythm is called **sinus rhythm**. An **arrhythmia** is any irregularity of the heart's rhythm, such as a slow or fast rate or extra beats. **Bradycardia** (less than 50 beats/minute) is a slower than normal heart rate, and **tachycardia** (more than 90 beats/minute) is a faster than normal rate. **Fibrillation** describes rapid, random, and ineffective contractions of the heart. Some

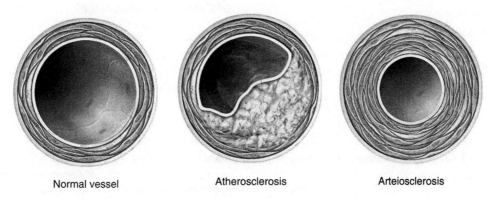

Normal vessel   Atherosclerosis   Arteiosclerosis

Figure 10.7 A comparison between atherosclerosis and arteriosclerosis.

arrhythmias are more serious than others. **Atrial fibrillation**, commonly shortened to "A-fib," occurs when the atria beat faster than the ventricles. This condition causes a quivering motion of the atria, which is usually not life threatening, although it can predispose the atria to thrombi formation. It affects many people and can often be controlled with drugs. Sustained **ventricular fibrillation**, a condition in which the ventricles ineffectively pump blood, can be fatal.

Hypertension

The term for high blood pressure is **hypertension** (HTN). It occurs when the systolic reading exceeds 140 mm Hg or the diastolic is more than 90 mm Hg. Over time, hypertension may lead to arteriosclerosis (hardening of the arteries) and/or **left ventricular hypertrophy** (oversized left ventricle). When hypertension is related to another medical problem, such as a kidney disorder, it is called **secondary hypertension**.

Are atherosclerosis and arteriosclerosis the same ailment? Not exactly. Both conditions exhibit similar symptoms; however, these symptoms occur for different reasons. A patient who has arteriosclerosis has hardening of the arteries caused by continuous high blood pressure. A patient with atherosclerosis has similar symptoms because their arteries have been narrowed by plaque buildup. So, a patient can have arteriosclerosis and not have atherosclerosis, and a patient can have atherosclerosis without arteriosclerosis. Both have the same symptoms, however, and some patients have both conditions.

Blood Disorders

Any abnormality of the blood may be called a **dyscrasia**. There are three major types: anemia, leukemia, and clotting disorders:

- **Anemia** is a condition marked by a deficiency of red blood cells or a low level of hemoglobin (Hb).
- **Leukemia** is characterized by an increased number of white blood cells (leukocytes).
- **Clotting disorders** include **hemophilia** (hereditary bleeding disorder), **thrombocytopenia** (an insufficient number of thrombocytes), and **disseminated intravascular coagulation** (DIC; extreme clotting caused by trauma or disease).

Diagnostic Tests, Treatments, and Surgical Procedures

Medications and surgical procedures are used to treat arrhythmias. **Antiarrhythmics**, such as amiodarone, are medications that affect calcium channels in the heart to regulate rhythm. Blood thinners are commonly used for patients with atrial fibrillation because these patients are at higher risk of developing blood clots due to blood pooling in the heart and not continuously flowing as it should. Blood thinners also help prevent blood clot formation in other parts of the body to ensure that blood flows freely. **Cardioversion**, a treatment for fibrillation, involves applying an electric current to restore a normal heart rhythm. **Cardiac ablation**, a treatment for cardiac arrhythmias, uses heat or cold energy to create tiny scars on the heart's interior to block irregular electrical signals and restore normal heart rhythm.

Surgical procedures for treating blockages in blood vessels include the following:

- **Percutaneous transluminal coronary angioplasty** (PTCA) involves the insertion of a balloon-tipped catheter to open a blocked coronary artery (see **Figure 10.8**).
- **Arterial stent** refers to the implantation of a stent, which is a mesh tube that is implanted into an artery to provide support (see **Figure 10.9**).
- **Coronary artery bypass graft** (CABG) is a surgical procedure in which a damaged section of a coronary artery is replaced or bypassed with a graft vessel (see **Figure 10.10**).
- **Endarterectomy** is the removal of the inner lining of a blocked artery.

Practice and Practitioners

The specialists who treat disorders of the cardiovascular system include cardiologists, cardiovascular surgeons, cardiothoracic surgeons, and hematologists. **Cardiologists** diagnose and treat heart disorders. Physicians who specialize in surgical procedures of the heart, lungs, esophagus, and other chest organs are called **cardiothoracic surgeons**. **Cardiovascular surgeons** surgically correct disorders of the cardiovascular system. **Hematologists** treat disorders of the blood.

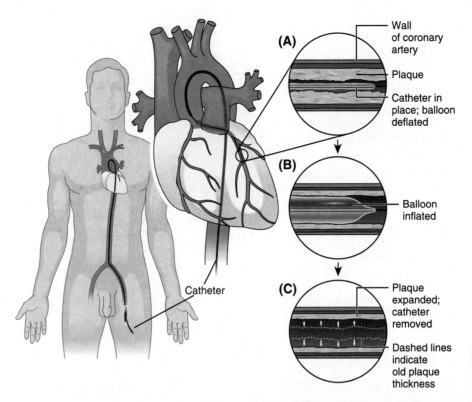

Figure 10.8 Percutaneous transluminal coronary angioplasty (PTCA). **(A)** Plaque deposits in the artery. **(B)** Plaque buildup narrows the coronary vessel, impeding blood flow to the myocardium. **(C)** The rough interior edges encourage clot formation in the artery.

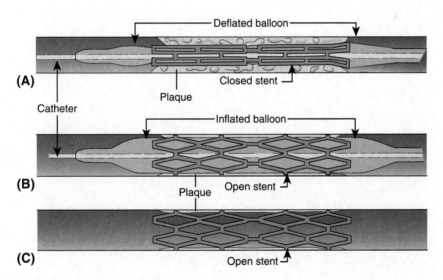

Figure 10.9 Arterial stent. **(A)** A balloon-tipped catheter is placed into the artery with the balloon deflated and the stent closed. **(B)** When the stent is in the proper position of the narrowed artery, the balloon is inflated, causing the stent to open. **(C)** The catheter is removed, and the stent remains in place.

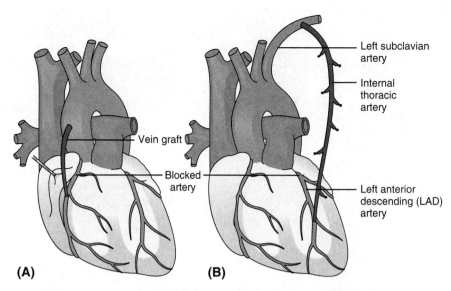

Figure 10.10 Coronary artery bypass graft (CABG). **(A)** A segment of the saphenous vein extracted from the leg is used to carry blood from the aorta to a part of the right coronary artery that is distal to the occlusion. **(B)** The internal thoracic artery from the chest is used to bypass an obstruction in the left anterior descending artery. The graft redirects the blood flow or "bypasses" the blocked artery.

Abbreviation Table The Cardiovascular System

Abbreviation	Meaning
A-fib	atrial fibrillation
AV	atrioventricular
BP	blood pressure
CABG	coronary artery bypass graft
CAD	coronary artery disease
CCU	cardiac care unit
CHF	congestive heart failure
DIC	disseminated intravascular coagulation
DVT	deep vein thrombosis
ECG	electrocardiogram, electrocardiograph, electrocardiography
EKG	electrocardiogram, electrocardiograph, electrocardiography
Hb	hemoglobin (protein in red blood cells that carries oxygen)

Abbreviation	Meaning
HDL	high-density lipoprotein
HR	heart rate
HTN	hypertension
LDL	low-density lipoprotein
MI	myocardial infarction
PA	physician assistant
PE	pulmonary embolism
PTCA	percutaneous transluminal coronary angioplasty
RBC	red blood cell
Rh⁺, Rh⁻	symbol for Rh blood group; Rh positive, Rh negative
SA	sinoatrial
SOB	shortness of breath
TIA	transient ischemic attack
US	ultrasound
WBC	white blood cell

Study Table The Cardiovascular System

Term and Pronunciation	Analysis	Meaning
Structure and Function		
aorta (ay-OR-tuh)	from the Greek word *aeirein* (to raise)	the main trunk of the systemic arterial system
aortic valve (ay-OR-tik VALV)	from the Greek word *aeirein* (to raise); from the Latin word *valva* (that which turns)	valve between the left ventricle to the aorta; also called *aortic semilunar valve*

Term and Pronunciation	Analysis	Meaning
Structure and Function		
apex (AY-peks)	from the Latin for summit or tip	the pointed inferior portion of the heart
arteries (AR-tur-reez)	from the Greek word *arteria* (windpipe)	the largest of the blood vessels that carry blood away from the heart
arterioles (ar-TEER-ee-olz)	from the Greek word *arteria* (windpipe)	the smallest arteries that connect with the capillaries
atria (AY-tree-uh)	a Latin word meaning "entry hall"	upper two of the four heart chambers, composed of the right atrium and left atrium
atrioventricular node (AY-tree-oh-ven-TRIK-you-lur NODE)	from the Latin word meaning "entry hall"; from the Latin *venter* (belly)	fibers located at the base of the right atrium near the ventricle that carry electrical stimulation to the atrioventricular bundle
atrioventricular valve (ay-tree-oh-ven-TRIK-you-lur VALV)	from the Greek word *arteria* (windpipe); from the Latin word *venter* (belly)	a valve between an atrium and a ventricle; there are two atrioventricular valves, a right and a left
basophil (BAY-zoh-fil)	from the Greek *basis* and *philein* (to love)	a white blood cell with granules that stain with basic dyes
bicuspid valve (by-KUS-pid VALV)	*bi-* (two); from the Latin *cuspidem* (cusp or point); from the Latin word *valva* (that which turns)	flap (valve) between the left atrium and left ventricle; also called *mitral valve*
bundle of His (BUHN-dul UV HIZ)	named for Swiss cardiologist Wilhelm His, Jr., who discovered the function of these cells in 1893	located at the top of the interventricular septum; carries electrical impulses from the atrioventricular node to Purkinje fibers
capillaries (KAP-ih-lair-eez)	from the Latin word *capillus* (hair)	the smallest of the blood vessels where gas and nutrient exchange occurs
cardiac cycle (KAR-dee-ak SIGH-kul)	*cardi/o* (heart); *-ac* (adjective ending)	a complete round of systole and diastole
conducting system of the heart (kun-DUCK-shun SIS-tem UV THE HART)	from the Latin word, *cunduct* (brought together)	system of muscle fibers comprising the sinoatrial (SA) node, internodal pathways, atrioventricular (AV) node and bundle, right and left bundle branches, and Purkinje fibers
coronary sinus (KOR-uh-nair-ee SIGH-nus)	from the Latin words *coronarius* (crown) and *sinus* (bend)	channel that receives blood from the coronary veins of the heart and empties into the right atrium of the heart
diastole (dye-AS-toh-lee)	from the Greek word *diastole* (dilation)	relaxation phase of the heart
endocardium (en-doh-KAR-dee-um)	*endo-* (within); *cardi/o* (heart)	the inner lining of the heart
eosinophil (ee-oh-SIN-oh-fil)	from the Greek words *eos* (dawn); *philein* (to love)	white blood cell that stains with certain dyes
epicardium (ep-ih-KAR-dee-um)	*epi-* (on, upon); *cardi/o* (heart)	the outer covering of the heart
erythrocytes (eh-RITH-roh-sites)	*erythr/o* (red); *-cyte* (cell)	red blood cells that carry oxygen

(continues)

Study Table The Cardiovascular System		*(continued)*
Term and Pronunciation	**Analysis**	**Meaning**
Structure and Function		
heartbeat (HART-beet)	from the Dutch word *hart* (heart) and the German word *Herz* (heart)	a complete cycle of heart contraction and relaxation
heart rate (HART RATE)	From the German word *Herz* (heart) and late Middle English *rate* (expressing something of estimated value)	the number of times per minute the heart contracts
hemoglobin (Hb) (hee-moh-GLOW-bin)	*hem-* (blood); from the Latin *globus* (globe)	the protein in red blood cells that transports oxygen
inferior vena cava (in-FEER-ee-ur VEE-nuh KAY-vuh)	from the Latin words *inferior* (lower), *vena* (vein), and *cava* (hollow)	large vein that collects blood from the smaller veins of the lower body
left atrium (LEFT AY-tree-um)	a Latin word meaning "entry hall"	upper left heart chamber
left ventricle (LEFT VEN-trih-kul)	from the Latin word *venter* (belly)	lower left heart chamber
leukocytes (LOO-koh-sites)	*leuk/o* (white); *-cyte* (cell)	white blood cells that play a role in immunity
lumen (LOO-men)	Latin for "light"; in anatomy used to describe an opening or passageway	the space in the interior of a hollow tubular structure like an artery
lymphocyte (LIM-foh-site)	from the Latin *lympho-* (lymph); *-cyte* (cell)	one of five types of white blood cell; distributed throughout lymphatic tissue
mitral valve (MY-trul VALV)	from the Latin word *mitra* (turban); from the Latin word *valva* (that which turns)	flap (valve) between the left atrium and the left ventricle; also called *bicuspid valve*
monocyte (MON-oh-site)	*mon/o* (single); *-cyte* (cell)	a relatively large white blood cell
myocardium (my-oh-KAR-dee-um)	*my/o* (muscle); *cardi/o* (heart)	the heart muscle, which includes nerves and blood vessels
neutrophil (NEW-troh-fil)	from the Latin word *neuter* (neither); from the Greek word *philein* (to love)	a mature white blood cell normally constituting more than half the total number of leukocytes
pericardium (pair-ih-KAR-dee-um)	*peri-* (surrounding); *cardi/o* (heart)	sac that surrounds the heart
plasma (PLAZ-muh)	a Greek word meaning "something molded" or "created"	the fluid portion of blood consisting mainly of water
platelets (PLATE-lets)	from the English word plate and the diminutive suffix *-let*	smallest of the formed elements; important in the clotting process; also called *thrombocytes*
pulmonary artery (PULL-mon-air-ee AR-tur-ree)	*pulmon/o* (lung); from the Greek word *arteria* (windpipe)	vessel that carries deoxygenated blood from the right ventricle to the lungs
pulmonary circuit (PULL-mon-air-ee SER-kit)	*pulmon/o* (lung); from the Latin word *circuitus* (going around)	passage of blood from the right ventricle through the pulmonary arteries to the lungs and back through the pulmonary veins to the left atrium
pulmonary valve (PULL-mon-air-ee VALV)	*pulmon/o* (lung); from the Latin word *valva* (that which turns)	valve between the right ventricle and lungs; also called *pulmonary semilunar valve*

Term and Pronunciation	Analysis	Meaning
Structure and Function		
pulmonary veins (PULL-mon-air-ee VAINZ)	*pulmon/o* (lung); from the Latin word *vena* (blood vessel)	vessels that carry oxygenated blood from the lungs to the left atrium
pulse (PULS)	from the Latin word *pulsus* (beating)	rhythmic expansion and contraction of an artery produced by pressure of the blood moving through the artery
Purkinje fibers (per-KIN-jee FIGH-berz)	named after Jan Evangelista Purkinje, who discovered them in 1839	fibers that carry stimulation throughout the ventricles
red blood cells (RED BLUD SELZ)	common English words	erythrocytes that contain hemoglobin for carrying oxygen
Rh factor (R-H FAK-tur)	from rh(esus), so-called because the blood group was discovered in rhesus monkeys	an antigen, first discovered in the rhesus monkey; a person is either Rh positive or Rh negative
right atrium (RITE AY-tree-um)	a Latin word meaning "entry hall"	upper right heart chamber
right ventricle (RITE VEN-trih-kul)	from the Latin word *venter* (belly)	lower right heart chamber
semilunar valve (sem-ee-LOO-nur VALV)	*semi-* (half); from the Latin word *luna* (moon)	a heart valve at the exit of a ventricle; pulmonary semilunar valve and aortic semilunar valve
septum (SEP-tum)	from the Latin word *saeptum* (a fence)	thin wall that separates cavities or masses; in the heart, septa separate the right atrium from the left atrium and the right ventricle from the left ventricle
sinoatrial node (SA node) (SYE-noh-AY-tree-ul NODE)	from the Latin words *sinus* (bend) and *atrium* (entry hall)	known as the pacemaker of the heart; electrical impulse originates here
sinus rhythm (SYE-nus RITH-um)	from the Latin word *sinus* (bend); from the Greek word *rhythmos* (measured flow or movement)	normal rhythm of the heartbeat
superior vena cava (sue-PEER-ee-ur VEE-nuh KAVE-uh)	from the Latin words *superior* (higher), *vena* (vein), and *cava* (hollow)	large vein that collects blood from the smaller veins of the upper body
systemic circuit (sis-TEM-ik SER-kit)	from the Greek word *systema* (an organized whole); from the Latin word *circuitus* (going around)	circulation of blood through the arteries, capillaries, and veins of the general circulation, from the left ventricle to the right atrium
systole (SIS-toe-lee)	a Greek word meaning "contraction"	contraction phase of the heart
thrombocyte (THROM-boh-site)	from the Greek word *thrombos* (clot of blood); *-cyte* (cell)	smallest of the formed elements; important in the coagulation process; also called *platelet*
tricuspid valve (try-KUS-pid VALV)	*tri-* (three); from the Latin *cuspidem* (cusp or point)	valve between the right atrium and the right ventricle; also called *right AV valve* or *right atrioventricular valve*
troponin (TROH-poh-nin)	from the Greek word *trepein* (to turn)	a muscle protein that is released into the bloodstream when a heart attack occurs

(continues)

Study Table The Cardiovascular System		*(continued)*
Term and Pronunciation	**Analysis**	**Meaning**
Structure and Function		
vascular (VASS-cue-lur)	*vascul/o* (blood vessel); *-ar* (adjective suffix)	adjectival form of *vessel*
vein (VANE)	from the Latin word *vena* (vein)	the blood vessel that returns blood from the tissues to the heart
venous (VEE-nus)	from the Latin word *vena* (vein)	adjectival form of *vein*
venules (VEEN-yoolz)	from the Latin *venula* (diminutive form of *vena* [vein])	small veins
ventricle (VEN-tri-kul)	from the Latin word *venter* (belly)	lower two of the four heart chambers, composed of the right ventricle and left ventricle
white blood cell (WHITE BLUD SELL)	common English words	formed element in the blood that protects the body against harmful bacteria
Disorders		
anemia (uh-NEE-mee-uh)	from the Greek word *anaimia* (without blood)	abnormally low red blood cell count
aneurysm (AN-yur-iz-um)	from the Greek word *aneurysmos* (to dilate)	a localized dilation of an artery, cardiac chamber, or other vessel
angina pectoris (an-JYE-nuh PEK-tor-is)	from the Greek word *agkhone* (a strangling); also *angere* (anguish); *pectoris*, a Latin word meaning "chest"	pain in the chest due to ischemia
angiitis (an-jee-EYE-tis)	from the Greek word *angeion* (vessel) and suffix -itis (inflammation)	inflammation of the blood vessels; also called *vasculitis*
angiospasm (AN-jee-oh-spaz-um)	*angi/o* (blood vessel); from the Greek word *spasmos* (spasm)	involuntary contraction in blood vessels
angiostenosis (AN-jee-oh-sten-OH-sis)	*angi/o* (blood vessel); *-stenosis* (a narrowing)	narrowing of a blood vessel
arrhythmia (uh-RITH-mee-uh)	a- (without); from the Greek word *rhythmos* (measured flow or movement); *-ia* (condition)	abnormal rhythm; irregular heartbeat
arteriosclerosis (ar-TEER-ee-oh-skle-ROH-sis)	from the Greek word *arteria* (windpipe); *scler/o* (hardness); *-osis* (abnormal condition of)	hardening of the arteries
arteriospasm (ar-TEER-ee-oh-spaz-um)	from the Greek word *arteria* (windpipe); from the Greek word *spasmos* (a spasm or convulsion)	involuntary contraction of an artery
arteriostenosis (ar-TEER-ee- oh-steh-NO-sis)	from the Greek word *arteria* (windpipe); *-steno* (narrow); *-osis* (abnormal condition)	narrowing of an artery
atheroma (ath-er-OH-muh)	from the Greek word *ather* (crushed grain, porridge); *-oma* (tumor)	fatty deposit or plaque within the arterial wall
atherosclerosis (ath-er-oh-skleh-ROH-sis)	*ather/o* (fatty); *scler/o* (hardening); *-osis* (abnormal condition of)	hardening and narrowing of the arteries

Term and Pronunciation	Analysis	Meaning
Disorders		
atrial fibrillation (A-fib) (AY-tree-ul fih-brih-LAY-shun)	from the Latin word *atrium* (entry hall) *-al* (adjective suffix); from the Latin word *fibra* (fiber, string, thread)	rapid, random, ineffective contractions of the atrium
atriomegaly (AY-tree-oh-MEG-uh-lee)	from the Latin word *atrium* (hall); *-megaly* (enlargement)	enlargement of an atrium
bradycardia (bray-dee-KAR-dee-uh)	*brady-* (slow); *cardi/o* (heart); *-ia* (condition)	abnormally slow heartbeat
cardiac arrest (KAR-dee-ak UH-rest)	*cardi/o* (heart); from the Latin words *ad + restare* (to stop, remain behind)	cessation of heart activity
cardiomegaly (kar-dee-oh-MEG-uh-lee)	*cardi/o* (heart); *-megaly* (enlargement)	enlargement of the heart
cardiomyopathy (kar-dee-oh-my-OP-uh-thee)	*cardi/o* (heart); *my/o* (muscle); *-pathy* (disease)	disease of the heart muscle (myocardium)
cardiopathy (kar-dee-OP-uh-thee)	*cardi/o* (heart); *-pathy* (disease)	any heart disease
cardiorrhexis (kar-dee-oh-REX-is)	*cardi/o* (heart); *-rrhexis* (rupture)	rupture in the heart wall
carditis (kar-DYE-tiss)	*cardi/o* (heart); *-itis* (inflammation)	inflammation of the heart
congestive heart failure (CHF) (kun-JEST-iv HART FALE-yur)	from the Latin word *congerere* (to bring together, pile up)	syndrome where the heart is unable to pump enough blood to meet the body's needs for oxygen and nutrients; as a result, fluid is retained and accumulates in the ankles and legs
coronary artery disease (CAD) (KOR-uh-nair-ee AR-ter-ree dih-ZEEZ)	from the Latin *coronarius* (of a crown); from the Greek word *arteria* (windpipe)	narrowing of the lumen of one or more coronary arteries, usually due to atherosclerosis
deep vein thrombosis (DVT) (DEEP VANE throm-BOH-sis)	related to Dutch *diep* (deep) + Latin *vena* (vein) + Greek *thrombos* (curdling, blood clot)	blood clot in a deep vein, usually the legs that develops when blood pools; blood thinners are prescribed to prevent further clot formation; risk for clot breaking loose and traveling in the bloodstream to the lungs, causing pulmonary embolism (PE)
disseminated intravascular coagulation (DIC) (dih-SEM-ihn-ay-ted in-truh-VASS-kyu-lur koh-AG-you-LAY-shun)	from the Latin *dis-* (in every direction); *seminare* (to plant, propagate); *intra-* (within); *vascul/o* (vessel); *-ar* (adjective suffix); coagulation (from the Latin verb *coagulo* [curdle])	widespread clotting and obstruction of blood flow to the tissues
dyscrasia (dys-KRAY-shuh)	*dys-* (bad, difficult); from the Greek word *krasis* (mingling)	general term for a blood disorder
embolism (EM-boh-liz-um)	from the Greek word *embolismos* (to insert)	obstruction of an artery from a traveling blood clot, air bubble, or fatty fragment
embolus (EM-boh-lis)	from the Greek word *embolus* (plug or stopper)	blood clot, air bubble, fatty fragment that is carried in the bloodstream

(continues)

Study Table The Cardiovascular System		*(continued)*
Term and Pronunciation	**Analysis**	**Meaning**
Disorders		
endocarditis (en-doh-kar-DYE-tiss)	*endo-* (within); *cardi/o* (heart); *-itis* (inflammation)	inflammation of the endocardium
fibrillation (fib-ruh-LAY-shun)	from the Latin word *fibrilla* (little fiber)	exceedingly rapid contractions or twitching of muscle fibers
hemolysis (hee-MOL-ih-sis)	*hem/o* (blood); *-lysis* (destruction)	change or destruction of red blood cells
hemophilia (hee-moh-FEE-lee-uh)	*hem/o* (blood); *-phil(ia)* (attraction)	congenital disorder impeding the coagulation process
hemorrhage (HEM-oh-rij)	*hem/o* (blood); *-rrhage* (burst forth)	discharge of blood; bleeding
hyperlipidemia (high-per- LIP-ih-DEE-mee-uh)	*hyper-* (above normal); *lip/o* (fat); *-demia* (from hema [blood])	elevated cholesterol, triglycerides, and lipoproteins in the blood
hypertension (high-per-TEN-shun)	*hyper-* (above normal); from the Latin word *tendere* (to stretch)	elevated blood pressure (>120/80 mm Hg)
hypertrophy (high-PUR-troh-fee)	*hyper-* (above normal); *-trophy* (nourishment)	increase in size of a part or organ
ischemia (is-KEE-mee-uh)	from the Greek word *iskhaimos* (a stopping of the blood); *-ia* (condition)	deficiency in blood supply and oxygen to the tissues
leukemia (loo-KEE-mee-uh)	leukos (Greek word for "white"); *-emia* (blood)	progressive proliferation of abnormal leukocytes (white blood cells)
murmur (MER-mer)	from Old French *murmure* (soft sound, murmur)	recurring heart sound heard through a stethoscope usually indicative of a faulty heart valve
myocardial infarction (MI) (my-oh-KAR-dee-uhl in-FARK-shun)	*my/o* (muscle); *cardi/o* (heart); *-al* (adjective suffix); from the Latin word *infractionem* (a breaking)	heart attack
myocarditis (my-oh-kar-DYE-tiss)	*my/o* (muscle); *cardi/o* (heart); *-itis* (inflammation)	inflammation of the heart muscle
pericarditis (pair-ih-kar-DYE-tiss)	*peri-* (surrounding); *cardi/o* (heart); *-itis* (inflammation)	inflammation of the pericardium
pulmonary embolism (PE) (pul-mun-AIR-ee em-buh-LIZ-um)	from Latin word *pulmonarius* (lung) and Greek word *embolismos* (to insert)	blood clot that develops in a blood vessel outside the lungs (usually in a leg) that travels to a lung artery, blocking blood flow; shortness of breath develops
secondary hypertension (SEK-uhn-der-ee high-per-TEN-shun)	*hyper-* (above normal); from the Latin word *tendere* (to stretch)	hypertension due to a known cause
tachycardia (tak-ih-KAR-dee-uh)	*tachy-* (fast); *cardi/o* (heart); *-ia* (condition)	abnormally rapid heartbeat
thrombocytopenia (THROM-boh-sigh-toh-PEE-nee-uh)	*thromb/o* (blood clot); *cyt/o* (cell); *-penia* (deficiency)	abnormal decrease in the number of thrombocytes (platelets)
thromboembolism (throm-boh-EM-boh-liz-um)	*thromb/o* (blood clot) and from the Greek word *embolismos* (to insert)	blood vessel obstruction caused by a traveling blood clot

Term and Pronunciation	Analysis	Meaning
Disorders		
thrombus (THROM-bus)	from the Latin and Greek *thrombos* (lump, blood clot)	blood clot within the vascular system
transient ischemic attack (TIA) (TRAN-see-ent is-KEE-mik uh-TAK)	isch: root from the Greek word for restricting or thinning; -emia, suffix referring to blood	sudden loss of neurologic function with complete recovery usually within 24 hours; referred to as a ministroke
thrombus (THROM-bus)	*thromb/o* (blood clot)	blood clot attached to an interior wall of a vein or artery
thrombosis (throm-BOH-sis)	Greek word for "a clumping or curdling"	formation or presence of a thrombus (blood clot)
valvulitis (valv-yu-LYE-tis)	from the Latin word *valva* (that which turns); -itis (inflammation)	inflammation of a heart valve
vasculitis (VAS-kyu-ligh-tis)	*vascul/o* (blood vessel); -itis (inflammation)	inflammation of a vessel; also called *angiitis*
vasoconstriction (VAZE-oh-kun-STRIK-shun)	*vas/o* (duct, blood vessel); from the Latin word *constingere* (to draw tight)	narrowing of blood vessels
vasodilation (VAZE-oh-dye-LAY-shun)	*vas/o* (vessel); from the Latin word *dilitare* (to make wider)	widening of blood vessels
ventricular fibrillation (ven-TRIK-yoo-lur fib-ruh-LAY-shun)	from the Latin word *venter* (belly); from the Latin word *fibrilla* (little fiber)	exceedingly rapid contractions or twitching of ventricular heart muscle that replaces normal contraction
Diagnostic Tests, Treatments, and Surgical Procedures		
angiogram (AN-jee-oh-gram)	*angi/o* (blood vessel); -gram (record or picture)	printed record obtained through angiography (radiography of blood vessels)
angiography (an-jee-OG-ruh-fee)	*angi/o* (blood vessel); -graphy (process of recording)	radiography of a blood vessel after injection of a contrast dye
angioplasty (AN-jee-oh-plass-tee)	*angi/o* (blood vessel); -plasty (surgical repair)	surgical repair of a blood vessel
antianginals (an-tee-AN-jye-nulz)	*anti-* (against); from the Greek *ankhone* (strangling); -al (adjective suffix)	drugs used to treat chest pain
antiarrhythmics (an-tee-uh-RITH-micks)	*anti-* (against); *a-* (without); from the Greek word *rhythmos* (measured flow or movement)	drug used to treat rhythm abnormalities
arterial stent (ar-TEER-ee-ul STENT)	English word *stenting* refers to the process of stiffening	a device implanted into an artery to open and provide support to the arterial wall
atrioseptoplasty (AY-tree-oh-SEP-toh-plass-tee)	from the Latin words *atrium* (entry hall) and *saeptum* (fence); -plasty (surgical repair)	surgical repair of an atrial septum
cardiac catheterization (KAR-dee-ak KATH-eh-tur-eye-zay-shun)	*cardi/o* (heart); -ac (pertaining to); from the Greek word *kathienai* (to let down, thrust in)	procedure where a catheter is inserted into an artery and guided into the heart; may be used for diagnosis of blockages or for treatment
cardiac ablation (KAR-dee-ak uh-BLAY-shun)	*cardi/o* (heart); -ac (pertaining to); from the Latin words *ab-* (away); and *latus* (brought)	partial destruction of the pathway of the electrical conducting system of the heart to treat irregular heart rhythms

(continues)

Study Table The Cardiovascular System		*(continued)*
Term and Pronunciation	**Analysis**	**Meaning**
Diagnostic Tests, Treatments, and Surgical Procedures		
cardiac glycosides (KAR-dee-ak GLYE-koh-sides)	*cardi/o* (heart); *-ac* (pertaining to); *glyc/o* (sugar) + *-ide*	drugs used to improve heart output by increasing the muscular contraction
cardiogram (KAR-dee-oh-gram)	*cardi/o* (heart); *-gram* (record or picture)	a graphic trace of electrical activity in the heart
cardiotomy (kar-dee-OT-uh-mee)	*cardi/o* (heart); *-tomy* (cutting operation)	incision into the heart or incision into the cardia of the stomach
cardioversion (KAR-dee-oh-VER-zhun)	*cardi/o* (heart); from the Latin word *vertere* (to turn)	use of electrical shock to restore the heart's normal rhythm
coronary artery bypass graft (CABG) (KOR-uh-nair-ee AR-tuh-ree BYE-pass GRAFT)	from the Latin *cor* (heart); from the Greek word *arteria* (windpipe); common English words	through an open chest, a graft (piece of vein or other heart artery) is implanted on the heart to bypass a blockage
diuretic (DYE-ur-et-ik)	from the Greek word *diouretikos* (prompting urine)	a drug used to increase urination and thereby decrease water content in blood to decrease blood pressure
echocardiography (EK-oh- KAR-dee-OG-ruh-fee)	from the Greek word *ekhe* (sound); *cardi/o* (heart); *-graphy* (process of recording)	ultrasonic procedure used to evaluate the structure and motion of the heart
electrocardiogram (ee-LEK-troh-KAR-dee-oh-gram)	*electro-* (electricity); Greek *kardia* (heart); *gramma* (drawing)	graphic record of the heart's electrical activity
electrocardiograph (ee-LEK-troh-KAR-dee-oh-graf)	*electro-* (electricity); *kardia* (heart); *graph* (instrument for recording)	an instrument for recording the electrical currents that traverse the heart
endarterectomy (end-ar-tur-ECK-toh-mee)	*endo-* (within); *arteri/o* (artery); *-ectomy* (excision)	surgical removal of the lining of an artery
nuclear stress test (NOO-klee-ur STRESS TEST)	common English words	assessment of blood flow through the heart using a nuclear tracer while the patient exercises
percutaneous transluminal coronary angioplasty (PTCA) (pur-kyoo-TAY- nee-us trans-LOO-min-uhl KOR-uh-nair-ee AN-jee-oh-plas-tee)	*per-* (through); *cutane/o* (skin); *trans-* (across, through); *lumen* (passage); *coron/o* (crown); *angi/o* (blood vessel); *-plasty* (surgical repair)	an operation for enlarging the narrowed lumen of a coronary artery by inflating and withdrawing a balloon on the tip of an angiographic catheter
pericardiotomy (PAIR-ih-kar-dee-OT-oh-mee)	*peri-* (surrounding); *cardi/o* (heart); *-tomy* (cutting operation)	incision into the pericardium
sphygmomanometer (SFIG-moh-mah-NOM-eh-tur)	from the Greek words *sphygmos* (pulse), *manos* (thin), *metros* (measure)	instrument used to measure BP

Term and Pronunciation	Analysis	Meaning
Diagnostic Tests, Treatments, and Surgical Procedures		
statins (STAT-inz)	from *static* (controlled state) and *-in* (suffix forming a pharmaceutical name)	a class of cholesterol-lowering drug
ultrasound (US) (UL-truh-sound)	from the Latin word *ultra* (beyond) and the Old Norse *sund* (swim)	Medical imaging procedure using sound vibrations
valvoplasty (VALV-oh-plass-tee)	from the Latin word *valva* (that which turns); *-plasty* (surgical repair)	surgical repair of a heart valve; also called *valvuloplasty*
valvotomy (valv-OT-oh-mee)	from the Latin word *valva* (that which turns); *-tomy* (cutting operation)	surgical removal of a blocked heart valve (stenosis of a heart valve) by cutting into it; also called *valvulotomy*
valvuloplasty (VALV-yu-loh-plass-tee)	from the Latin word *valva* (that which turns); *-plasty* (surgical repair)	surgical repair of a heart valve; also called *valvoplasty*
valvulotomy (VALV-yu-lot-oh-mee)	from the Latin word *valva* (that which turns); *-tomy* (cutting operation)	surgical removal of a blocked heart valve (stenosis of a heart valve) by cutting into it; also called *valvotomy*
Practice and Practitioners		
cardiologist (kar-dee-OL-oh-jist)	*cardi/o* (heart); *-logist* (one who specializes)	heart specialist
cardiology (kar-dee-OL-oh-jee)	*cardi/o* (heart); *-logy* (study of)	medical specialty dealing with the heart
cardiothoracic surgeon (kar-dee-oh-thor-ASS-ik SUR-jun)	from the Greek words *kardia* (heart) and *thorax* (chest); from the French word *surgien* (surgery, handiwork)	physician who specializes in surgical procedures of organs in the chest cavity, such as the heart, lungs, and esophagus
cardiovascular surgeon (kar-dee-oh-VAS-kyoo-lur SUR-jun)	*cardi/o* (heart); *vas/o* (vessel)	a medical practitioner who surgically corrects disorders of the cardiovascular system
hematologist (HEE-muh-tol-oh-gist)	*hemat/o* (blood); *-logist* (one who specializes)	blood specialist
hematology (HEE-muh-TOL-oh-jee)	*hemat/o* (blood); *-logy* (study of)	medical specialty dealing with blood
physician assistant (PA) (fuh-ZISH-un uh-SIST-ent)	from Old French word *fisicien*, based on Latin *physica* (things relating to nature) and the Latin word *assistant* (taking one's stand beside)	medical professional licensed to diagnose, treat, prescribe medications, and manage patient care; training is less than that for a physician and most have graduate degrees

CASE STUDY WRAP-UP

At the hospital, the emergency medicine physician on staff told Brian that he had a blood clot and was diagnosed with acute deep vein thrombosis (DVT). He was immediately injected with Lovenox and sent home with a prescription for warfarin. Brian was also given oral and written instructions for clot treatment, including wearing compression stockings. Goals were to prevent further clot formation or causing an embolism.

Case Study Application Questions

1. What is the difference between a physician assistant and a physician?
2. Describe a deep vein thrombosis (DVT).
3. Why types of drugs are Lovenox and warfarin?
4. Define embolism and explain the risk of embolism development.

END-OF-CHAPTER EXERCISES

Exercise 10.1 Labeling

Using the following list, choose the terms to label the diagram correctly.

aorta	left AV (mitral) valve	right atrium
aortic valve	pulmonary arteries	right ventricle
left atrium	pulmonary valve	superior and inferior vena cava
left ventricle	pulmonary veins	right AV (tricuspid) valve

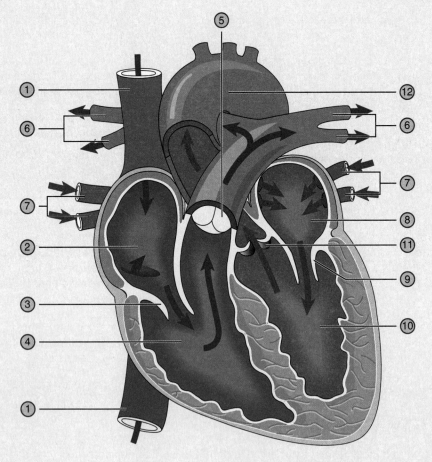

1. _____   5. _____   9. _____

2. _____   6. _____   10. _____

3. _____   7. _____   11. _____

4. _____   8. _____   12. _____

Exercise 10.2 Word Parts

Break each of the following terms into its word parts: prefix, root, or suffix. Give the meaning of each word part and then define the term.

1. *erythrocyte*

    root: _____

    suffix: _____

    definition: _____

2. *atherosclerosis*

    root: _____

    root: _____

    suffix: _____

    definition: _____

3. *cardiomyopathy*

    root: _____

    root: _____

    suffix: _____

    definition: _____

4. *endocarditis*

    prefix: _____

    root: _____

    suffix: _____

    definition: _____

5. *thrombocytopenia*

    root: _____

    root: _____

    suffix: _____

    definition: _____

6. *angiogram*

    root: _____

    suffix: _____

    definition: _____

7. *hematology*

    root: _____

    suffix: _____

    definition: _____

8. *pericardiotomy*

prefix: _____

root: _____

suffix: _____

definition: _____

Exercise 10.3 Word Building

Use the word parts listed to build the terms defined.

a-, an-	-dilation	inter-	peri-	valv/o
angio/o	-ectomy	leuk/o	-philia	vas/o
arteri/o	-emia	-lysis	-rhythm	ven/o
ather/o	erythr/o	-megaly	-spasm	ventricul/o
atri/o	-genic	my/o	-stenosis	
cardi/o	hem/o; hemat/o	-oma	thromb/o	
-cyte	-ic, -ia, -ac, -al, -ar, -ary -ous, -um	-penia	-tomy	

1. originating in the heart _____

2. an incision into the atrium _____

3. a red blood cell _____

4. hereditary bleeding disorder caused by a deficiency of a clotting factor _____

5. spasm of a vein _____

6. removal of a blood clot _____

7. dilation of a vessel _____

8. enlargement of the heart _____

9. narrowing of an artery _____

10. fatty plaque _____

11. a white blood cell _____

12. the surgical removal of a valve _____

13. pertaining to the heart _____

14. destruction of RBCs _____

15. between the ventricles _____

16. an abnormally low level of hemoglobin _____

17. heart muscle _____

18. removal of a fatty plaque _____

19. abnormal heart rhythm _____

Exercise 10.4 Matching

Match the term with its definition.

1. _____ ischemia
2. _____ anemia
3. _____ cardioversion
4. _____ SA node
5. _____ Hb
6. _____ vasoconstriction
7. _____ tricuspid valve
8. _____ endarterectomy
9. _____ platelets
10. _____ dyscrasia

a. pacemaker of the heart
b. electric current used to restore normal sinus rhythm
c. surgical removal of the inner lining of an artery
d. abnormality of the blood
e. thrombocytes
f. a protein in the RBC
g. deficiency of blood flow to an organ
h. vessels are narrowed
i. low level of Hb in the blood
j. between the right atrium and right ventricle

Exercise 10.5 Multiple Choice

Choose the correct answer for the following multiple-choice questions.

1. Which of the following is a type of white blood cell?
   a. thrombocyte
   b. eosinophil
   c. erythrocyte
   d. platelet
2. What is the term that describes the destruction of bacteria by special white blood cells?
   a. phagocytosis
   b. leukocytosis
   c. erythrocytosis
   d. neutrophilosis
3. Platelets are also referred to as _____.
   a. erythrocytes
   b. thrombocytes
   c. basophils
   d. neutrophils
4. Oxygen-carrying pigment of red blood cells is called_____.
   a. hematocrit
   b. Hb
   c. leukemia
   d. gamma globulin
5. Which of the following is a malignant disease of the blood?
   a. leukemia
   b. leukopenia
   c. erythropenia
   d. thrombosis

6. Which of the following terms describes hardened tissue?
   a. sclerotic
   b. thrombotic
   c. occluded
   d. fibrillated
7. The heart muscle is supplied with blood vessels called _____.
   a. capillaries
   b. coronary arteries
   c. corpuscles
   d. carpals
8. What is the function of a leukocyte?
   a. transports O_2
   b. manufactures Hgb
   c. initiates coagulation
   d. defends against disease
9. Which is the smallest blood vessel?
   a. artery
   b. arteriole
   c. vein
   d. capillary
10. Which of the following is characteristic of the artery in arteriostenosis?
    a. hardened
    b. soft
    c. dilated
    d. narrowed

Exercise 10.6 Fill in the Blank

Fill in the blank with the correct answer.

1. The term for low blood pressure is _____.
2. The term for a rapid pulse rate is _____.
3. A(n) _____ is medical specialist who deals with blood.
4. The artery that carries blood out of the heart to the lung is the _____ artery.
5. The "universal donor" is the blood type _____ while the "universal recipient" is the blood type _____.
6. The study of the heart and heart conditions is _____.
7. An incision into a vein is a(n) _____.
8. Elevated blood fat is called _____.
9. The mitral valve is also called the left AV valve and the _____ valve.
10. The two veins that carry blood into the right atrium are the _____ and the _____.

Exercise 10.7 Abbreviations

Write out the term for the following abbreviations.

1. _____ BP
2. _____ A-fib
3. _____ LDL
4. _____ SOB
5. _____ WBC
6. _____ AV
7. _____ CAD
8. _____ CHF
9. _____ HR
10. _____ Hb
11. _____ MI
12. _____ TIA

Write the abbreviation for the following terms.

13. _____ hemoglobin
14. _____ atrial fibrillation
15. _____ red blood cell
16. _____ sinoatrial
17. _____ congestive heart failure
18. _____ electrocardiogram
19. _____ coronary artery bypass graft
20. _____ hypertension
21. _____ disseminated intravascular coagulation
22. _____ high-density lipoprotein
23. _____ percutaneous transluminal coronary angioplasty

Exercise 10.8 Spelling

Select the correct spelling of the medical term.

1. The _____ BP reflects the arterial pressure during relaxation of a cardiac chamber.
   a. distolic
   b. diastolic
   c. diatolic
   d. diastollic

2. An adjective meaning "related to the myocardium" is _____.
   a. myocardial
   b. mycardial
   c. myocardal
   d. miocardial

3. A deficiency in blood supply to the tissues is
   _____.
   a. ichemia
   b. iscemia
   c. ischemia
   d. ishemia

4. The condition that exhibits both hardening and narrowing of the arteries is called
   _____.
   a. athrosclersis
   b. atheroclerosis
   c. atheroscleris
   d. atherosclerosis

5. A _____ is a WBC.
   a. leukocyte
   b. lukocyte
   c. luekocyte
   d. leukosite

6. An abnormal decrease in the number of thrombocytes or platelets is called
   _____.
   a. thrombocytpenia
   b. thrombocytopenia
   c. throbcytopenia
   d. thombecytpenia

7. The smallest blood vessel that connects the arterial and venous systems is known as a
   _____.
   a. capilary
   b. cappilary
   c. capillarie
   d. capillary

8. An abnormally rapid heartbeat is called
   _____.
   a. tachicardia
   b. tachycardia
   c. tacycardia
   d. tachycarda

9. A blood disorder characterized by an excessive increase in the number of WBCs is
   _____.
   a. lukemia
   b. lukimia
   c. leukemia
   d. luekemia

10. A drug used to treat heart rhythm abnormalities is called an _____.
    a. antiarrhythmic
    b. antarhythmic
    c. antiarhythmic
    d. antiarythmic

Exercise 10.9 Medical Report

Read the case and answer the questions that follow.

BRIEF HISTORY: The patient is a 56-year-old male with recurrent chest pain when performing mild activities at home. The chest pain subsides when he lies down. He also has experienced SOB when carrying in the groceries and climbing up one set of stairs. He has a history of high BP.

EMERGENCY ROOM VISIT: The patient arrives at the emergency room with angina pectoris that is relieved by rest, a BP of 180/110 mm Hg, and SOB. An EKG is performed, which indicates that the patient is having atrial arrhythmias and an MI. He is given aspirin and started on antiarrhythmics, diuretics, vasodilators, and oxygen. He is admitted to the CCU for observation and treatment.

DIAGNOSIS: Hypertension, an MI, and atrial fibrillation.

1. Define angina pectoris. _____
2. What does the acronym SOB stand for? _____
3. What is hypertension? _____
4. What is an EKG? _____
5. What type of pharmacologic intervention is used with this patient? Define each drug classification. _____
   _____
6. What is an MI? What are the two roots in myocardial, and what do they mean? _____
   _____
7. Define atrial fibrillation. _____

Exercise 10.10 Reflection

1. Using the Figures 10.1 and 10.3, could you trace a drop of blood throughout your body?
2. If blood clots develop from inactivity, what could you do to prevent blood clot formation?
3. As of this writing, there are nearly 8 billion people on the planet and only four different blood types, A, B, AB, and O in the world. Given this information, consider what this means in terms of being human.

CHAPTER 11

The Lymphatic System and Immunity

LEARNING OUTCOMES

Upon completion of this chapter, you should be able to:

- Name the organs that make up the lymphatic system.
- Understand the relationship between the cardiovascular system and the lymphatic system.
- Name the types of immunity.
- Pronounce, spell, and define medical terms related to the lymphatic system and its disorders.
- Pronounce, spell, and define medical terms related to immunity and immune disorders.
- Interpret abbreviations associated with the lymphatic system.
- Apply knowledge gained to case study questions.

CASE STUDY

Piano Playing Petra

Petra had a long career has a professional pianist, traveling the world from one concert stage to the next. She loved the challenge of learning new music and experiencing some of the world's most renowned venues. During the past year, she noticed that when she woke up in the morning, she was stiff and her body ached, which was irritating because sleep was supposed to be restorative. The pain and stiffness went away throughout the day as she became more active. She was also tired, but she attributed that to her unrelenting travel schedule. When her fingers couldn't glide across the keys as nimbly as necessary while playing the piano, she became concerned. Her hand joints looked a little swollen, and her hands felt tight, so she took ibuprofen, which seemed to help. But when her hands started to hurt all day, she became quite concerned. Piano playing was her life. What was she going to do?

Introduction

The lymphatic system and immunity are considered together because each supports the other. The **lymphatic system** is a network of tissues, organs, nodes, and lymphatic vessels (lymphatics) spread throughout the body. Interstitial fluid that has entered a lymphatic vessel is called **lymph**, and lymph empties into the right lymphatic duct and the thoracic duct (also called the left lymphatic duct.) These ducts connect to veins, the left subclavian vein and the right subclavian vein, which return lymph to the bloodstream (see **Figure 11.1**). Lymph contains a type of white blood cells called **lymphocytes**, which are groups of B cells (B lymphocytes) and T cells (T lymphocytes) important to immune function. Medically speaking, **immunity** refers to the

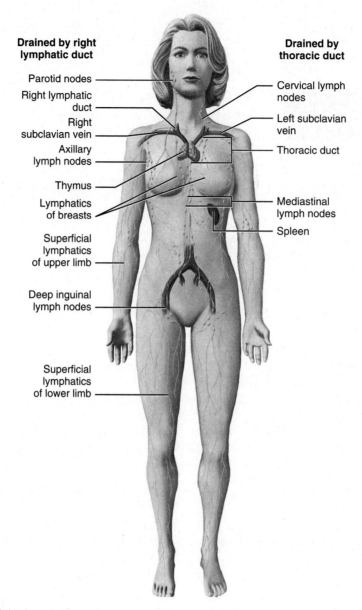

Drained by right lymphatic duct

Parotid nodes

Right lymphatic duct

Right subclavian vein

Axillary lymph nodes

Thymus

Lymphatics of breasts

Superficial lymphatics of upper limb

Deep inguinal lymph nodes

Superficial lymphatics of lower limb

Drained by thoracic duct

Cervical lymph nodes

Left subclavian vein

Thoracic duct

Mediastinal lymph nodes

Spleen

Figure 11.1 An overview of the lymphatic system.

body's ability to resist disease, and people gain immunity either actively (through contact with a disease or by vaccinations) or passively (from our biological mothers while in utero, from breast milk, or through injection of antibodies). **Vaccines** are substances used to stimulate the production of antibodies and to provide immunity against disease without inducing the disease.

What is lymph? Like plasma, which is the fluid part of blood, lymph is a fluid that consists mostly of water. Lymph also contains a low concentration of proteins and lymphocytes. The word lymph is also used as an adjective in naming lymph vessels and lymph nodes. A second adjective, lymphatic, is most often used when referring either to the whole system or to some specific part of the system, such as the "right lymphatic duct." Either adjective, however, is acceptable.

The lymphatic system works closely with the immune response to ensure defense against **pathogens** (disease-causing agents). In addition to protecting the body from infection, the lymphatic system also maintains fluid balance and absorbs recently digested fats that are broken down in the digestive tract.

Word Parts Related to the Lymphatic System and Immunity

The term *lymph* is derived from the Latin word *lympha* meaning water. The roots that come from this word are lymph/o and lymphat/o. The root word immun/o comes from the Latin word *immunis*, which means exempt from. In the medical sense, immun/o means the body is "exempt" from illness. **Table 11.1** lists word parts related to the lymphatic system and immunity.

Table 11.1 Word Parts Related to the Lymphatic System and Immunity

Word Part	Meaning
an-	without
immun/o	immune system
lymph/o	lymph or lymphatic system
lymphaden/o	lymph nodes
lymphangi/o	lymph vessels
lymphat/o	lymph or lymphatic system
-megaly	enlargement
-oid	resembling
path/o	disease
phag/o	ingest or engulf
-phylaxis	protection
splen/o	spleen
thym/o	thymus
tonsill/o	tonsil

Word Parts Exercise

After studying Table 11.1, write the meaning of each word part.

1. immun/o	1. _____
2. phag/o	2. _____
3. -phylaxis	3. _____
4. -megaly	4. _____
5. tonsill/o	5. _____
6. splen/o	6. _____
7. an-	7. _____
8. lymphaden/o	8. _____
9. lymphangi/o	9. _____
10. lymph/o, lymphat/o	10. _____
11. thym/o	11. _____
12. -oid	12. _____
13. path/o	13. _____

Structure and Function

Lymphatic tissues include *tonsils*, the *thymus*, *spleen*, *lymph nodes*, *lymphoid nodules of the small intestine* (Peyer's patches), and the *appendix* (see Figure 1.1). **Tonsils** are masses of lymphatic tissue in the pharynx that help filter bacteria and other germs to prevent infection. The **thymus** is a lymphatic organ located in the chest deep to the sternum. The **spleen** is a large mass of lymphatic tissue in the upper left quadrant of the abdomen involved with destroying bacteria by **phagocytosis** (ingestion by lymphocytes) and removing old blood cells by **hemolysis** (red blood cell rupture). Cells able to complete phagocytosis are called **phagocytes** and include **macrophages**, **microphages**, **neutrophils**, and **monocytes**.

Bean-shaped masses of lymphatic tissue distributed along lymphatic vessels are called **lymph nodes**. Collections of closely packed lymphoid nodules in the wall of the small intestine, known as **Peyer's patches**, are involved with intestinal immunity. The **appendix**, a worm-like structure that extends from the intestine, contains immune system cells that protect the "good bacteria" living in the gut.

Whereas the cardiovascular system circulates blood within a closed system, the lymphatic system distributes lymph on a one-way path via lymphatic vessels. Lymphatic vessels, which are positioned alongside blood vessels, begin where lymphatic capillaries interlace with the blood capillaries of the cardiovascular system, forming networks. Recall that lymph is similar to blood in that it contains special cells called *lymphocytes*, which are a type of white blood cell that fights disease and infection.

How does blood become lymph? Blood travels from arterioles to venules through capillary beds. Some of the fluid that leaks out of the blood capillaries is left in the tissues. This fluid is now called interstitial fluid. Interstitial fluid is picked up by the open-ended lymph capillaries and circulates in the lymphatic system as lymph (see **Figure 11.2**). Lymph continues to flow in the lymphatic system until it re-enters the bloodstream at collecting ducts.

How does lymph return to the bloodstream? Lymph is picked up by the lymph vessels, filtered by the lymph nodes, and propelled back into the venules and then into the veins. The lymphatic vessels from bigger structures called lymphatic trunks, which merge into the thoracic duct on the left side of the body or the right lymphatic duct on the right sides of

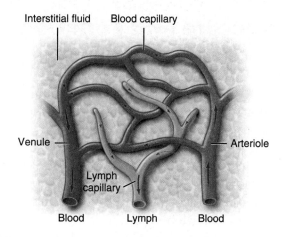

Interstitial fluid   Blood capillary

Venule

Arteriole

Lymph
capillary

Blood   Lymph   Blood

Figure 11.2 Lymph flow. This figure shows the structural relationship between the blood capillaries and the lymph capillaries.

the body. These ducts then empty into the left or right subclavian vein (see Figure 11.1).

All these structures play important roles in the body's immune responses. An immune response is the body's reaction to an **antigen** (a substance that induces an immune response in the body). An **antibody** is a soldier-like protein that protects the body and inactivates antigens.

Immunity is classified as innate immunity or adaptive immunity. **Innate immunity** (natural immunity) is genetically determined resistance that a person is born with. **Adaptive immunity** is a type of resistance that is acquired only after a person has been exposed to a particular antigen. Adaptive immunity is then broken down into two categories, each with two subcategories. The two types of adaptive immunity are *active immunity* (resistance that results from previous exposure to an antigen)

and *passive immunity* (resistance that results from the transfer of antibodies). The two types of active immunity are *naturally acquired* (results from contact with the disease) and *artificially acquired* (results from vaccination). The two types of passive immunity are *naturally acquired* (resistance that results through the placenta or from breast milk) and *artificially acquired* (resistance that results from injection of antibodies) (see **Figure 11.3**).

QUICK CHECK

Fill in the blanks.

1. Besides fighting infection, the lymphatic system maintains _____ balance and absorbs recently digested _____.

2. Name the tissues and organs of the lymphatic system. _____

3. A(n) _____ is a substance that induces an immune response.

Disorders Related to the Lymphatic System and Immunity

A primary function of the lymphatic system is to filter out harmful organisms. When bacteria spread into the lymphatic system or when an injury to the body is not treated effectively, an infection can result, causing **lymphadenitis**, which is swelling of a lymph node. Swelling of lymph tissue is called **lymphedema** (see **Figure 11.4**). Lymphedema is the result of infection or obstruction of the lymph vessels.

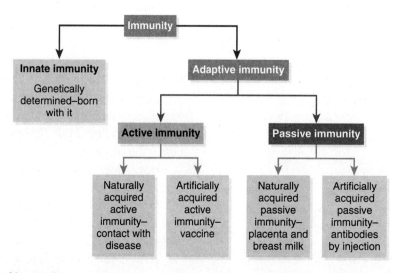

Immunity

Innate immunity
Genetically determined—born with it

Adaptive immunity

Active immunity

Passive immunity

Naturally acquired active immunity—contact with disease

Artificially acquired active immunity—vaccine

Naturally acquired passive immunity—placenta and breast milk

Artificially acquired passive immunity—antibodies by injection

Figure 11.3 The types of immunity.

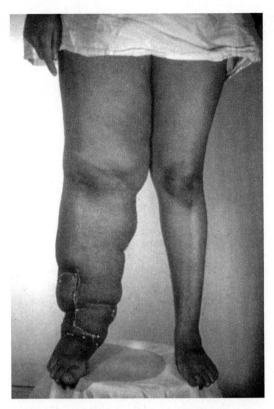

Figure 11.4 Lymphedema of the right lower extremity in a patient with elephantiasis. Elephantiasis is a parasitic infection that causes lymphatic vessel obstruction.

Lymphadenopathy, any disease process affecting lymph nodes, is an indicator of possible infection. **Autoimmune diseases** are disorders in which normal body tissues are destroyed when the body's immune response is directed against itself. An **allergy** is a hypersensitivity reaction to a particular antigen (allergen), such as pollen, a particular food, or dust. Lymph and immune disorders include the following:

- **Acquired immunodeficiency syndrome** (AIDS) is caused by the human immunodeficiency virus (HIV) and is an infectious process characterized by swollen lymph glands or lymphadenopathy.
- **Infectious mononucleosis** is an acute infection caused by the Epstein–Barr virus (EBV) and is characterized by fever, enlarged cervical lymph nodes, and fatigue.
- **Splenomegaly**, enlargement of the spleen, is indicative of infectious disease.
- **Anaphylaxis** is a systemic, life-threatening reaction to a foreign substance.
- **Hodgkin's lymphoma** is a malignant disease of the lymph nodes.
- **Rheumatoid arthritis** (RA) is an autoimmune disorder that affects joints.

- **Systemic lupus erythematosus** (SLE) is a chronic inflammatory disorder that affects connective tissue throughout the body and is marked by fever, weakness, joint pain, and lymphadenopathy.

Diagnostic Tests, Treatments, and Surgical Procedures

A range of treatments exists for treating lymphatic and immune system disorders. They include **corticosteroids** for relief of inflammation, **immunosuppressants** to dampen the immune response, **antivirals** to thwart virus infections, and **vaccinations** (*immunizations*) to offer artificially acquired immunity.

Surgical procedures may be necessary. The spleen is especially fragile, making it susceptible to rupturing. This makes it difficult to repair and instead a **splenectomy** (excision of the spleen) occurs. Other removal procedures may include a **lymphadenectomy** (removal of a lymph node), **lymphangiectomy** (removal of a lymph vessel), **thymectomy** (removal of the thymus), or **tonsillectomy** (removal of a tonsil).

Practice and Practitioners

Allergists specialize in diagnosing and treating altered immunologic and allergic conditions, and **hematologists** provide diagnosis and treatment of blood and blood-forming tissue disorders. **Immunology** is the study of the immune system. An **immunologist** is a specialist who studies, diagnoses, and treats problems associated with immunity. **Oncologists** may become involved in the care of patients with tumors.

Abbreviation Table	The Lymphatic System and Immunity
Abbreviation	**Meaning**
AIDS	acquired immunodeficiency syndrome
CRP test	C-reactive protein test
EBV	Epstein–Barr virus
HIV	human immunodeficiency virus
RA	rheumatoid arthritis
SLE	systemic lupus erythematosus

Study Table The Lymphatic System and Immunity

Term and Pronunciation	Analysis	Meaning
Structure and Function		
acquired immunity (uh-KWI-erd ih-MYOO-nih-tee)	from Old French *aquerre* (get in addition) and Latin *immunitas* (immune, resistant)	resistance resulting from previous exposure to an infectious agent
allergen (AL-ur-jen)	from the Greek word *allos* (other); *-gen* (producing)	an antigen that induces an allergic or hypersensitive response
antibody (AN-tuh-bod-ee)	*anti-* (against) + body	a molecule generated in specific opposition to an antigen
antigen (AN-tuh-jen)	*anti-* (against); *-gen* (producing)	agent or substance that provokes an immune response
appendix (uh-PEN-dicks)	from the Latin verb *appendum* (attach)	tube-shaped sac attached to an opening into the large intestine that plays a role in immunity
artificial immunity (ar-tuh-FISH-ul ih-MYOO-nih-tee)	from the Latin words *artificialis* (handcraft) and *immunitas* (immune, resistant)	immunization; immunity acquired from a vaccination
autoimmunity (aw-toh-ih-MYOO-nih-tee)	*auto-* (self) + the Latin word *immunitas* (immune, resistant)	antibodies or lymphocytes produced against antigens normally present in the body; literally, immune to oneself
B cell (BEE sell)	B refers to the fact that these cells are derived from bone marrow	nonthymus-dependent, short-lived lymphocyte; also called *B lymphocyte*
B lymphocyte (BEE LIM-foh-site)	B refers to the fact that these cells are derived from bone marrow; *lymph/o* (lymph); *-cyte* (cell)	nonthymus-dependent, short-lived lymphocyte; also called *B cell*
immunity (ih-MYOO-nih-tee)	from the Latin word *immunis* (exempt)	protection against disease
inflammation (in-fluh-MAY-shun)	from Latin *inflammation* (inflame)	redness and swelling caused by injury or abnormal stimulation by a physical, chemical, or biologic agent
leukocyte (LOO-koh-site)	*leuk/o* (white); *-cyte* (cell)	white blood cell
lymph (LIMF)	*lymph/o* (lymph)	a fluid collected from tissues throughout the body that contains mostly white blood cells and flows through the lymphatic vessels
lymph node (LIMF NODE)	*lymph/o* (lymph); from the Latin word, *nodus* (knot)	small, bean-shaped mass of lymphatic tissue that filters bacteria and foreign material from the lymph; located on larger lymph vessels in the cervical, mediastinal, axillary, and inguinal regions
lymphatic system (lim-FAT-tik SIS-tum)	*lymph/o* (lymph); *-atic* (adjective suffix)	collectively, the vessels, nodes, and capillaries that carry lymph and its disease-fighting cells to the areas in which they are needed

Term and Pronunciation	Analysis	Meaning
lymphocyte (LIM-foh-site)	*lymph/o* (lymph); *-cyte* (cell)	white blood cell in the lymphatic system
lymphoid nodules of the small intestine (LIMF-oid NOD-yulz UV THE SMALL in-TES-tin)	*lymph/o* (lymph); -oid (forming adjective for resembling) and from the Latin *intestinum* (within)	collections of spherical masses of lymphoid cells closely packed together; also called *Peyer's patches*
macrophage (MAK-roh-fayj)	*macro-* (large); *phag/o* (ingest or engulf)	large phagocyte
microphage (MIKE-roh-fayj)	*micro-* (small); *phag/o* (ingest or engulf)	small phagocyte
monocyte (MON-oh-site)	*mono-* (single); *-cyte* (cell)	a type of white blood cell that is also a phagocyte
natural immunity (NACTH-er-uhl ih-MYOO-nih-tee)	from the Latin words *natura* (birth) and *immunis* (exempt)	resistance manifested by an individual who has not been immunized; immunity passed on from biological mother to fetus or to baby in breast milk
neutrophil (NU-troh-fil)	*neutr/o* (neutral); *-phil* (love)	a type of white blood cell that is also a phagocyte
pathogen (PATH-oh-jen)	*path/o* (disease); *-gen* (produce)	substance that produces disease
Peyer's patches (PEY-erz PACH-ez)	named after Swiss anatomist Johann Peyer	collections of spherical masses of lymphoid cells closely packed together; also called *lymphoid nodules of the small intestine*
phagocyte (FAG-oh-site)	*phag/o* (ingest or engulf); *-cyte* (cell)	white blood cell that clears away pathogens and debris
phagocytosis (FAG-oh-sigh-toh-sis)	*phag/o* (ingest or engulf); *cyt/o* (cell); *-osis* (condition of)	process of ingestion and digestion carried out by white blood cells
reaction (ree-AK-shun)	from medieval Latin *reaction* (done against)	an action of an antibody on a specific antigen; also, in reference to immune responses, an abnormal or unwanted reaction
spleen (SPLEEN)	*splen/o* (spleen)	immune system organ that gets rid of damaged red blood cells and reclaims and stores iron
T cell (TEE SELL)	T (stands for thymus); from Old French *celle* or Latin *cella* (storeroom or chamber)	thymus-dependent, long-lived lymphocyte; also called *T lymphocyte*
T lymphocyte (TEE LIM-foh-site)	T (stands for thymus); *lymph/o* (lymph); *-cyte* (cell)	thymus-dependent, long-lived lymphocyte; also called *T cell*
thymus (THIGH-mus)	*thym/o* (thymus)	immune system gland located behind (deep to) the sternum
tonsil (TON-sul)	*tonsill/o* (tonsil)	collection of lymph tissue; in common understanding, the lingual, pharyngeal, and (especially) palatine tonsils

(continues)

Study Table The Lymphatic System and Immunity		(continued)
Term and Pronunciation	**Analysis**	**Meaning**
Disorders		
allergy (AL-ur-jee)	From the Greek word, *allos* (other) + *ergon* (work)	extreme sensitivity reaction to a normally harmless substance
anaphylaxis (an-uh-FIL-ax-iss)	*ana-* (without); from the Greek word *phylaxis* (protection)	life-threatening reaction to a foreign substance; symptoms include blockage of air passages, decreased blood pressure, generalized edema
acquired immunodeficiency syndrome (AIDS) (uh-KWIGH-erd im-yoo-no-dee-FISH-un-see SIN-drome)	from the Latin word *acquirere* (gain); *immunis* (exempt); *deficere* (to desert, fail)	a deficiency of cellular immunity induced by infection with the human immunodeficiency virus (HIV)
autoimmune disease (aw-toh- ih-MEWN dih-ZEEZ)	*auto-* (self) + *immunis* (exempt from) and from Old French *desaise* (lack of ease)	disorder in which the immune response is directed against the body's own tissues
elephantiasis (el-eh-fan-TYE-uh-sis)	from the Greek word, *elephas* (elephant) and *-iasis* (suffix forming the name of the disease)	lymphatic disease caused by filaria (parasitic roundworm) that is characterized by swelling of the legs and male scrotum
hemolysis (hee-MAWL-ih-sis)	*hem/o* (blood); *-lysis* (destruction)	change or destruction of red blood cells
Hodgkin's disease (HODJ-kinz dih-ZEEZ	named after English physician Thomas Hodgkin (1798–1866) who first described it; and from Old French *desaise* (lack of ease)	chronic malignant disease of the lymph nodes; also called *Hodgkin's lymphoma*
Hodgkin's lymphoma (HODJ-kinz lim-FOH-muh)	named after English physician Thomas Hodgkin (1798–1866) who first described it; *lymph/o* (lymph or lymphatic system); *-oma* (tumor)	chronic malignant disease of the lymph nodes; also called *Hodgkin's disease*
immunodeficiency (IM-yoo-noh-dee-FISH-un-see)	*immun/o* (immune system) + deficiency	impairment of the immune system
infectious mononucleosis (in-FEK-shus mon-oh-noo-klee-OH-sis)	from the Latin word *infectionem* (infection); *mono-* (one); Latin *nucleus* (kernel); *-osis* (abnormal condition)	an acute illness of young adults caused by the Epstein–Barr virus (EBV); spread by saliva transfer; characterized by fever, sore throat, enlargement of lymph nodes and spleen
lymphadenitis (lim-FAD-eh-NYE-tiss)	*lymph/o* (lymph or lymphatic system); *aden/o* (gland); *-itis* (inflammation)	inflammation of a lymph node or lymph nodes
lymphadenopathy (lim-fad-en-OP-uh-thee)	*lymph/o* (lymph or lymphatic system); *aden/o* (gland); *-pa- thy* (disease)	chronic or excessively swollen lymph nodes; any disease of the lymph nodes
lymphangiitis (lim-FAN-jee-EYE-tiss)	*lymphangi/o* (lymph vessel); *-itis* (inflammation)	inflammation of lymph vessels; also called *lymphangitis and lymphatitis*
lymphangitis (lim-fan-JYE-tiss)	*lymphangi/o* (lymph vessel);	inflammation of lymph vessels; also called *lymphangiitis and lymphatitis*

Term and Pronunciation	Analysis	Meaning
Disorders		
lymphatitis (lim-fuh-TYE-tiss)	*lymph/o* (lymph or lymphatic system); *-itis* (inflammation)	inflammation of the lymph vessels or nodes; also called *lymphangiitis* and *lymphangitis*
lymphedema (lim-fuh-DEE-muh)	*lymph/o* (lymph or lymphatic system); from the Greek word *oidema* (a swelling tumor)	swelling of the subcutaneous tissues due to obstruction of lymph vessels or nodes
lymphoma (lim-FOH-muh)	*lymph/o* (lymph or lymphatic system); *-oma* (tumor)	tumor of lymph tissue
lymphopathy (limf-OP-uh-thee)	*lymph/o* (lymph or lymph gland); *-pathy* (disease)	disease of the lymph vessels or nodes
rheumatoid arthritis (RA) (ROO-muh-toid ar-THRIGH-tiss)	from the Greek word *rheuma* (flux); *-oid* (resemblance of)	systemic autoimmune disease that affects the connective tissue; involves many joints, especially those of the hands and feet
splenitis (splen-EYE-tiss)	*splen/o* (spleen); *-itis* (inflammation)	inflammation of the spleen
splenomegaly (splen-oh-MEG-uh-lee)	*splen/o* (spleen); *-megaly* (enlargement)	enlargement of the spleen
splenopathy (splen-OP-uh-thee)	*splen/o* (spleen); *-pathy* (disease)	any disease of the spleen
systemic lupus erythematosus (SLE) (sis-TEM-ik LOO-pus er-ih-THEE-muh-toh-sus)	adjective form of the English word *system*; *lupus* (a Latin word meaning "wolf"); *erythematosus* (from the Greek word *erythema* meaning "flush")	an inflammatory, autoimmune connective tissue disorder with variable features; diffuse erythematous (red) butterfly rash on face; oftentimes shortened to lupus
thymitis (thye-MY-tiss)	*thym/o* (thymus); *-itis* (inflammation)	inflammation of the thymus
tonsillitis (TAWN-sih-LYE-tiss)	*tonsill/o* (tonsils); *-it is* (inflammation)	inflammation of a tonsil (commonly, the palatine tonsil)
Diagnostic Tests, Treatments, and Surgical Procedures		
antiviral (an-tee-VYE-ruhl)	*anti-* (against); from the Latin word *virus* (poison, sap of plants, slimy liquid)	drug used to treat various viral infections or conditions
chemotherapy (KEE-moh-ther-uh-pee)	*chem/o* (chemical) + therapy, a common English word	treatment of malignancies using chemical agents and drugs (usually reserved for treatment of cancer)
corticosteroids (kor-tih-koh-STAIR-oyds)	from the Latin word *cortex* (bark); from the Greek *steros* (solid, stable)	hormone-like preparations used as anti-inflammatory agents; topical agents used for their immunosuppressive and anti-inflammatory properties
C-reactive protein (CRP) CEE-ree-ACK-tiv PRO-teen	from the Greek *protos* (first)	Blood test used to diagnose inflammatory disorders; this protein is elevated in chronic inflammatory diseases and can also be used to determine heart disease risk
ibuprofen (eye-byoo-PRO-fen)	named for the chemical elements in its makeup	synthetic drug used as an over-the-counter analgesic (pain reliever) and inflammation reducer

(continues)

Study Table The Lymphatic System and Immunity		*(continued)*
Term and Pronunciation	**Analysis**	**Meaning**
Diagnostic Tests, Treatments, and Surgical Procedures		
immunization (IM-yoo-nuh-zay-shun)	*immun/o* (immune system); *-ization* (noun suffix)	protection from communicable diseases by administration of a weakened or killed pathogen, or a protein of a pathogen, to cause the immune system to create antibodies for future protection; also called *vaccination*
immunosuppressant (IM-yoo-noh-suh-PRESS-ant)	*immun/o* (immune system) + suppressant	something that interferes with the immune system
lymphangiography (limf-AN-jee-OG-ruh-fee)	*lymphangi/o* (lymph vessel); *-graphy* (process of recording)	radiography of the lymph vessels
lymphadenectomy (limf-ad-en-EK-tuh-mee)	*lymphaden/o* (lymph gland); *-ectomy* (excision)	removal of lymph nodes
lymphangiectomy (limf-AN-jee-EK-tuh-mee)	*lymphangi/o* (lymph vessel); *-ectomy* (excision)	removal of a lymph vessel
lymphangiotomy (limf-AN-jee-OT-uh-mee)	*lymphangi/o* (lymph vessel); *-tomy* (cutting operation)	incision of a lymph vessel
lymphography (limf-OG-ruh-fee)	*lympho-* (lymph) + *grapho* (to write)	visualization of lymphatics (lymphangiography) and lymph nodes (lymphadenography) by radiography after injecting a contrast dye (usually iodized oil) into a lymphatic vessel
splenectomy (splen-EK-toh-mee)	*splen/o* (spleen); *-ectomy* (excision)	removal of the spleen
splenorrhaphy (splen-OR-uh-fee)	*splen/o* (spleen); *-rraphy* (rupture)	suture of a ruptured spleen
splenotomy (splen-OT-oh-mee)	*splen/o* (spleen); *-tomy* (cutting operation)	incision of the spleen
thymectomy (thigh-MEK-toh-me)	*thym/o* (thymus); *-ectomy* (excision)	removal of the thymus
tonsillectomy (TAWN-sih-LEK-toh-mee)	*tonsill/o* (tonsil); *-ectomy* (excision)	removal of a tonsil
vaccination (vak-sih-NAY-shun)	from the Latin word *vaccinus* (relating to a cow); so named because of its early use of the cowpox virus against smallpox	protection from communicable diseases by administration of a weakened or killed pathogen, or a protein of a pathogen, to cause the immune system to create antibodies for future protection; also called *immunization*
vaccine (VAK-seen)	from the Latin word *vaccinus*, from *vacca* (cow); so named because of its early use of the cowpox virus against smallpox	substance used to stimulate antibody production and to provide immunity against a disease without causing the disease

Term and Pronunciation	Analysis	Meaning
Practice and Practitioners		
allergist (AL-er-jist)	from the Greek words *allos* (other, different, strange) and *ergon* (activity); *-ist* (one who specializes)	a medical practitioner who specializes in the diagnosis and treatment of allergies
hematologist (hee-muh-TOL-oh-jist)	*hemat/o* (blood); *-logist* (one who specializes)	a medical practitioner who specializes in the diagnosis and treatment of blood disorders
immunologist (im-yoo-NOL-oh-jist)	*immun/o* (immune system); *-logist* (one who specializes)	a medical practitioner specializing in the immune system
immunology (IM-yoo-NOL-oh-jee)	*immun/o* (immune system); *-logy* (study of)	the medical specialty dealing with the immune system
oncologist (on-KOL-oh-jist)	from the Greek word *onkos* (mass, bulk); *-logist* (one who specializes)	a medical practitioner who specializes in the diagnosis and treatment of malignant tumors (cancer)
rheumatologist (roo-muh-TOL-oh-jist)	*rheumat/o* (flux); *-logist* (one who studies a certain field)	physician who treats musculoskeletal disorders, joints, and connective tissue disease such as arthritis

CASE STUDY WRAP-UP

By the time Petra was able to see her family physician, both hands were tender, and swollen joints were developing in her fingers. Her elbows and shoulders were also stiff and sore. The family physician examined the swollen joints for redness and warmth, checked her reflexes, and evaluated her muscle strength. The physician suspected rheumatoid arthritis and ordered a C-reactive protein (CRP) test and hand X-rays to confirm the suspicion. Petra was advised to follow up with a rheumatologist.

Case Study Application Questions

1. How would ibuprofen help Petra?
2. What is a C-reactive protein (CRP) test?
3. Describe rheumatoid arthritis.
4. Why was a rheumatologist recommended for Petra?

END-OF-CHAPTER EXERCISES

Exercise 11.1 Labeling

Using the following list, choose the terms to label the diagram correctly.

axillary lymph nodes	mediastinal lymph nodes	superficial lymphatics of lower limb
cervical lymph nodes	spleen	thymus

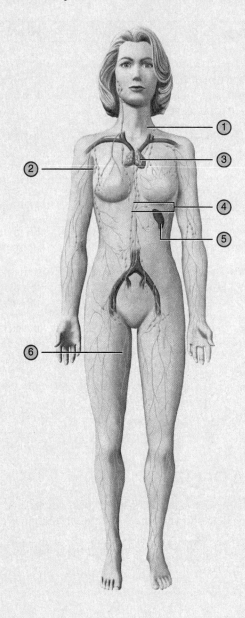

1. _____   4. _____

2. _____   5. _____

3. _____   6. _____

Exercise 11.2 Word Parts

Break each of the following terms into its word parts: prefix, root, or suffix. Give the meaning of each word part and then define the term.

1. *lymphocyte*

   root: _____

   suffix: _____

   definition: _____

2. *phagocytosis*

    root: _____

    root: _____

    suffix: _____

    definition: _____

3. *anaphylaxis*

    prefix: _____

    root: _____

    definition: _____

4. *hemolysis*

    root: _____

    suffix: _____

    definition: _____

5. *lymphoma*

    root: _____

    suffix: _____

    definition: _____

6. *splenectomy*

    root: _____

    suffix: _____

    definition: _____

7. *thymectomy*

    root: _____

    suffix: _____

    definition: _____

8. *immunology*

    root: _____

    suffix: _____

    definition: _____

Exercise 11.3 Word Building

Use the word parts listed to build the terms defined.

aden/o	immun/o	lymph/o	-pathy	thym/o
angi/o	-itis	-megaly	phag/o	-graphy
-cytosis	-logist	-oma		

1. inflammation of a lymph gland
    _____

2. tumor of a lymph gland
    _____

3. enlargement of the thymus
    _____

4. inflammation of a lymph vessel
    _____

5. disease of a lymph gland
    _____

6. specialist who studies and treats the immune system _____

7. radiographic procedure of the lymphatic system _____

8. process of a WBC engulfing a harmful organism _____

Exercise 11.4 Matching

Match the term with its definition.

1. _____ lymphadenopathy

2. _____ lymphedema

3. _____ phagocytosis

4. _____ autoimmune

5. _____ splenomegaly

6. _____ lymphocyte

7. _____ immunology

8. _____ anaphylaxis

9. _____ appendix

10. _____ immunization

a. enlarged spleen

b. specialty that deals with immune disorders

c. artificially acquired immunity

d. life-threatening allergic reaction to a foreign substance

e. disease of the lymph glands

f. accumulation of fluid in the intercellular tissues

g. the process of engulfing foreign materials

h. protective lymph organ that is attached to the proximal end of the large intestine

i. the body reacts to its own tissues

j. specialized WBC of the immune system

Exercise 11.5 Multiple Choice

Choose the correct answer for the following multiple-choice questions.

1. The lymphatic organ that removes old blood cells by means of hemolysis is the
    _____.
    a. tonsils
    b. spleen
    c. thymus
    d. appendix

2. Peyer's patches are found in the
    _____.
    a. respiratory system
    b. cardiovascular system
    c. digestive system
    d. muscular system

3. Immunizations are a type of _____.
    a. naturally acquired immunity
    b. naturally acquired passive immunity
    c. artificially acquired immunity
    d. innate immunity

4. Lymphocytes are a type of _____.
    a. white blood cell
    b. red blood cell
    c. platelet
    d. thrombocyte

5. The tonsils are found in the _____.
    a. larynx
    b. abdomen
    c. lungs
    d. pharynx

6. A practitioner who specializes in blood disorders is a(n) _____.
   a. allergist
   b. hematologist
   c. immunologist
   d. oncologist
7. A treatment used to treat inflammation is a(n) _____.
   a. antiviral
   b. chemotherapy
   c. corticosteroid
   d. immunosuppressant
8. A molecule that is generated in specific opposition to an antigen is a(n) _____.
   a. allergen
   b. antibody
   c. pathogen
   d. leukocyte
9. The type of immunity passed down from mother to child is called _____.
   a. naturally acquired active immunity
   b. artificially acquired active immunity
   c. naturally acquired passive immunity
   d. autoimmunity
10. The root lymphaden/o means _____.
   a. lymph
   b. immune
   c. lymph vessel
   d. lymph node

Exercise 11.6 Fill in the Blank

Fill in the blank with the correct answer.

1. Lymph contains white blood cells, called _____, that fight infection.
2. The functions of the immune system are to protect the body from infection, absorb fats that are broken down in the digestive tract, and _____.
3. After lymph is picked up by the lymph vessels and filtered by the _____, it is propelled into venules and then into veins.
4. _____ immunity is genetically determined.
5. The _____ are masses of lymphatic tissue located in the pharynx to filter out bacteria.
6. Swelling caused by obstruction of lymphatic vessels is called _____.
7. Surgical removal of the spleen is called a(n) _____.
8. The medical professional who specializes in diagnosing and treating altered immunologic and allergic conditions is known as a(n) _____.
9. The "T" in T cell stands for _____.
10. Failure of the immune system to adequately protect the body from infection is known as _____.

Exercise 11.7 Abbreviations

Write out the term for the following abbreviations.

1. _____ SLE

2. _____ RA

3. _____ EBV

Write the abbreviation for the following terms.

4. _____ acquired immunodeficiency syndrome
5. _____ human immunodeficiency virus

Exercise 11.8 Spelling

Select the correct spelling of the medical term.

1. A _____ is a type of white blood cell that is distributed throughout lymphatic tissue.
   a. lymphocyte
   b. limphocyte
   c. lymfocyte
   d. lymphosite
2. A _____ is a type of mature, phagocytic white blood cell.
   a. nuetrophil
   b. nutrophil
   c. neutrophil
   d. neutraphil

3. _____ is the process of ingestion and digestion by white blood cells.
   a. Pagocytosis
   b. Phagecytosis
   c. Phagocytosis
   d. Phageocytosis

4. Protection against infectious disease is called _____.
   a. immunity
   b. imunity
   c. imunnity
   d. ammunity

5. Some signs of the life-threatening reaction to a foreign substance, called _____, are blockage of air passages, decreased blood pressure, and generalized edema.
   a. anephylaxis
   b. anaphilaxis
   c. aniphylaxis
   d. anaphylaxis

6. An impairment of the immune system is called an _____.
   a. imunodeficiency
   b. immunodeficiency
   c. immunedeficiency
   d. immunodeficency

7. _____ is the process by which resistance to an infectious disease is induced.
   a. Imunization
   b. Immunisation
   c. Immunizasion
   d. Immunization

8. Treatment of malignancies using chemical agents and drugs is called _____.
   a. kemotherapy
   b. cemotherapy
   c. chemotherapy
   d. chematherapy

9. A _____ is a medical practitioner who specializes in the diagnosis and treatment of blood disorders.
   a. hemtologist
   b. hematologist
   c. hemetologist
   d. hemitologist

10. An _____ is a substance that induces sensitivity or an immune response in the form of antibodies.
    a. antigen
    b. antugen
    c. antegin
    d. antegen

Exercise 11.9 Medical Report

Read the case and answer the questions that follow.

BRIEF HISTORY: A 16-year-old male complained to his parents of being extremely fatigued. He was not able to keep up with his school schedule or after school sports. His throat was sore, and he noticed "lumps" in his neck and groin. He had a fever and loss of appetite. He recently began to complain of pain in his upper left belly.

OFFICE VISIT: A physician examined the patient and ordered blood tests. He noted lymphadenopathy in the cervical, axillary, and inguinal areas. He also observed an erythematous throat and determined that the spleen was enlarged.

DIAGNOSIS AND TREATMENT PLAN: The diagnosis was mononucleosis, an infectious disease caused by a virus. The prescribed treatment consisted of over-the-counter analgesics to reduce the abdominal pain, along with fluids and rest. Throat lozenges were prescribed to ease sore throat discomfort.

1. What does "lymphadenopathy" mean? _____
2. What is the medical term for an "enlarged spleen"? _____
3. What is mononucleosis? _____

Exercise 11.10 Reflection

1. Could you relate anything you learned in this chapter to the COVID-19 pandemic?
2. Would you be able to describe the various types of immunity to a young child?
3. What is one thing you think you will always remember from this chapter?

CHAPTER 12

The Respiratory System

LEARNING OUTCOMES

Upon completion of this chapter, you should be able to:

- Name the structures that make up the respiratory system.
- Pronounce, spell, and define medical terms related to the respiratory system and its disorders.
- Interpret abbreviations associated with the respiratory system.
- Apply knowledge gained to case study questions.

CASE STUDY

My Child Tastes Salty

Amelia was a typical teenager. She excelled in school, played video games, and enjoyed spending time with friends. Throughout her young life, she had a persistent cough and wheezed while riding her bicycle. Lately, Amelia was more tired than usual and had been hospitalized twice within the past year for a lung infection. Her parents were concerned because throughout her 13 years, she was relatively healthy, although she was diagnosed early in life with an inherited disorder. Her parents were alerted that something was "different" about their daughter one night after reading her nightly bedtime story. When her mother kissed her goodnight, she tasted salt. What condition might Amelia have?

Introduction

The respiratory system includes all the air passages from the nose to the pulmonary alveoli in the lungs. It is divided into an *upper respiratory tract* and a *lower respiratory tract*. The upper respiratory tract is made up of the **paranasal sinuses**, **nasal cavity**, **nose**, and **pharynx**. The lower respiratory tract is made up of the **larynx, lungs, trachea, bronchi, bronchioles**, and **alveoli** (see **Figure 12.1**). The respiratory system allows humans to inhale oxygen (O_2) and

exhale carbon dioxide (CO_2). Oxygen is a gas needed by body cells, and carbon dioxide is a gaseous metabolic waste that needs to be eliminated. **Figure 12.2** shows the process of this gas exchange, which is accomplished through external and internal respiration. **External respiration** is the process in which air is brought into the lungs where oxygen and carbon dioxide are exchanged in the bloodstream at the capillaries surrounding the alveoli. **Internal respiration** is the process where oxygen and carbon dioxide move between the bloodstream and the body's cells.

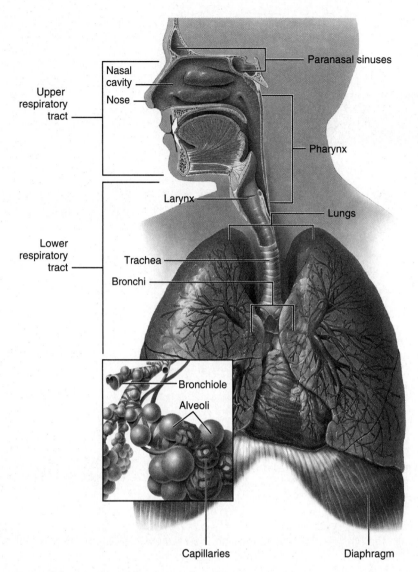

Figure 12.1 The structures of the upper and lower respiratory system.

Word Parts Related to the Respiratory System

The word part spir/o (which is a root) and the suffix -*pnea* are both used to describe breathing. Pulmon/o means lung and is the root of the word **pulmonary** (an adjective used to describe the lungs). Similarly, nas/o means nose and provides the root for **nasal** (an adjective used to describe the nose). Another root meaning nose is rhin/o. Nasal comes from the Latin word for nose, *nasus*, while rhin/o comes from the Greek word for nose, *rhis*. Pneum/o comes from the Greek word *pneumon* (lung) and can refer to the lungs or air. Pneum/o is the root for the lung infection, pneumonia. **Table 12.1** shows common word parts related to the respiratory system.

Structure and Function

The respiratory system begins with the paranasal sinuses, nasal cavity, and nose and then descends to the pharynx, larynx, and trachea. Inferior to the trachea, the system splits into the right and left side. This inferior portion consists of the bronchi and bronchioles that branch in the lungs, and the tiny air sacs called alveoli. A dome-shaped muscle important for breathing, called the **diaphragm**, is located at the base of the lungs.

The Nose, Nasal Cavity, and Paranasal Sinuses

Air enters the nose through openings called **nostrils**. The **nose** is lined with small hairs that trap particles and prevent them from entering the respiratory tract.

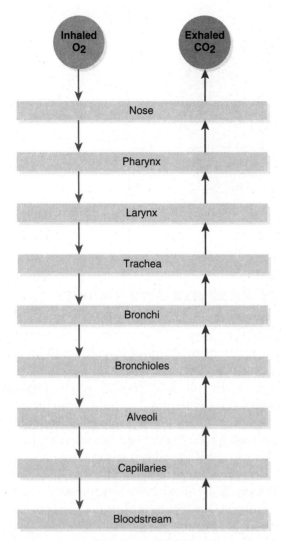

Word Part	Meaning
or/o	mouth, opening
-oxia	oxygen
pharyng/o	pharynx
-phonia	voice
phren/o	diaphragm
pleur/o	rib, side, pleura
-pnea	breathing
pneumo-, pneumon/o	lungs, air
pulmon/o	lung
rhin/o	nose
sinus/o	sinus cavity
spir/o	breathing
thorac/o, thorac/i, thoracic/o	thorax, chest
tonsill/o	tonsil
trache/o	trachea

Figure 12.2 Pathway of inhaled/exhaled air. *Red arrows* indicate oxygenated air and *blue arrows* represent deoxygenated air. Oxygen (O_2) enters the respiratory system through the nose and travels down through the pharynx, larynx, and trachea then into the bronchi, bronchioles, and alveoli of the lungs where a gas exchange takes place at the alveolar capillaries. Oxygen moves into the bloodstream where it is carried to the cells and is exchanged with carbon dioxide (CO_2). The carbon dioxide passes back up through the respiratory structures and is exhaled.

Table 12.1 Common Word Parts Related to the Respiratory System

Word Part	Meaning
adeno-	glandlike
bronch/o, bronchi/o	bronchus
laryng/o	larynx
lob/o	lobe
nas/o	nose

Word Parts Exercise

After studying Table 12.1, write the meaning of each word part.

Word Part	Meaning
1. -phonia	1. _____
2. trache/o	2. _____
3. thorac/o, thorac/i, thoracic/o	3. _____
4. bronch/o, bronchi/o	4. _____
5. -pnea	5. _____
6. laryng/o	6. _____
7. sinus/o	7. _____
8. pleur/o	8. _____
9. pneumo-, pneumon/o	9. _____
10. nas/o	10. _____
11. -oxia	11. _____
12. pharyng/o	12. _____
13. phren/o	13. _____
14. pulmon/o	14. _____
15. or/o	15. _____

Anterior view   Lateral view

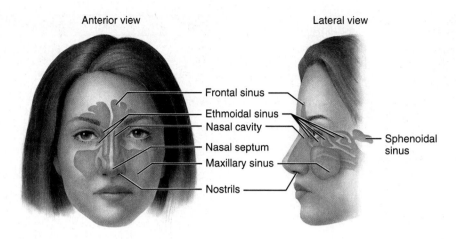

Figure 12.3 The nasal cavity and paranasal sinuses.

Air then passes into the **nasal cavity**, a space on each side of a wall called the **nasal septum**. The nasal septum divides the nose into left and right halves. Here, the air is warmed and moistened. **Mucus**, a clear sticky secretion, coats the lining of the nasal cavity to filter out particles. The **paranasal sinuses** are air-filled cavities in the bones of the face that are connected to the nasal cavity. These sinuses include the frontal, ethmoidal, maxillary, and sphenoidal (see **Figure 12.3**).

What is the difference between *mucus* and *mucous*? Mucus is a noun, and mucous is an adjective. Mucus is the sticky, slimy substance secreted by mucous membranes.

The Pharynx and Tonsils

The **pharynx**, also known as the throat, has three regions: the *nasopharynx*, *oropharnyx*, and *laryngopharynx*. The **nasopharynx** is posterior to the nasal cavity, the **oropharynx** is the middle portion located posterior to the oral cavity (mouth), and the **laryngopharynx** is the lower portion posterior to the larynx (see **Figure 12.4**). Lymphatic tissue called **tonsils** that aid in filtering bacteria are associated with the pharynx. The **pharyngeal tonsils** are in the nasopharynx, the **palatine tonsils** are in the oropharynx, and the **lingual tonsils** are at the base of the posterior portion of the tongue (see **Figure 12.5**). When referring to the tonsils in general, clinicians usually mean the palatine tonsils. The **adenoids** are the pharyngeal tonsils that

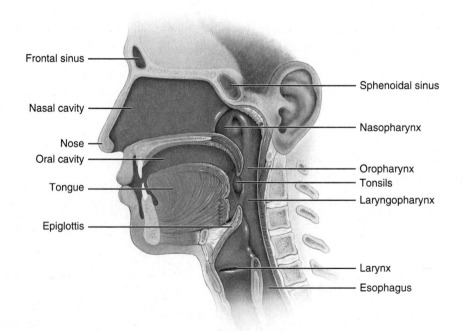

Figure 12.4 The regions of the pharynx.

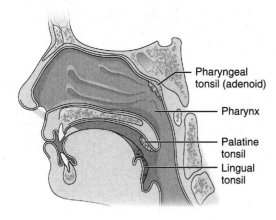

Figure 12.5 The pharynx and tonsils.

are located high in the throat behind the nose. These are not easily viewed and require an angled mirror. Removal of the tonsils and adenoids is referred to as a *tonsillectomy and adenoidectomy*; this is abbreviated as T and A.

The Larynx and Trachea

The **larynx**, or *voice box*, is the organ that produces sound. Located between the pharynx and trachea, it is made up of cartilages and elastic membranes that contain the vocal cords (vocal folds) and the muscles that control them (see Figure 12.4 and **Figure 12.6**). Air enters the larynx through a slit-like opening called the **glottis**. A flap of cartilage known as the **epiglottis** protects the glottis during swallowing to prevent food or liquids from entering the respiratory tract. As air flows over the **vocal cords**, they vibrate to produce sound (see Figure 12.6).

The Trachea, Bronchi, Bronchioles, and Alveoli

The **trachea** (windpipe) is a cartilaginous tube that conducts air from the larynx to the bronchial tree. The **bronchial tree** consists of air-passage tubes that lead from the trachea to the lungs. It begins with two major airways called the **left bronchus** and **right bronchus**. The plural form of *bronchus* is *bronchi*. Air passes through the bronchi, which subdivide into increasingly smaller branches called **bronchioles**. The flow of air terminates in the bronchial tree in tiny air sacs called **alveoli**. Alveoli are structures where gas exchange of oxygen and carbon dioxide occurs (see Figure 12.1 and **Figure 12.7**).

The Lungs

The **lungs** are paired, spongy organs of breathing located in the thoracic (chest) cavity. They are enclosed in the **pleura**, which is a membrane composed of two

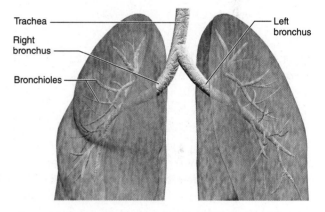

Figure 12.7 The trachea and bronchial tree.

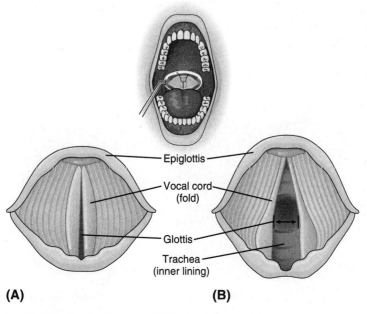

(A) **(B)**

Figure 12.6 The vocal cords with **(A)** glottis closed and **(B)** glottis open.

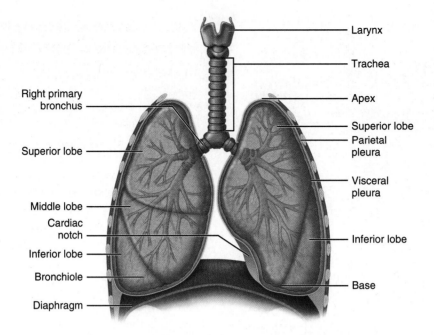

Figure 12.8 The lungs are paired organs of breathing located in the thoracic cavity. They are enclosed by an outer parietal pleura and an inner visceral pleura.

layers called the **parietal pleura** and the **visceral pleura** (see **Figure 12.8**). The parietal (outer) pleura lines the thoracic cavity and forms the sac containing each lung. The visceral (inner) pleura closely surrounds each lung. The right lung is slightly larger than the left and has three lobes called the **superior lobe**, **middle lobe**, and **lower lobe**. The left lung has only two lobes, the **superior lobe** and **inferior lobe**. The left lung also has a medial indentation called the **cardiac notch**, which provides room for the heart. Each cone-shaped lung has an upper **apex** and a lower **base**, which rests on the diaphragm. The lungs and airways bring in fresh, oxygen-enriched air and get rid of carbon dioxide waste made by the body's cells.

The Diaphragm

The **diaphragm** is a sheet of muscle that separates the upper thoracic cavity (which encloses the lungs) from the lower abdominal cavity. The diaphragm is a major muscle used in breathing. When the diaphragm contracts, it moves inferiorly, the chest expands, and inhalation (inspiration or breathing in) occurs. When the diaphragm relaxes, it moves superiorly, the chest contracts, and exhalation (expiration or breathing out) occurs (see **Figure 12.9**). Two adjectives that mean the same thing and are used to describe the diaphragm are *diaphragmatic* and *phrenic*.

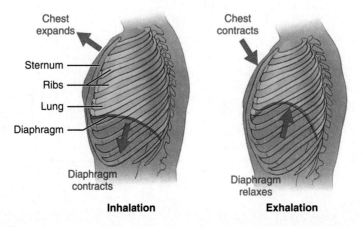

Figure 12.9 The process of breathing.

QUICK CHECK

1. Another name for the voice box is the _____.

2. Another name for the windpipe is the _____.

3. Another name for the throat is the _____.

Disorders Related to the Respiratory System

The pathway through which air moves in and out of the lungs has to be **patent** (open) for proper oxygen and carbon dioxide exchange to take place. When this pathway becomes partially blocked, the body's normal response is a sneeze or cough, which may produce **sputum** (mucus from the lower respiratory system); **hemoptysis**, which is spitting or coughing up blood; or other secretions that need to be removed for optimal airway **patency** (state of being freely open).

Abnormal breath sounds are other indications of respiratory disease. **Rales**, also known as crackles, are high-pitched popping sounds usually originating in the smaller airways. **Rhonchi** are low-pitched sounds that come from the larger airways. **Wheezing** or whistling sounds may indicate excessive secretions or partially obstructed airways. **Stridor** is a high-pitched squeaking sound that occurs when one breathes in, which is a sign of respiratory obstruction, especially in the trachea or larynx. Respiratory diseases may also alter breathing patterns and rates. Normal breathing, **eupnea**, should be regular and effortless. The following is a list of abnormalities in breathing:

- **Tachypnea**: rapid breathing rate (it is normal to have tachypnea during exercise)
- **Bradypnea**: abnormally slow breathing rate
- **Apnea**: cessation of breathing; short periods of apnea may occur during sleep
- **Dyspnea**: difficult or labored breathing
- **Orthopnea**: difficulty breathing while lying flat; difficulty is relieved by sitting up
- **Cheyne-Stokes respiration**: a cyclical breathing pattern in which breathing gradually decreases to a complete stop and then returns to normal
- **Kussmaul respiration**: rapid, deep breathing; characteristic of diabetic acidosis or other causes of acidosis

Many disorders affect the respiratory system. Some result in **rhinitis**, inflammation of the nasal mucous membrane, or **dysphonia**, altered voice production, which is usually painful or difficult (seen commonly in laryngitis). Disorders are discussed under the following broad categories: infectious disorders, obstructive lung diseases, and expansion disorders.

Infectious Disorders

Infectious disorders are diseases that are transmitted from person to person without actual contact. An upper respiratory infection (URI) typically presents with a runny nose, sore throat, and cough. Here are some common upper respiratory system infectious disorders:

Common cold virus: any virus strain associated with the common cold, chiefly rhinoviruses

> Although rhinoviruses most frequently cause the common cold, more than 200 other viruses, including the human coronavirus and the respiratory syncytial virus, can also cause the common cold. Coronaviruses also cause bird bronchitis, mouse hepatitis, and newborn calf diarrhea.

Sinusitis: inflammation of any sinus mucous membrane

Croup: acute obstruction of the upper respiratory tract (upper airway) in infants and children resulting in a barking cough with difficult and noisy breathing; also called **laryngotracheobronchitis**

Epiglottitis: inflammation of the epiglottis, which may cause respiratory obstruction

Influenza (flu): acute infectious respiratory disease caused by influenza viruses

Pneumonia: inflammation of the lung parenchyma (lung tissue of bronchioles, bronchi, blood vessels, and alveoli); may be caused by bacterial or viral infection

Laryngitis: inflammation of the larynx mucous membrane

Pertussis (whooping cough): acute inflammation of the larynx, trachea, and bronchi caused by *Bordetella pertussis*

Tuberculosis (TB): infection caused by *Mycobacterium tuberculosis*; symptoms include fatigue, anorexia, weight loss, fever, chronic cough, and hemoptysis

Obstructive Lung Diseases

Obstructive disease impairs airflow through the bronchial tree. The obstruction may be caused by increased secretion production or lung tissue destruction. Well-known disorders within this category include the following:

Asthma: lung disease characterized by reversible inflammation and constriction

Cystic fibrosis (CF): genetic disorder in which the lungs become clogged with excessive amounts of abnormally thick mucus

Chronic obstructive pulmonary disease (COPD): an umbrella term that includes both emphysema and chronic bronchitis (described next)

Emphysema: condition in which the alveoli are enlarged and inefficient, leading to shortness of breath (SOB)

Chronic bronchitis: inflammation of the bronchial mucous membranes

Expansion Disorders

Adequate lung expansion is necessary for proper gas exchange. Some diseases cause restrictions on lung capacity, thereby causing inadequate exchange between the atmosphere and the lungs. **Atelectasis** (collapsed lung) and **pneumothorax** (accumulation of air in the pleural cavity) are two such disorders.

Diagnostic Tests, Treatments, and Surgical Procedures

Both noninvasive and invasive procedures are used to diagnose respiratory system disorders. The noninvasive procedures include chest X-ray (CXR), lung scan, pulse oximetry, arterial blood gas (ABG), and computed tomography (CT) scans. **Pulse oximetry** measures the oxygen saturation of arterial blood, whereas an **arterial blood gas** measures the amount of oxygen and carbon dioxide dissolved in arterial blood. Invasive procedures may include thoracentesis and bronchoscopy. A **thoracentesis** (*pleural tap*) is an insertion of a needle into the pleural cavity to withdraw fluid. A **bronchoscopy** is an examination of the trachea and bronchial tree through a viewing instrument called a bronchoscope (see **Figure 12.10**). Respiratory therapists perform **pulmonary function tests** (PFT) on patients to assess breathing. A **spirometer** is an instrument used for measuring the air capacity of the lungs. Examples of air volumes and lung capacities measured by spirometry are presented in **Table 12.2**.

Treatment of lung conditions commonly includes medication. **Antihistamines** are drugs used to treat acute allergic reactions, like the signs and symptoms observed in common pollen allergies.

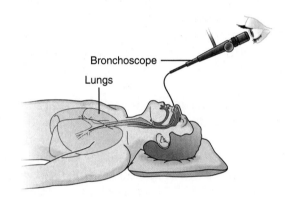

Figure 12.10 Bronchoscopy. Introduction of a bronchoscope through the nose that is then guided down into the bronchi. Visual examination (suffix -scopy means "visual examination") can be made of the bronchial tree, biopsies may be taken from the bronchi, and secretions may be removed for analysis or to reduce respiratory distress.

Table 12.2 Pulmonary Volumes and Capacities

Volume	Description	Average Value
tidal volume (TV)	volume of air entering or exiting the lungs during normal breathing	500 mL
inspiratory reserve volume (IRV)	volume of air entering the lungs plus the tidal volume during forced inhalation	300 mL
expiratory reserve volume (ERV)	volume of air exiting the lungs plus the tidal volume during forced exhalation	1,000 mL
vital capacity (VC)	maximum volume of air that can be exhaled after taking the deepest possible breath	4,500 mL
residual volume (RV)	volume of air in the lungs at all times	1,500 mL
total lung capacity (TLC)	volume of air that the lungs can hold	6,000 mL

Decongestants are used to treat congestion. There are multiple types of drugs that one inhales. For example, a **bronchodilator** is used to expand the bronchi. Another example is an inhaled corticosteroid, which is used to reduce respiratory system inflammation.

Practice and Practitioners

Several different healthcare professionals diagnose and treat respiratory system disorders. A **pulmonologist** is a physician who specializes in **pulmonology**, which is the study of the lungs and their related structures. Both **otolaryngologists** and **otorhinolaryngologists** diagnose and treat disorders of the ears, nose, and throat. **Respiratory therapists** are allied healthcare professionals who specialize in airway management, mechanical ventilation (breathing), and managing blood acid–base balance.

Abbreviation Table The Respiratory System

Abbreviation	Meaning
ABG	arterial blood gas
BP	blood pressure
CF	cystic fibrosis
c/o	complains of
CO_2	carbon dioxide
COPD	chronic obstructive pulmonary disease
CT	computed tomography
CXR	chest X-ray
ERV	expiratory reserve volume
F	Fahrenheit
ICU	intensive care unit
IRV	inspiratory reserve volume
O_2	oxygen
P	pulse
PFT	pulmonary function test
R	respiration
RV	residual volume (as measured with test equipment)
SOB	shortness of breath
T	temperature
T and A	tonsillectomy and adenoidectomy
TB	tuberculosis
TLC	total lung capacity
TV	tidal volume
URI	upper respiratory infection
VC	vital capacity
WBC	white blood cell

Study Table The Respiratory System

Term and Pronunciation	Analysis	Meaning
Structure and Function		
adenoids (AD-en-oidz)	from the Greek word *adenoeides* (gland)	epithelial and lymphatic structure located on the posterior wall of the nasopharynx; also called pharyngeal tonsils
alveoli (al-VEE-oh-lye); singular: alveolus (al-VEE-oh-luss)	diminutive of the Latin word *alveus* (cavity, hollow)	tiny air sacs in the lungs where the exchange of oxygen and carbon dioxide occurs between the lungs and blood
apex (AY-pex)	a Latin word meaning "summit," "peak," "tip"	upper tip of each lung
base (BASE)	from the Latin word *basis* (base, pedestal)	word used to describe the bottom of each lung
bronchi (BRON-kye); singular: bronchus (BRON-kus)	*bronch/o-, bronch/i-* (bronchus)	tubes (right and left) branching from the trachea and into the lungs
bronchiole (BRON-kee-ole)	*bronch/o-, bronch/i-* (bronchus)	very small branches of bronchi that extend into the lungs
cilia (SIL-ee-uh)	plural of the Latin word *cilium* (eyelash, eyelid)	small hairs in the upper respiratory tract that sweep foreign matter and mucus out of the respiratory tract
diaphragm (DYE-uh-fram)	from the Greek word *diaphragma* (partition, barrier)	the dome-shaped major muscle of breathing located at the base of the lungs within the thoracic cavity
epiglottis (ep-ih-GLOT-I)	*epi-* (upon) + the Greek *glottis* (tongue, mouth of the windpipe)	a mucous membrane-covered, leaf-shaped piece of cartilage at the root of the tongue
external respiration (eks-TUR-nul res-puh-RAY-shun)	from the Latin words *externus* (outside) and *respirationem* (breathing)	process in which air is brought into the lungs where oxygen and carbon dioxide are exchanged in the bloodstream at the capillaries surrounding the alveoli
glottis (GLOT-is)	a Greek word meaning "tongue," "mouth of the windpipe"	part of the larynx consisting of the vocal folds (vocal cords) and the slit-like opening between the folds
internal respiration (in-TUR-nul res-puh-RAY-shun)	from the Latin words *internus* (internal) and *respirationem* (breathing)	process where oxygen and carbon dioxide move between the bloodstream and the body's cells
laryngopharynx (luh-RIN-go-FAIR-inks)	*laryng/o* (larynx); *-al* (adjective suffix); *pharyng/o* (pharynx)	lower portion of the pharynx
larynx (LAIR-inx)	*laryng/o* (larynx)	air passageway between the pharynx and the trachea that holds the vocal cords; commonly called the *voice box*
lingual tonsils (LING-gwuhl TON-sulz)	from the Latin words *lingua* (tongue) and *tonsillae* (tonsil)	collection of lymphatic tissue on the under surface of the tongue
lobe (LOBE)	from the Latin word *lobus* (lobe)	a subdivision of the lung; the left lung has a *superior lobe*, *middle lobe*, and *lower lobe*; the right lung has a *superior lobe* and *inferior lobe*

Term and Pronunciation	Analysis	Meaning
Structure and Function		
lungs (LUNGZ)	from the German word *lunge* (lung)	organs of breathing located in the pulmonary cavities of the thorax
mediastinum (MEE-dee-uh-STYE-num)	from the Latin word *mediastinus* (midway)	partition between the lungs that contains the heart, aorta, trachea, esophagus, and bronchi
mucus (MYU-kus)	a Latin word meaning "slime," "mold"	clear secretion produced by the mucous membranes of the respiratory tract
nasal (NAY-zul)	*nas/o* (nose); *-al* (adjective suffix)	adjective referring to the nose
nasal cavity (NAY-zul KAV-ih-tee)	from the Latin words *nasus* (nose) and *cavus* (hollow)	the space on each side of the nasal septum that extends from the nostril to the pharynx
nasal septum (NAY-zul SEP-tum)	*nas/o* (nose); *-al* (adjective); from the Latin word *saeptum* (partition)	the wall dividing the nasal cavity into halves
nasopharynx (NAY-zoh-FAIR-inks)	*nas/o* (nose); *pharyng/o* (pharynx)	upper portion of the pharynx
nose (NOZE)	from the Latin word *nasus* (nose)	specialized organ at the entrance of the respiratory system
oropharynx (or-oh-FAIR-inks)	from the Latin word *oris* (mouth); *pharyng/o* (pharynx)	middle portion of the pharynx
palatine tonsils (PAL-uh-teen TON-sulz)	from the Latin word *tonsillae* (tonsil)	a mass of lymphatic tissue embedded in the lateral wall of the oral pharynx
paranasal sinuses (pair-uh-NAY-zul SIGH-nuh-sez)	*para-* (alongside); *nas/o* (nose); *-al* (adjective); from the Latin word *sinus* (cavity)	paired air-filled cavities in the bones of the face that are connected to the nasal cavity; these include the frontal, sphenoidal, maxillary, and ethmoidal sinuses
patency (PAT-en-see)	from the Latin word *patere* (lie open, be open)	the state of being open
patent (PAT-ent)	from the Latin word *patere* (lie open, be open)	open; adjective form of patency
pharyngeal tonsils (fuh-RIN-jee-uhl TON-sulz)	from the Latin words *pharyngeus* (pharyx) and *tonsillae* (tonsil)	epithelial and lymphatic structure located on the posterior wall of the nasopharynx; also called *adenoids*
pharynx (FAIR-inks)	a Greek word meaning "throat"	passageway just inferior to the nasal cavity and mouth
phrenic (FREN-ik)	from the Greek word *phren* (diaphragm, mind)	adjective referring to the diaphragm; synonymous with diaphragmatic
pleura (PLUR-uh)	a Greek word meaning "side of the body," "rib"	serous membrane that surrounds the lung; *parietal pleura* is the outer layer; *visceral pleura* is the inner layer
pulmonary (PULL-mun-air-ee)	*pulmon/o* (lung); *-ary* (adjective suffix)	adjective meaning relating to the lungs
sputum (SPYOU-tum)	from the Latin word *spuere* (to spit)	thick mucus ejected through the mouth
tonsils (TON-silz)	from the Latin word *tonsillar* (a stake)	lymphatic structures including the pharyngeal tonsils (adenoids), palatine tonsils, and lingual tonsils

(continues)

Study Table The Respiratory System		(continued)
Term and Pronunciation	**Analysis**	**Meaning**
Structure and Function		
trachea (TRAY-kee-uh)	from the Greek word *trakheia* (windpipe)	air passage extending from the larynx into the thorax; *windpipe*
ventilation (ven-ti-LAY-shun)	from the Latin word *ventilo* (the wind)	movement of gases into and out of the lungs
vocal cords (VO-kul kords)	from the Latin words *vocalis* (speaking) and *chorda* (string)	folds of mucus membranes that are used in speech production
Disorders		
apnea (APP-nee-uh)	*a-* (without); *-pnea* (breathing)	absence of breathing
asthma (AZ-muh)	a Greek word meaning "a panting"	a lung disease characterized by reversible inflammation and constriction
atelectasis (at-eh-LEK-tuh-sis)	from the Greek word *ateles* (incomplete); *ectasis* (expansion)	collapse of a lung or part of a lung, leading to decreased gas exchange
bradypnea (BRAY-dip-NEE-uh)	*brady-* (slow); *-pnea* (breathing)	abnormally slow breathing
bronchial pneumonia (BRAWN-kee-ul new-MONE-yuh)	*bronchi/o* (bronchus); *-al* (adjective suffix); *pneumon/o* (air, lung)	inflammation of the smaller bronchial tubes; also called *bronchopneumonia*
bronchiectasis (BRON-kee-EK-tay-sis)	*bronchi/o* (bronchus); *-ectasis* (expansion)	chronic dilation of the bronchi
bronchiolitis (bron-kee-oh-LYE-I)	*bronchi/o* (bronchus); *-itis* (inflammation)	inflammation of the bronchioles
bronchiostenosis (BRON-kee-oh-steh-NO-sis)	*bronchi/o* (bronchus); *sten/o* (narrowing); *-osis* (abnormal condition of)	narrowing of the bronchial tubes
bronchitis (bron-KYE-I)	*bronchi/o* (bronchus); *-itis* (inflammation)	inflammation of the mucous membranes of the bronchial tubes
bronchoconstriction (BRON- koh-kon-STRIK-shun)	*bronch/o* (bronchus); from the Latin word *constrictus* (compress)	the bronchi become narrowed or constricted
bronchodilation (BRON-koh-DYE-lay-shun)	*bronch/o* (bronchus); from the Latin word *dilatare* (make wider, dilate)	the bronchi become more open or dilated
bronchopneumonia (BRON-koh-new-MONE-yuh)	*bronch/o* (bronchus); *pneumon/o* (air, lung); *-ia* (condition)	inflammation of the smaller bronchial tubes; also called *bronchial pneumonia*
bronchospasm (BRON-koh-spaz-um)	*bronch/o* (bronchus); from the Latin word *spasmus* (a spasm)	abnormal contraction of bronchi
Cheyne-Stokes respiration (SHANE STOKES res-puh-RAY-shun)	named after John Cheyne, British physician, and William Stokes, Irish physician, who first described the disorder in the 19th century	a rhythmic respiratory pattern where there is a variation in depth of respirations alternating with periods of apnea
common cold virus (KOM-un COLD VYE-rus)	*virus* is the Latin word for poison	any virus associated with the common cold, chiefly rhinoviruses

Term and Pronunciation	Analysis	Meaning
Disorders		
croup (KRUPE)	from the Old French word *kroupe* (to croak)	a viral infection that causes swelling of the larynx and epiglottis; a barking noise is characteristic; also called *laryngotracheobronchitis*
cyanosis (sigh-uh-NO-sis)	from the Greek, *kyanos* (dark blue color)	dark bluish discoloration of the skin and mucous membranes due to deficient oxygenation of the blood
cystic fibrosis (SIS-tik FYE-broh-sis)	from the Greek word *kystis* (bladder, pouch); from the Latin word *fibra* (fiber); *-osis* (abnormal condition)	genetic disorder in which the lungs become clogged with excessive amounts of abnormally thick mucus
dysphonia (DIS-fone-yuh)	*dys-* (difficult); *phon/o* (sound); *-ia* (condition)	difficult or painful speech
dyspnea (DISP-nee-uh)	*dys-* (difficult); *-pnea* (breathing)	difficulty breathing
emphysema (em-fuh-SEE-muh)	a Greek word meaning "swelling"	condition in which the alveoli are inefficient because of distension
epiglottitis (ep-ih-GLOT-eye-tis)	*epiglottis* (Latin for epiglottis); *-itis* (inflammation)	inflammation of the epiglottis
eupnea (yoop-NEE-uh)	*eu-* (good, normal); *-pnea* (breathing)	normal breathing while resting
flu (FLEW)	abbreviated form of *influenza*	highly contagious viral infection of the upper respiratory tract that is spread by droplets; also called *influenza*
hemoptysis (HEE-mop-ti-sis)	*hem/o* (blood); *-ptysis* (spitting)	spitting or coughing up blood
hypercapnia (high-pur-KAP-nee-uh)	from the Greek words *huper* (over, beyond) and *kapnos* (smoke)	excessive carbon dioxide in the bloodstream, usually caused by inadequate respiration; also called *hypercarbia*
hypercarbia (high-pur-KAR-bee-uh)	from the Greek word *huper* (over, beyond) and the Latin word *carbon* (coal)	excessive carbon dioxide in the bloodstream, usually caused by inadequate respiration; also called *hypercapnia*
influenza (IN-flew-EN-zuh)	an Italian word meaning "influence" (of planets or stars)	highly contagious viral infection of the upper respiratory tract that is spread by droplets; also called *flu*
Kussmaul respiration (KUHS-mowl res-puh-RAY-shun)	named after 19th-century German physician who first noted it among patients with advanced diabetes mellitus	rapid deep respirations that are characteristic of an acid–base imbalance (frequently seen in uncontrolled diabetes)
laryngitis (LAIR-in-jye-tis)	*laryng/o* (larynx); *-itis* (inflammation)	inflammation of the larynx
laryngospasm (luh-RIN-go-spaz-um)	*laryng/o* (larynx); from the Latin word *spasmus* (a spasm)	involuntary contraction of the larynx
laryngostenosis (luh-RIN-go-sten-NO-sis)	*laryng/o* (larynx); *sten/o* (narrowing); *-osis* (abnormal condition)	a narrowing of the larynx

(continues)

Study Table The Respiratory System		*(continued)*
Term and Pronunciation	**Analysis**	**Meaning**
Disorders		
laryngotracheobronchitis (LUH-rin-go-TRAY-kee-oh-bron-KYE-tis)	*laryng/o* (larynx); *trache/o* (trachea); *bronchi/o* (bronchus)	a viral infection that causes swelling of the larynx and epiglottis; a barking noise is characteristic; also called *croup*
orthopnea (or-THOP-nee-uh)	*ortho-* (straight, correct); *-pnea* (breathing)	difficulty breathing while lying flat; difficulty is relieved by sitting up
pertussis (per-TUSS-is)	from the Latin *per-* (through); *tussis* (cough)	an acute infectious inflammation of the larynx, trachea, and bronchi caused by *Bordetella pertussis*
pharyngitis (fair-in-JYE-tis)	*pharyng/o* (pharynx); *-itis* (inflammation)	inflammation of the pharynx
pharyngospasm (fuh-RIN-go-spaz-um)	*pharyng/o* (pharynx); from the Latin word *spasmus* (a spasm)	involuntary contraction of the pharynx
phrenoplegia (fren-oh-PLEE-jee-uh)	*phren/o* (diaphragm); *-plegia* (paralysis)	paralysis of the diaphragm
pleurisy (PLUR-ih-see)	from the Latin word *pleurisis* (side of the body)	inflammation of the pleura (membrane that surrounds the lungs and lines the walls of the thoracic cavity)
pneumolith (NEW-mo-lith)	*pneum/o* (air, lung); from the Greek word *lithos* (stone)	calculus (stone) in a lung
pneumonia (new-MONE-yuh)	*pneumon/o* (air, lung); *-ia* (condition)	inflammation of a lung caused by infection, chemical inhalation, or trauma; also called *pneumonitis*
pneumonitis (new-moh-NYE-tis)	*pneumon/o* (air, lung); *-itis* (inflammation)	inflammation of a lung caused by infection, chemical inhalation, or trauma; also called *pneumonia*
pneumothorax (NEW-moh-thor-ax)	*pneumon/o* (air, lung); from the Greek word *thorakos* (breastplate, chest)	accumulation of air in the pleural cavity
rales (RALZ)	from the French word *raler* (to make a rattling sound in the throat)	abnormal breath sound; crackles
rhinitis (rye-NYE-tis)	*rhin/o* (nose); *-itis* (inflammation)	inflammation of the inner lining of the nasal cavity
rhinopathy (rye-NO-path-ee)	*rhin/o* (nose); *-pathy* (disease)	any disease of the nose
rhinorrhea (rye-no-REE-uh)	*rhin/o* (nose); *-rrhea* (discharge)	discharge from the nose
rhonchi (RON-kye)	from the Greek *rhonchos* (snore)	abnormal breath sound; low-pitched sonorous sounds
sinusitis (sigh-nuh-SYE-tis)	*sinus/o* (sinus); *-itis* (inflammation)	inflammation of the respiratory sinuses
stridor (STRYE-dor)	a Latin word meaning "harsh, high pitched"	high-pitched squeaking sound frequently associated with croup
tachypnea (tack-IP-nee-uh)	*tachy-* (rapid); *-pnea* (breathing)	abnormal rapid respiration

Term and Pronunciation	Analysis	Meaning
Disorders		
tracheitis (tray-kee-EYE-tis)	*trache/o* (trachea); *-itis* (inflammation)	inflammation of the trachea
tracheostenosis (TRAY-kee-oh-sten-OH-sis)	*trache/o* (trachea); *sten/o* (narrowing); -sis (condition)	abnormal narrowing of the trachea
tuberculosis (too-BURK-yu-loh-sis)	from the Latin word- *tuberculum* (small swelling, pimple); *-osis* (abnormal condition)	disease caused by presence of *Mycobacterium tuberculosis*, most commonly affecting the lungs
wheezing (WE-zing)	common English word; from Old Norse *hvaesa* (to hiss)	abnormal breath sounds; whistling sounds heard with upper airway obstruction
Diagnostic Tests, Treatments, and Surgical Procedures		
antihistamine (an-tee-HISS-tuh-MEEN)	*anti-* (against); from the Greek word *histos* (tissue); from the Latin *amine* (ammonia, compound)	drug used to treat acute allergic reactions
antipyretic (an-tee-PYE-ret-ik)	*anti-* (against); from the Greek *pyretos* (fever); *-ic* (adjective suffix)	drug used to reduce fever
arterial blood gas (ar-TEER-ee-ul BLUD GAS)	*arteri/o* (artery) + blood + gas, common English words	measures the partial pressures of oxygen and carbon dioxide in the arterial blood
bronchodilator (bron-koh-DYE-lay-tur)	*bronch/o* (bronchus); from the Latin word *dilatare* (make wider)	drug used to expand the bronchial passages
bronchoplasty (BRON-koh-plass-tee)	*bronch/o* (bronchus); *-plasty* (surgical repair)	surgical repair of a bronchus
bronchoscope (BRON-koh-skope)	*bronch/o* (bronchus); *-scope* (instrument for viewing)	device for visually inspecting the interior of a bronchus
bronchoscopy (bron-KOSS-koh-pee)	*bronch/o* (bronchus); *-scopy* (use of instrument for viewing)	inspection of the bronchial tree using a bronchoscope
decongestant (DEE-kon-jes-tent)	*de-* (away from, cessation); from the Latin word *congerere* (to bring together)	drug used to reduce congestion
laryngectomy (LAIR-en-JEK-toh-mee)	*laryng/o* (larynx); *-ectomy* (excision)	excision of the larynx
laryngoscope (luh-RIN-go-skope)	*laryng/o* (larynx); *-scope* (instrument for viewing)	instrument with a light at the tip to aid in visual inspection of the larynx
laryngoplasty (luh-RIN-go-plass-tee)	*laryng/o* (larynx); *-plasty* (surgical repair)	surgical repair of the larynx
laryngoscopy (LAIR-in-GOSS-koh-pee)	*laryng/o* (larynx); *-scopy* (use of instrument for viewing)	visual inspection of the larynx with the aid of a laryngoscope
laryngotomy (lair-in-GOT-oh-mee)	*laryng/o* (larynx); *-tomy* (cutting operation)	incision into the larynx
mucolytic (myu-koh-LIT-ik)	from the Latin *mucus* and the Greek word *lutikos* (able to loosen)	drug that thins mucus to aid in coughing up the mucus and clearing the lungs to improve lung function
pharyngoplasty (fuh-RIN-go-plass-tee)	*pharyng/o* (pharynx); *-plasty* (surgical repair)	surgical repair of the pharynx

(continues)

Study Table The Respiratory System		(continued)
Term and Pronunciation	**Analysis**	**Meaning**
Diagnostic Tests, Treatments, and Surgical Procedures		
pharyngoscope (fuh-RIN-go-skope)	*pharyng/o* (pharynx); *-scope* (instrument for viewing)	instrument with a light at the tip to aid in the visual inspection of the pharynx
pharyngoscopy (FUH-rin-GOS-koh-pee)	*pharyng/o* (pharynx); *-scopy* (use of instrument for viewing)	visual inspection of the pharynx with aid of a pharyngoscope
pharyngotomy (FAIR-in-GOT-oh-mee)	*pharyng/o* (pharynx); *-tomy* (cutting operation)	surgical incision into the pharynx
pneumonectomy (NOO-moh-NEK-tuh-mee)	*pneumon/o* (air, lung); *-ectomy* (excision)	removal of pulmonary lobes from a lung
pneumonorrhaphy (noo-moh-NOR-uh-fee)	*pneumon/o* (air, lung); *-rrhaphy* (surgical suturing)	suturing of a lung
pneumonotomy (noo-moh-NOT-uh-mee)	*pneumon/o* (air, lung); *-tomy* (cutting operation)	incision into a lung
postural drainage (POS-chur-ul DRAIN-ej)	from the Italian word *postura* (position) and the Old English word *drehnian* (strain)	a physical therapy technique where patients lie on their sides on a decline to help drain the lungs
pulmonary function test (PULL-muh-nair-ee FUNK-shuhn TEST)	*pulmon/o* (lung); *-ary* (adjective suffix); function test, common English words	measurement of lung volumes to assess breathing and ventilation; instrument used is a spirometer
pulse oximeter (PULS ock-SIM-eh-tur)	from the Latin word *pellere* (to push, drive); from the Greek words *oxys* (sharp) and *metron* (measure)	a device that measures the oxygen saturation of arterial blood by reference to light
pulse oximetry (PULS ock-SIM-eh-tree)	from the Latin word *pellere* (to push, drive); from the Greek words *oxys* (sharp) and *metron* (measure)	a small instrument placed on a finger or thin body part that measures the oxygen saturation of arterial blood
rhinoplasty (RYE-noh-plass-tee)	*rhin/o* (nose); *-plasty* (surgical repair)	surgery performed on the nose
rhinoscope (RYE-noh-skope)	*rhin/o* (nose); *-scope* (instrument for viewing)	a small mirror with a thin handle; used in rhinoscopy
rhinoscopy (rye-NOS-koh-pee)	*rhin/o* (nose); *-scopy* (use of instrument for viewing)	visual inspection of the nasal areas
rhinotomy (rye-NOT-uh-mee)	*rhin/o* (nose); *-tomy* (cutting operation)	surgical incision into the nose
sinusotomy (sigh-nus-OT-oh-mee)	*sinus/o* (sinus); *-tomy* (cutting operation)	incision into a sinus
spirometer (spy-ROM-eh-tur)	from the Latin word *spirare* (breath, blow, live); from the Greek word *metron* (measure)	a device used to measure respiratory gases
thoracentesis (THOR-uh-sen-TEE-sis)	*thorac/o* (thorax); *-centesis* (surgical puncture)	insertion of a needle into the pleural cavity to withdraw fluid for diagnostic purposes, to drain excess fluid, or to re-expand a collapsed lung

Term and Pronunciation	Analysis	Meaning
Diagnostic Tests, Treatments, and Surgical Procedures		
tracheoplasty (TRAY-kee-oh-plass-tee)	*trache/o* (trachea); *-plasty* (surgical repair)	surgical repair of the trachea
tracheostomy (tray-kee-OS-toh-mee)	*trache/o* (trachea); from the Greek *stoma* (mouth)	surgical creation of an opening into the trachea to form an airway or to prepare for the insertion of a tube for ventilation
tracheotomy (tray-kee-OT-oh-mee)	*trache/o* (trachea); *-tomy* (cutting operation)	incision into the trachea for purpose of restoring airflow to the lungs
Practice and Practitioners		
otolaryngologist (oh-toh-LAIR-in-GOL-oh-jist)	*ot/o* (ear); *laryng/o* (larynx); *-logist* (one who specializes)	physician who specializes in diagnosis and treatment of ear, nose, and throat diseases
otolaryngology (oh-toh-LAIR-in-GOL-oh-jee)	*ot/o* (ear); *laryng/o* (larynx); *-logy* (study of)	branch of medical study concerned with the ear, nose, and throat and diagnosis and treatment of its diseases
otorhinolaryngologist (oh-toh-RYE-no-lair-in-GOL-oh-jist)	*ot/o* (ear); *rhin/o* (nose); *laryng/o* (larynx); *-logist* (one who specializes)	physician who specializes in diagnosis and treatment of ear, nose, and throat diseases
pulmonologist (PULL-mun-OL-oh-jist)	*pulmon/o* (lung); *-logist* (one who specializes)	physician who specializes in diagnosing and treating respiratory disorders
pulmonology (PULL-mun-OL-oh-jee)	*pulmon/o* (lung); *-logy* (study of)	medical specialty of diagnosing and treating respiratory disorders
respiratory therapist (RES-per-uh-tor-ee THER-uh-pist)	from the Latin word *respirare* (breathe, blow back, blow again) + therapist	allied health care professional who specializes in airway management, mechanical ventilation, and managing blood acid–base balance

CASE STUDY WRAP-UP

Amelia was diagnosed with cystic fibrosis (CF), an inherited disorder that affects cells that produce mucus. Her skin tasted salty because the chloride channels in cells are faulty. Salt is made of sodium and chloride. If chloride cannot be reabsorbed, this leads to a loss of sodium on the skin surface and thick, sticky mucus. This thickened mucus clogs respiratory passages and digestive organs, leading to damage. Today, newborns are screened for CF, but when Amelia was born, these tests were not available. Amelia's pulmonologist specializes in treating cystic fibrosis, and Amelia will take medications, including bronchodilators, antibiotics to treat infections, mucolytics, and pancreatic enzymes, throughout her life.

Case Study Application Questions

1. Describe wheezing.
2. What is cystic fibrosis (CF)?
3. Why was Amelia under the care of a pulmonologist?
4. Of the medications Amelia was taking, which one is used to thin mucous secretions and which one expands air passages?

END-OF-CHAPTER EXERCISES

Exercise 12.1 Labeling

Using the following list, choose the terms to label the diagram correctly.

alveoli   lungs   trachea

bronchi   paranasal   sinuses

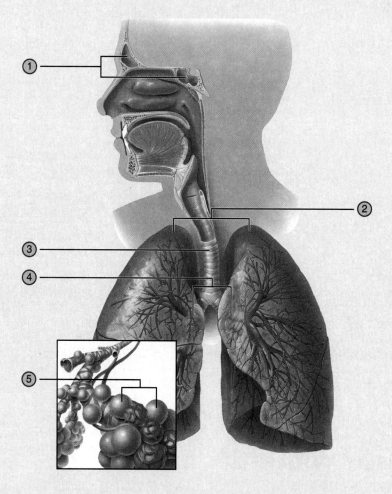

1. _____   3. _____   5. _____

2. _____   4. _____

Exercise 12.2 Word Parts

Break each of the following terms into its word parts: prefix, root, or suffix. Give the meaning of each word part and then define the term.

1.   *nasopharynx*

     root: _____

     root: _____

     definition: _____

2. *pulmonary*

   root: _____

   suffix: _____

   definition: _____

3. *dysphonia*

   prefix: _____

   root: _____

   suffix: _____

   definition: _____

4. *hemoptysis*

   root: _____

   suffix: _____

   definition: _____

5. *laryngostenosis*

   root: _____

   root: _____

   suffix: _____

   definition: _____

6. *antipyretic*

   prefix: _____

   root: _____

   suffix: _____

   definition: _____

7. *rhinoplasty*

   root: _____

   suffix: _____

   definition: _____

8. *otolaryngologist*

   root: _____

   root: _____

   suffix: _____

   definition: _____

Exercise 12.3 Word Building

Use bronch/o or bronchi/o to build the medical words meaning:

1. inflammation of the bronchi _____
2. chronic dilation of the bronchioles _____

Use the suffix -itis to build the medical words meaning:

3. inflammation of the larynx _____
4. inflammation of a sinus _____
5. inflammation of the epiglottis _____

Use the suffix -pnea to build the medical words meaning:

6. rapid breathing _____
7. slow breathing _____
8. painful or difficulty breathing _____
9. difficulty breathing while lying down _____

Exercise 12.4 Matching

Match the term with its definition.

1. _____ alveoli
   a. the lid or flap that helps prevent food and drink from entering the trachea

2. _____ diaphragm
   b. the "voice box"

3. _____ pulmonary
   c. indicating something in or associated with the lungs

4. _____ trachea
   d. the major muscle of the respiratory system

5. _____ epiglottis
   e. tiny "sacs" in the lungs that receive oxygen from the bronchioles and transfer it to the capillaries

6. _____ pneumonia, pneumonitis
   f. the "windpipe"; air flows through it to the bronchi

7. _____ larynx
   g. inflammation of a lung, caused by infection, chemical inhalation, or trauma

8. _____ bronchioles
   h. incision into the trachea

9. _____ asthma
   i. inner lining of the lung

10. _____ pharynx
    j. the smallest extensions of the bronchi, which pass air directly to the alveoli

11. _____ emphysema
    k. a lung disease characterized by reversible inflammation and constriction

12. _____ bronchitis
    l. throat

13. _____ dyspnea
    m. narrowing of a bronchial tube

14. _____ tracheotomy
    n. inflammation of the mucous membrane of the bronchial tubes

15. _____ bronchiostenosis
    o. difficulty breathing

16. _____ apnea
    p. inspection using a bronchoscope

17. _____ visceral pleura
    q. absence of breathing

18. _____ bronchoscopy
    r. condition in which the alveoli are inefficient due to distension

Exercise 12.5 Multiple Choice

Choose the correct answer for the following multiple-choice questions.

1. Pertussis is the medical term for_____.
   a. strep throat
   b. diphtheria
   c. whooping cough
   d. Lyme disease

2. What is the uppermost part of the pharynx?
   a. oropharynx
   b. laryngopharynx
   c. nasopharynx
   d. hypopharynx

3. What is the serous membrane that lines the walls of the pulmonary cavity?
   a. visceral pleura
   b. parietal pleura
   c. visceral peritoneum
   d. parietal peritoneum

4. Which procedure involves making an opening in the trachea to facilitate breathing?
   a. intubation
   b. tracheocentesis
   c. tracheoplasty
   d. tracheostomy

5. Which of the following would probably cause dysphonia?
   a. rhinitis
   b. laryngitis
   c. otitis
   d. ophthalmodynia

6. Which of the following is the same as pharyngitis?
   a. sore lung
   b. inflammation of the pharynx
   c. examination of the throat
   d. a fungal condition of the pharynx

7. Which term means the drawing of air into the lungs?
   a. respiration
   b. orthopnea
   c. inhalation
   d. hypoxia

8. What is another term for *pneumonia*?
   a. pleuropneumonia
   b. pneumonitis
   c. pulmonary edema
   d. pulmonary insufficiency

9. What is a collapse of part of a lung called?
   a. asthma
   b. atelectasis
   c. SIDS
   d. CF

10. What is a lobectomy?
    a. incision of the lung
    b. excision of a lung
    c. excision of a lobe of a lung
    d. bilateral incision of the skull

Exercise 12.6 Fill in the Blank

Fill in the blank with the correct answer.

1. Expectoration of blood is called _____.
2. The term for slow breathing is _____.
3. A surgical puncture of the lung is called a(n) _____.
4. Pleurisy is _____.
5. The membrane that surrounds the lung is the _____.
6. The term for difficulty breathing while lying down is _____.
7. Chronic dilation of the bronchi is called _____.
8. Discharge from the nose is known as _____.
9. The abnormal breathing condition that describes alternating periods of apnea and dyspnea is _____.

Exercise 12.7 Abbreviations

Write out the term for the following abbreviations.

1. _____ COPD

2. _____ ABG

3. _____ TLC

4. _____ CF

5. _____ T and A

6. _____ URI

Write the abbreviation for the following terms.

7. _____ tuberculosis

8. _____ oxygen

9. _____ carbon dioxide

10. _____ pulmonary function test

11. _____ residual volume

12. _____ shortness of breath

Exercise 12.8 Spelling

Select the correct spelling of the medical term.

1. The _____ is the major muscle responsible for breathing, located at the base of the thoracic cavity.
   a. diafram
   b. diaphram
   c. diagphram
   d. diaphragm

2. The _____ is more commonly known as the throat.
   a. pharinx
   b. pharynx
   c. pherinx
   d. pherynx

3. The _____, which is also called the windpipe, is the tube that connects the larynx to the bronchi.
   a. tracea
   b. trachia
   c. trachea
   d. traychea

4. Abnormally rapid breathing is called _____.
   a. tachypnea
   b. tachynea
   c. tachypnia
   d. tacypnia

5. Inflammation of a lung commonly caused by infection is called _____.
   a. pneumonia
   b. pnuemonia
   c. neumonia
   d. numonia

6. Discharge from the nasal mucous membrane is called _____.
   a. rinorea
   b. rhinorrhea
   c. rinoria
   d. rhinorhea

7. A _____ is a drug used to expand the bronchi.
   a. broncodilator
   b. bronchodilater
   c. bronkodilator
   d. bronchodilator

8. Inserting a needle into the pleural cavity to withdraw fluid, drain fluid, or re-expand a collapsed lung is called _____.
   a. thorcentesis
   b. thoracensis
   c. thoracentesis
   d. thoracenteesys

9. An _____ is a physician who specializes in the diagnosis and treatment of ear, nose, and throat diseases.
   a. otolaringologist
   b. otolaryngologist
   c. otolaryngolist
   d. otalaringologist

10. _____ is a Greek word that means "short breath" or "a panting."
    a. Asthma
    b. Asma
    c. Azma
    d. Azthma

Exercise 12.9 Medical Report

Analyze the following medical record and answer the questions that follow.

MEDICAL RECORD

HISTORY: A 30-year-old female who c/o a nonproductive cough, dyspnea, and a fever of 3 days; patient has a negative history for smoking and has otherwise been in good health.

PHYSICAL EXAM: T 102°F, BP 104/65, R 26, P 108
Tachypnea is accompanied by mild cyanosis, and inspiratory rales are noted during a stethoscope exam. WBC is elevated, CXR shows diffuse infiltrates at the bases of both lungs. An ABG taken while the patient was breathing room air was abnormal and showed the patient had low oxygen content in the blood. A sputum specimen contained WBCs.

DIAGNOSIS: Pneumonia of unknown etiology.

TREATMENT PLAN: Admit patient to the ICU. Administer antibiotics and oxygen by face mask and monitor patient's status.

1. What are the findings on physical examination?
   a. Fast breathing, blue skin, and crackles heard in the lungs as the patient inhales
   b. Slow breathing, blue skin, and rales heard in the lungs as the patient holds her breath
   c. Slow breathing, blue skin, and rhonchi heard in the lungs as the patient exhales
   d. Fast heart rate, blue skin, and rales heard in the lungs as the patient inhales
   e. Fast breathing, blue skin, and wheezing heard in the lungs as the patient inhales

2. What is the patient's chief complaint?
   a. Cannot breathe, fever, and coughing up material from lungs
   b. Dry cough and difficulty breathing
   c. Fever, coughing up sputum, and breathing fast
   d. Hoarse throat, dry cough, and fever
   e. Fever with a dry cough and difficulty breathing

Exercise 12.10 Reflection

1. What respiratory disorders were you already familiar with?
2. Think about the anatomy of the lungs and their position in the body. Why does standing up make it easier to breathe?

CHAPTER 13

The Digestive System

LEARNING OUTCOMES

Upon completion of this chapter, you should be able to:

- Name the major organs and accessory organs that make up the digestive system.
- Pronounce, spell, and define medical terms related to the digestive system and its disorders.
- Interpret abbreviations associated with the digestive system.
- Apply knowledge gained to case study questions.

CASE STUDY

Mario's Malaise

Mario was a 25-year-old male with a slight build who had frequent bouts of abdominal pain and diarrhea for as long as he could remember. Sometimes, the pain was so severe that he would double over and lay on the bathroom floor. One evening, the cramping was so painful that he could not sit up straight, and so he rocked in a fetal position. When he was able to sit up, it was to make a mad dash to the toilet. He had taken an over-the-counter antidiarrheal, but he still had explosive diarrhea that looked bloody. After several hours, his cramping resolved, but he felt nauseous. He hoped he would feel well enough in the morning to go to work.

Introduction

The digestive system is composed of organs whose job is to ingest food, change that food into a usable form, and then eliminate wastes. The **digestive tract** is a continuous tube beginning with the mouth and ending at the anus. This tract is also called the **gastrointestinal (GI) tract** or **alimentary canal**. Organs of the digestive system include the mouth, pharynx, esophagus, stomach, small intestine, and large intestine. Accessory organs of the digestive system include

salivary glands, the liver, gallbladder, and pancreas (see **Figure 13.1**). The three main functions of the digestive system are digestion, absorption, and elimination. **Digestion** is the physical, chemical, and enzymatic processes in which ingested food is converted into substances the body can use. **Absorption** is taking in these substances by the body's cells. The removal of wastes from the body is called **elimination**.

The gastrointestinal tract is divided into an upper gastrointestinal (UGI) tract and a lower gastrointestinal (LGI) tract. The upper gastrointestinal tract

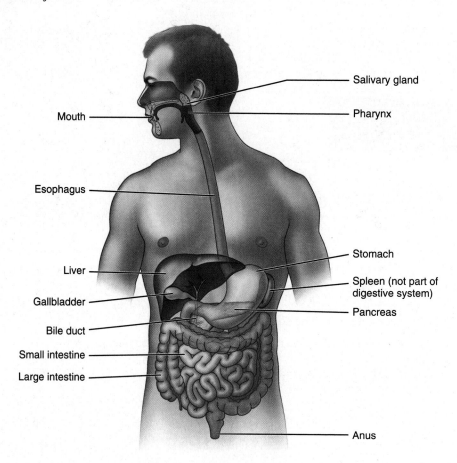

Figure 13.1 Structures of the digestive system.

consists of the mouth, esophagus, and the stomach. The pyloric sphincter at the distal end of the stomach marks the end of the upper GI tract. Past this point, the GI tract is called the lower gastrointestinal tract. The lower GI tract consists of the small intestine and the large intestine. The small intestine is subdivided into three different regions. The large intestine is also divided into three different regions.

Word Parts Related to the Gastrointestinal System

The term *gastrointestinal* is made up of two words from two different languages. "Gastr/o" is the root word for stomach and comes from the Greek language, whereas *intestinum* is the Latin word for gut. The other name this tract is known by is alimentary canal. The root word "aliment/o" means nutrition. Eating or swallowing can be designated by either the root phag/o or the suffix-phagia, which both refer to eating. Many of the word parts related to the digestive system are listed in **Table 13.1**.

Table 13.1 Word Parts Related to the Digestive System

Word Part	Meaning
abdomin/o	abdomen
aliment/o	nutrition
bucc/o	cheek
cheil/o	lip
chol/e, chol/o	bile, gall
cholangi/o	bile duct
cholecyst/o	gallbladder
choledoch/o	common bile duct
col/o, colon/o	colon
dent/i, dent/o	teeth
diverticul/o	diverticulum
duoden/o	duodenum
-emesis	vomiting
enter/o	intestine

Table 13.1 Word Parts Related to the Digestive System *(continued)*

Word Part	Meaning
esophag/o	esophagus
gastr/o	stomach
gingiv/o	gums
gloss/o	tongue
hepat/o	liver
ile/o	ileum
jejun/o	jejunum
lapar/o	abdomen
-lith	stone
pancreat/o	pancreas
-pepsia	digestion
phag/o	eating, swallowing
-phagia	eat or swallow
proct/o	anus and rectum
pylor/o	pylorus
rect/o	rectum
-scope	instrument used for viewing
-scopy	visual examination
sial/o	salivary glands
sigmoid/o	sigmoid colon
stomat/o	mouth

Word Parts Exercise

After studying Table 13.1, write the meaning of each the word parts.

1. -phagia	1. _____
2. choledoch/o	2. _____
3. stomat/o	3. _____
4. sigmoid/o	4. _____
5. abdomin/o	5. _____
6. enter/o	6. _____
7. lapar/o	7. _____
8. rect/o	8. _____
9. -lith	9. _____

Word Parts Exercise *(continued)*

10. sial/o	10. _____
11. hepat/o	11. _____
12. pylor/o	12. _____
13. chol/e, chol/o	13. _____
14. cholangi/o	14. _____
15. esophag/o	15. _____
16. -emesis	16. _____
17. -scope	17. _____
18. gloss/o	18. _____
19. jejun/o	19. _____
20. gastr/o	20. _____
21. cheil/o	21. _____
22. ile/o	22. _____
23. pancreat/o	23. _____
24. bucc/o	24. _____
25. cholecyst/o	25. _____
26. -pepsia	26. _____
27. col/o, colon/o	27. _____
28. dent/i, dent/o	28. _____
29. phag/o	29. _____
30. duoden/o	30. _____
31. proct/o	31. _____
32. gingiv/o	32. _____
33. -scopy	33. _____
34. aliment/o	34. _____

Structure and Function

The food we eat needs to be converted into a form our bodies can use. The digestive tract and associated organs are responsible for that conversion.

Major Organs of the Digestive Tract

The major organs of the digestive tract are those that make up the one-way tube. These structures include the mouth, pharynx, esophagus, stomach, small intestine, and large intestine.

The Mouth (Oral Cavity)

Digestion begins in the mouth (oral cavity), where food is broken apart by **mastication**, which is a technical term for chewing. A slightly acidic fluid called *saliva* is produced by the salivary glands. Saliva moistens the food and forms a **bolus**, a small ball of masticated food that is pushed back and downward with the tongue.

> Why *bolus* and not simply *ball* or *mass*? That is a good question, especially as the Latin word *bolus*, which means ball, has a more common medical meaning that has no direct connection to the digestive system. Bolus can simply mean "a large pill" or a dose of medication given intravenously for a special purpose. Within the GI system, it refers to a ball of chewed food.

The Pharynx and Esophagus

Next, the bolus enters the pharynx (throat), which, as you know from Chapter 12, is also part of the respiratory tract. From the pharynx, the bolus passes into the **esophagus**, a tube that connects the throat to the stomach. Within the esophagus, the bolus is lubricated with mucus before being carried into the stomach by **peristalsis** (wavelike muscular contractions). The **lower esophageal sphincter** (LES), also called the *cardiac sphincter*, is a ring of muscle that controls the flow from the esophagus into the stomach (**Figure 13.2**).

The Stomach

The **stomach** is a J-shaped organ that physically and chemically digests food. The regions of the

stomach include the *cardia*, *fundus*, *body*, and *pylorus*. Its first job is storing food temporarily, while its second job is secreting hydrochloric acid and enzymes to help break down proteins, fats, and carbohydrates. Digestion includes physical changes, such as reducing particle size and converting solids to liquids. Digestion also includes chemical changes needed to produce fuel for the body's cells. Within 3 to 4 hours, gastric juices and partially digested food form a pasty substance called **chyme**, which enters the small intestine. Chyme passes through the **pyloric sphincter**, a ring of muscle at the distal end of the stomach, and into the **duodenum**, the first region of the small intestine. At times, a *nasogastric tube*, which is a narrow tube passed into the stomach via the nose, is used short term to supply nutrition or it can be used to aspirate (suction fluid from) the stomach. Nutrition that is maintained entirely by venous injection or by other nongastrointestinal routes is termed *total parenteral nutrition* (TPN). Shorthand for "nothing by mouth" is NPO, derived from the Latin non per os. Figure 13.2 shows the esophagus, stomach, and duodenum.

The Small Intestine

The lower gastrointestinal tract begins with the small intestine, which extends from the stomach's pyloric sphincter to the first region of the large intestine. Although it is about 20 feet in length, it is known as the small intestine because it is smaller in diameter than the large intestine. The small intestine is divided into three regions: **duodenum**, **jejunum**, and **ileum**. From the duodenum, chyme moves into the jejunum and from there into the ileum. The **ileocecal sphincter** (not shown) controls the flow from the ileum into the cecum, the first region of the large intestine (see **Figure 13.3**).

> Isn't the ileum also the name of one of the three bones making up the hip? No, that's the ilium. Although both words are pronounced the same, they have one letter that is different. If you remember that hip and ilium both have an "i" in the middle, you will be able to distinguish these two terms, which have different roots.

The Large Intestine

The large intestine extends from the ileocecal valve to the anus. It is divided into three regions: **cecum**, **colon**, and **rectum**. The cecum is the beginning segment of the large intestine. Attached to the cecum is a tube-shaped sac called the **appendix**.

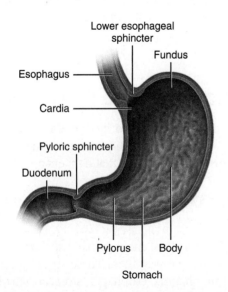

Lower esophageal sphincter

Fundus

Esophagus

Cardia

Pyloric sphincter

Duodenum

Pylorus   Body

Stomach

Figure 13.2 The esophagus, stomach, and duodenum.

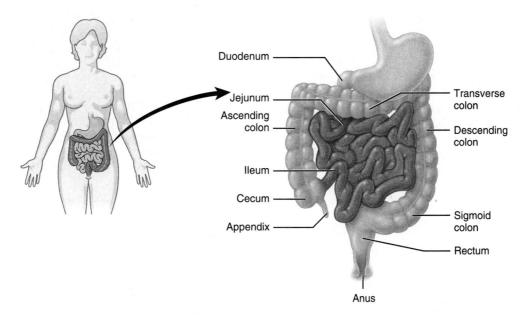

Figure 13.3 The small and large intestines. The small intestine, illustrated in *dark pink*, is made up of the duodenum, jejunum, and ileum. The large intestine, illustrated in *light pink*, is divided into the ascending colon, transverse colon, and descending colon. The intestinal tract ends at the anus.

This structure is sometimes called the *vermiform appendix*. Vermiform, which means wormlike, is usually omitted, and the single word *appendix* is the preferred term. The appendix consists of lymphatic tissue and is, functionally speaking, part of the lymphatic system.

The colon is subdivided into four regions: **ascending colon**, **transverse colon**, **descending colon**, and **sigmoid colon** (see Figure 13.3). The last part, the sigmoid colon, continues from the descending colon and connects to the rectum. The rectum takes up approximately the last 6 inches of the large intestine and terminates at the **anus**, through which wastes are eliminated. **Figure 13.4** illustrates the pathway of food through the gastrointestinal tract.

Accessory Organs

Although the *salivary glands, liver, gallbladder,* and *pancreas* are not part of the gastrointestinal tract, they play key roles in digestion. Because they are not part of the one-way canal, they are referred to as **accessory organs** of the digestive system (see **Figure 13.5**).

Salivary Glands

Salivary glands are any of the saliva-secreting glands (*parotid, submandibular,* and *sublingual*) of the oral cavity. The senses of taste and smell stimulate the salivary glands to secrete **saliva**, a watery liquid that contains enzymes that begin digestion. Saliva also helps flush bacteria in the mouth and keeps the teeth and tongue clean. Figure 13.1 shows the location of the parotid salivary gland.

Liver

The liver, located in the upper right quadrant of the abdomen deep to the diaphragm, plays many important roles in digestion, metabolism, and detoxification of harmful substances. One of its main digestive functions is to manufacture and secrete **bile**, a liquid that breaks down fat into droplets. This breaking down process is called *emulsification*. Our bodies need bile to process fats before they are released into the bloodstream. Once bile is produced in the liver, it travels down the **bile duct** to the gallbladder for storage. The liver is an important organ whose functions are integrated into many body systems.

Gallbladder

Although the liver produces and recycles bile, the **gallbladder**, which is in a depression under the liver, stores, condenses, and delivers the bile to the small intestine, specifically the duodenum (see Figure 13.5).

Pancreas

The pancreas is an elongated feather-shaped organ that lies posterior to the stomach. It has both digestive and endocrine functions. It produces digestive enzymes that aid in processing carbohydrates and fats in foods as well as secreting hormones directly into the bloodstream (see Figure 13.5).

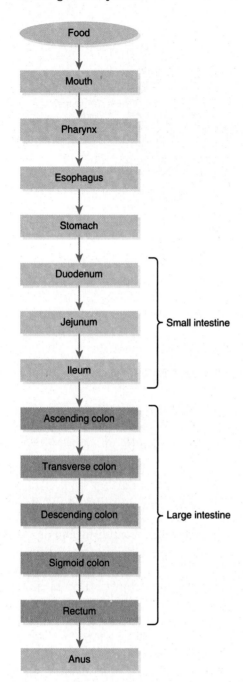

Figure 13.4 Pathway of food through the gastrointestinal tract.

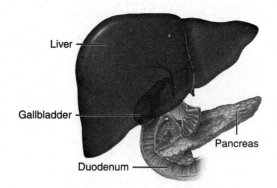

Figure 13.5 Accessory organs of the digestive system.

involuntary clenching or grinding of teeth) can occur in the mouth.

The following are a few common disorders of the upper digestive tract:

1. **Dysphagia**: difficulty in swallowing
2. **Esophagitis**: inflammation of the esophagus
3. **Hiatal hernia**: stomach protrusion through the esophageal hiatus (opening) of the diaphragm into the thoracic cavity (see **Figure 13.6**)
4. **Gastroesophageal reflux disease** (GERD): upward flow of stomach acid into the esophagus
5. **Gastritis**: inflammation of the stomach (gastric) mucous membranes.

QUICK CHECK

Fill in the blanks.

1. A small ball of masticated food is called a(n) _____.
2. The stomach has two main jobs. The first is the temporary storage of food. What is the other one? _____
3. The three regions of the small intestine are the _____, _____, and _____.

Disorders Related to the Digestive System

Disorders of the upper gastrointestinal tract may involve oral cavity infections, such as **stomatitis** (inflammation of the mucous membranes in the mouth) and **gingivitis** (inflammation of the gums). **Parotiditis** (also known as *parotitis*) is an inflammation of the parotid gland, which is the largest of the salivary glands. (See Figure 13.1 for the location of the parotid salivary gland). Other abnormal conditions such as **dental caries** (cavities) and **bruxism** (an

Disorders of the Lower Gastrointestinal Tract

Disorders of the lower gastrointestinal tract include obstructions, inflammation, or structural abnormalities. These conditions are listed later. A common procedure for studying the lower intestinal tract is a *barium enema* (BE). With this procedure, barium sulfate, a radiopaque dye, is injected into the rectum for X-ray imaging.

1. **Crohn's disease**: inflammation in the mucosal lining of the intestine (usually the ileum)
2. **Appendicitis**: inflammation of the appendix

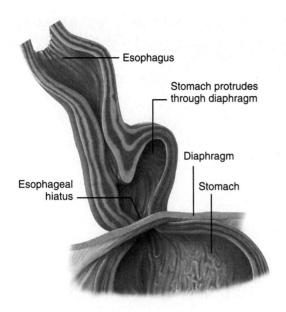

Figure 13.6 Hiatal hernia.

3. **Peritonitis**: inflammation of the peritoneum, which is the sac that lines the abdominal cavity
4. **Diverticula**: pouches in the intestinal wall that form as increased pressure pushes the wall of the colon outward at weakened points
5. **Diverticulosis**: condition characterized by the presence of diverticula
6. **Diverticulitis**: inflammation of diverticula, which fill with stagnant fecal matter and become inflamed
7. **Inguinal hernia**: protrusion of a small loop of intestine through a weak spot in the lower abdominal wall or groin
8. **Intestinal obstruction**: refers to a lack of movement of the intestinal contents through the intestine
9. **Intussusception**: telescoping of a section of bowel inside an adjacent section
10. **Volvulus**: twisting of the bowel
11. **Ulcerative colitis** (UC): immune disorder causing inflammation and sores (ulcers) on the large intestine inner lining
12. **Inflammatory bowel disease** (IBD): group of disorders causing inflamed digestive system organs. Two common types are ulcerative colitis and Crohn's disease.

Disorders of the Accessory Organs of the Digestive System

Many of the conditions that affect the digestive system accessory organs are obstructions caused by stones, tumors, or inflammatory processes. A few of these are described as follows:

1. **Cholelithiasis**: a condition in which calculi (stones) reside in the gallbladder or bile ducts
2. **Cholecystitis**: inflammation of the gallbladder
3. **Cholangiolitis**: inflammation of a bile duct
4. **Choledocholithiasis**: obstruction of the biliary tract by gallstones
5. **Hepatitis**: inflammation of the liver
6. **Irritable bowel syndrome** (IBS): a condition characterized by abdominal pain, constipation (infrequent bowel movements with hardened feces), diarrhea, gas, and bloating
7. **Jaundice** (also called **icterus**): a symptom of hepatitis characterized by a yellowing of the skin and eyes resulting from bile accumulation
8. **Cirrhosis**: chronic liver disease characterized by inflammation and scar tissue formation; typically results from alcoholism or hepatitis

Additional conditions, signs, symptoms, and disorders of the digestive system include **anorexia** (loss of appetite), **bulimia** (binge eating followed by self-induced vomiting and misuse of laxatives), **eructation** (belching or burping gas), **hyperemesis** (excessive vomiting), **dyspepsia** (indigestion), and **hemorrhoids** (enlarged veins in or near the anus).

Diagnostic Tests, Treatments, and Surgical Procedures

To view different parts of the gastrointestinal tract, different tools are required. An **enteroscope** is an instrument for inspecting the inside of the intestine; the procedure is called an **enteroscopy**. Visual examination of the duodenum is called **duodenoscopy**. A **gastroscope** is an instrument for viewing the stomach, and the procedure is called **gastroscopy**. A **colonoscope** is a long, flexible fiber-optic endoscope used to perform a **colonoscopy** (visual examination of the colon). Endoscopic examination of the esophagus, stomach, and duodenum performed using a fiber-optic instrument is called an **esophagogastroduodenoscopy** (EGD), whereas a radiographic contrast study using dye is called an **upper gastrointestinal series** (UGIS).

Sometimes, a surgical procedure is necessary. An **ostomy** (or **stoma**) is a surgical opening into the gastrointestinal tract. Patients with an ostomy have a section of their intestines removed, so instead of waste exiting through the rectum, an artificial opening is established, and waste exits into a bag or pouch the patient wears. A **colostomy** is an opening into the colon. A **duodenostomy** is an opening into the duodenum, an **ileostomy** is an opening into the ileum, and a **gastrostomy** is an opening into the stomach. Notice that -ostomy looks very similar to -otomy, which is an incision (cutting), not the establishment of an opening.

Practice and Practitioners

Apart from specialists, such as dentists, who treat the oral cavity, the specialists concerned with the digestive system are **gastroenterologists** (physicians specializing in disorders of the stomach and intestines) and **proctologists** (physicians specializing in disorders of the anus and rectum). The specialties are **gastroenterology** and **proctology**, respectively. In the hospital setting, many GI disorders are diagnosed and treated by an **internist**, a nonsurgical specialist in internal medicine.

Abbreviation Table The Digestive System	
Abbreviation	**Meaning**
BE	barium enema
BP	blood pressure
BM	bowel movement
EGD	esophagogastroduodenoscopy
GERD	gastroesophageal reflux disease

Abbreviation Table The Digestive System (continued)	
Abbreviation	**Meaning**
GI	gastrointestinal
GP	general practitioner
HCl	hydrochloric acid
HTN	hypertension
IBS	irritable bowel syndrome
IBD	inflammatory bowel disease
LES	lower esophageal sphincter
LGI	lower gastrointestinal
NG	nasogastric
NPO	non per os (Latin for "nothing by mouth")
PO	per os (Latin for "by mouth")
SOB	shortness of breath
TPN	total parenteral nutrition
UC	ulcerative colitis
UGI	upper gastrointestinal
UGIS	upper gastrointestinal series
WBC	white blood cell

Study Table The Digestive System		
Term and Pronunciation	**Analysis**	**Meaning**
Structure and Function		
accessory organs (ak-SES-uh- ree OR-gunz)	from the Latin word *accessorius* (that which is subordinate to something else)	in the gastrointestinal system: the salivary glands, liver, gallbladder, and pancreas
alimentary canal (al-ih-MEN-tuh-ree)	from the Latin word *alimentarius* (pertaining to food) + canal	passage leading from the mouth to the anus through the pharynx, esophagus, stomach, and intestines; *digestive tract* or *GI tract*
appendix (uh-PEN-diks)	Latin word for "something attached"	tube-shaped sac attached into the cecum of the large intestine; also called *vermiform appendix*
bile (BILE)	from the Latin word *bilis* (fluid secreted from the liver)	yellow-brown or green liquid secreted by the liver into the duodenum to emulsify fats
bile duct (BILE DUKT)	from the Latin words *bilis* (fluid secreted from the liver) and *ductus* (a leading)	tube that transports bile from the liver to the gallbladder
bilirubin (BILL-ee-ROO-bin)	from the Latin *bilus* (bile) and *ruber* (red)	waste produced by worn out red blood cells breaking down
bowel movement (BM) (BOW-el MOOV-ment)	from the Latin *botellus*, a diminutive of *botulus* (sausage)	defecation

Term and Pronunciation	Analysis	Meaning
Structure and Function		
cardiac sphincter (KAR-dee-ak SFINGK-tur)	*cardi/o* (heart); *-ac* (adjective suffix); from the Greek word *sphingein* (to bind tight)	the ringlike muscle between the esophagus and stomach that controls food flow; also called *lower esophageal sphincter* (LES)
cecum (SEE-kum)	from the Latin word *caecus* (hidden)	a pouch connected to the junction of the small and large intestines, forming the first part of the large intestine
chyme (KIME)	from the Latin word *chymus* (juice produced by digestion)	the semifluid mass of partly digested food passed from the stomach into the duodenum
colon (KOH-lun)	from the Greek word *kolon* (large intestine)	the large intestine, divisible into the ascending, transverse, descending, and sigmoid colons
deglutition (dee-gloo-TISH-un)	from the Latin word *deglutire* (swallow down)	swallowing
digestive tract (dye-JES-tiv TRAKT)	from the Latin word *digero* + *-gestus* (to force apart, divide, dissolve)	passage leading from the mouth to the anus through the pharynx, esophagus, stomach, and intestines; also called *alimentary canal* or *GI tract*
duodenal (doo-OD-en-ul)	from the Greek word *dodekadaktylon* (literally "12 fingers long"; named by Greek physician Herophilus) + *-al* (adjective suffix)	adjective form of duodenum used in the terms naming some digestive system disorders
duodenum (doo-OD-en-um)	from the Greek *dodekadaktylon* (12 fingers long)	segment of the small intestine connecting with the stomach
esophagus (ee-SOF-uh-gus)	from the Greek *oisophagos* (gullet, literally "what carries and eats")	the part of the digestive tract between the pharynx and stomach
gallbladder (GAWL-blad-ur)	from Old English *galla* (to shine, yellow); from Old English *bledre* (to blast, blow up, swell up)	small pear-shaped organ that stores bile
gastric (GAS-trik)	*gastr/o* (stomach); *-ic* (adjective suffix)	adjective form of stomach
gastrointestinal tract (GAS-troh-in-TES-tin-ul TRAKT)	*gastr/o* (stomach); from Latin *intestina*, plural of *intestinus* (internal, inward, intestine) + tract	passage leading from the mouth to the anus through the pharynx, esophagus, stomach, and intestines; also called *alimentary canal* or *digestive tract*
ileocecal sphincter (ILL-ee-oh-see-kul SFINGK-tur)	*ile/o* (ileum); from the Latin *caecum* (blind); *-al* (adjective suffix); *sphincter* (from the Greek word *sphingein*: to bind tight)	muscular ring that separates the distal portion of the ileum (small intestine) and the beginning of the cecum (large intestine)
ileum (ILL-ee-um)	a Latin word meaning flank or groin	the longest segment of the small intestine, which leads into the large intestine
intestine (in-TESS-tin)	from Latin *intestina*, plural of *intestinus* (internal, inward, intestine)	the small intestine is divisible into the duodenum, jejunum, and ileum; the large intestine comprises the cecum, colon, rectum, and anus
jejunum (jeh-JOO-num)	from the Latin word *jejunus* (empty, fasting, abstinent, hungry)	eight-foot-long segment of the small intestine between the duodenum and the ileum

(continues)

Study Table The Digestive System		*(continued)*
Term and Pronunciation	**Analysis**	**Meaning**
Structure and Function		
liver (LIV-ur)	from the Old English word *lifer* (liver)	the largest glandular organ of the body, lying beneath the diaphragm in the upper part of the gastric region, involved in many metabolic processes
lower esophageal sphincter (LES) (LOW-ur eh-sof-uh-JEE-ul SFINGK-ter)	from the Greek word *sphingein* (to bind tight)	the ringlike muscle between the esophagus and stomach that controls food flow; also called *cardiac sphincter*
lower gastrointestinal tract (LOH-er GAS-troh-in-TES-tin-ul TRAKT)	*gastr/o* (stomach); from Latin *intestina*, plural of *intestinus* (internal, inward, intestine) + tract	the small intestine and large intestine
mastication (MAS-ti-kay-shun)	from the Latin verb *masticare* (to chew)	the process of chewing food
oral cavity (OR-ul KAV-ih-tee)	from the Latin words *os* (mouth) and *cavus* (hollow)	the mouth
pancreas (PAN-kree-us)	from the Greek words *pan* (all) and *kreas* (flesh, meat)	organ of the digestive system that has both exocrine and endocrine functions; secretes enzymes that aid in digestion
pancreatic (pan-kree-AT-ik)	*pancreat/o* (pancreas); *-ic* (adjective suffix)	adjective for pancreas
peristalsis (pear-ih-STAL-sis)	from the Greek word *peristaltiko* (clasping and compressing)	wavelike muscular contractions that move food along in the digestive tract
pharynx (FAIR-inks)	from the Greek word *pharunx* (throat)	passageway just below the nasal cavity and mouth
pyloric sphincter (pye-LOR-ik SFINGK-tur)	*pylor/o* (pylorus); *-ic* (adjective suffix); sphincter (from the Greek word *sphingein*: to bind tight)	ring of muscle between the stomach and duodenum
rectum (REK-tum)	Latin word for "straight"	the terminal portion of the digestive tract
saliva (suh-LYE-vuh)	Latin word for "spittle"	a clear, tasteless, slightly acidic fluid secreted from the salivary glands
salivary glands (SAL-ih-vair-ee GLANDZ)	from the Latin word *salivarius* (slimy, clammy) + gland from the Latin word *glans* (acorn)	collectively, the parotid, sublingual, and submandibular glands that secrete saliva
stoma (STOH-muh)	a Greek word meaning "mouth," "opening"	an artificial opening
stomach (STUM-eck)	from the Latin word *stomachus* (throat, gullet, stomach)	digestive organ composed of four regions (cardia, fundus, body, and pylorus)
upper gastrointestinal tract (UP-ur GAS-troh-in-TES-tin-ul TRAKT)	*gastr/o* (stomach); from Latin *intestina*, plural of *intestinus* (internal, inward, intestine) + tract	the oral cavity, pharynx, esophagus, and stomach
vermiform appendix (VUR-muh-form uh-PEN-diks)	from Latin word *vermis* (worm) and *appendere* (hang upon)	tube-shaped sac attached into the cecum of the large intestine; also called *appendix*

Term and Pronunciation	Analysis	Meaning
Disorders		
anorexia (an-or-ECKS-ee-uh)	from the Greek *an* (without) + *orexis* (appetite, desire)	loss of appetite
appendicitis (uh-PEN-dih-SIGH-tis)	from the Latin word *appendix* (something attached); *-itis* (inflammation)	inflammation of the appendix
ascites (uh-SIGH-teez)	from the Greek word *askos* (bag)	abnormal accumulation of fluid in the peritoneal cavity
bruxism (BRUKS-iz-um)	from the Greek word *brukhein* (gnash the teeth) + *-ism* (condition)	involuntary grinding of the teeth that usually occurs during sleep
bulimia (bull-EE-mee-uh)	from the Greek word *boulemia* (hunger)	eating disorder characterized by episodes of binge eating followed by self-induced vomiting and misuse of laxatives
cholangiolitis (KOH-lan-jee-oh-LYE-tis)	*cholangi/o* (bile, duct); *-itis* (inflammation)	inflammation of the bile ducts
cholecystitis (KOH-lee-siss-TYE-tis)	*cholecyst/o* (gallbladder); *-itis* (inflammation)	inflammation of the gallbladder
cholecystopathy (KOH-lee-siss-TOP-uh-thee)	*cholecyst/o* (gallbladder); *-pathy* (disease)	any disease of the gallbladder
choledocholithiasis (koh-LED-oh-koh-lith-EYE-uh-sis)	*choledoch/o* (common bile duct); *-lithiasis* (condition of having stones)	inflammation of the bile duct
cholelithiasis (KOH-lee-lih-THIGH-uh-sis)	*chol/e* (bile, gall); *-lithiasis* (condition of having stones)	formation or presence of stones in the gallbladder or bile duct
cirrhosis (sir-OH-sis)	from the Greek word *kirrhos* (tawny), named for the orange-yellow appearance of a diseased liver	chronic disease of the liver
colitis (koh-LYE-tis)	*col/o* (colon); *-itis* (inflammation)	inflammation of the colon
constipation (kon-stih-PAY-shun)	from the Latin word *constipare* (to press or crowd together)	decrease in the frequency of bowel movements; difficulty in passing stools and/or hard, dry stools
Crohn's disease (KRONZ dih-ZEEZ)	named after American B.B. Crohn (1884–1983), one of the team that described it in 1932	autoimmune disorder characterized by chronic inflammation of the intestines, particularly the ileum and colon
dental caries (DEN-tul KAIR-eez)	*dent/i* (tooth); *-al* (adjective suffix) + *caries*, a Latin word meaning "rot," "rottenness," "corruption"	tooth decay
diverticulum (dye-ver-TIK-yoo-lum); diverticula (plural form) (dye-ver-TIK-yoo-luh)	Latin word for "a byway"	a pouch or sac opening from a tube, such as the gut
diverticulitis (dye-ver-tik-yoo-LYE-tis)	from the Latin word *diverticulum* (a byway, side road); *-itis* (inflammation)	inflammation of a diverticulum or sac in the intestinal tract
diverticulosis (dye-ver-tik-yoo-LOH-sis)	*diverticulum* (byway); *-osis* (abnormal condition)	presence of several diverticula of the intestine

(continues)

Study Table The Digestive System		(continued)
Term and Pronunciation	**Analysis**	**Meaning**
Disorders		
duodenitis (doo-odd-en-EYE-tis)	*duoden/o* (duodenum); *-itis* (inflammation)	inflammation of the duodenum
dyspepsia (dis-PEP-see-uh)	from the Greek word *dyspeptos* (hard to digest); *-ia* (condition of)	impairment of digestion
dysphagia (dis-FAY-jee-uh)	*dys-* (difficulty); *phag/o* (eating, swallowing); *-ia* (condition of)	difficulty swallowing
enteritis (en-tuh-RYE-tis)	*enter/o* (intestine); *-itis* (inflammation)	inflammation of the intestine
enterohepatitis (EN-teh-roh-hep-uh-TYE-tiss)	*enter/o* (intestine); *hepat/o* (liver); *-itis* (inflammation)	inflammation of the intestine and liver
enteropathy (en-ter-OP-uh-thee)	*enter/o* (intestine); *-pathy* (disease)	any intestinal disease
eructation (ee-RUK-tay-shun)	from the Latin verb *eructo* (belch)	belching or burping gas up from the stomach
esophagitis (ih-SOF-uh-jye-tiss)	*esophag/o* (esophagus); *-itis* (inflammation)	inflammation of the esophagus
gastric ulcers (GAS-trik UL-surz)	*gastr/o* (stomach); *-ic* (adjective suffix) + ulcer, from the Latin *ulcus*, related to the Greek word *helkos* (wound, sore)	erosion of the gastric mucosa
gastritis (gas-TRY-tiss)	*gastr/o* (stomach); *-itis* (inflammation)	inflammation of the stomach
gastroduodenitis (GAS-troh-doo-oh-den-EYE-tis)	*gastr/o* (stomach); *duoden/o* (duodenum); *-itis* (inflammation)	inflammation of the stomach and duodenum
gastroenteritis (GAS-troh-en-tuh-RYE-tiss)	*gastr/o* (stomach); *enter/o* (intestine); *-itis* (inflammation)	inflammation of the stomach and intestine
gastroesophageal reflux disease (GERD) (GAS-troh-ee-sof-a-JEE-ul REE-flucks dih-ZEEZ)	*gastr/o* (stomach); *esophag/o* (esophagus); *-al* (adjective suffix); + reflux disease	backward flow of stomach acid into the esophagus
gingivitis (JIN-jeh-vye-tiss)	*gingiv/o* (gums); *-itis* (inflammation)	inflammation of the gums
hemorrhoids (HEM-oh-roydz)	from the Greek word *haimorrhoides* derived from *haima* (blood); and *rhoos* (a flowing)	enlarged veins in or near the anus that may cause pain or bleeding
hepatitis (hep-uh-TYE-tisss)	*hepat/o* (liver); *-itis* (inflammation)	inflammation of the liver
hepatogenic (heh-pat-oh-JEN-ick)	*hepat/o* (liver); *-genic* (originating)	originating in the liver
hepatomegaly (heh-PAT-oh-MEG-uh-lee)	*hepat/o* (liver); *-megaly* (enlargement)	enlarged liver

Term and Pronunciation	Analysis	Meaning
Disorders		
hiatal hernia (HYE-ay-tuhl HER-nee-uh)	from the Latin word *hiatus* (gaping, opening); *-al* (adjective suffix) + the Latin word *hernia* (rupture)	protrusion of the stomach
hyperemesis (hy-per-EM-ih-sis)	*hyper-* (excessive); *-emesis* (vomit)	excessive vomiting
icterus (ICK-tur-us)	from Greek word *icterus* (jaundice); also a yellowish-green colored bird that was thought to cure jaundice	jaundice; skin yellowing caused by accumulation of the pigment, bilirubin, typically because of bile duct obstruction; also called *jaundice*
inflammatory bowel disease (IBD) (in-FLAM-ih-tor-ee BOW-el dih-ZEEZ)	from the Latin words *inflammatio* (inflame) and *botellus*, diminutive of *botulus* (sausage) + Old French *desaise* (lack of ease)	chronic inflammation of all or part of the digestive tract; common types include Crohn's disease and ulcerative colitis
inguinal hernia (ING-gwi-nuhl HER-nee-uh)	from the Latin word *inguinalis* (of the groin) + the Latin word *hernia* (rupture)	outpouching of intestines into the inguinal or groin region
intestinal obstruction (in-TES-tih-nul ob-STRUK-shun)	from the Latin words *intestinum* (gut); *-al* (adjective suffix); *obstructionem* (a barrier)	an obstruction in the intestine
intussusception (in-tuh-suh-SEP-shun)	from the Latin word *intus* (within); from the Latin word *suscipere* (undertake; support, accept)	one part of the intestine slipping or telescoping over another
irritable bowel syndrome (IBS) (IR-ih-tuh-bul BOW-el SIN-drome)	from the Latin *irritabilis* (irritate) + from the Latin *botellus*, diminutive of *botulus* (sausage) + from the Greek *sundrome*, from *sun-* (together) + *dramein* (to run)	condition characterized by abdominal pain, constipation, diarrhea, gas, and bloating
jaundice (JAWN-dis)	from Middle French word *jaunisse* (yellow)	yellowish cast to the skin, sclera (white part of the eye), and mucous membranes caused by bile deposits; also called *icterus*
jejunitis (jeh-joo-NYE-tiss)	*jejun/o* (jejunum); *-itis* (inflammation)	inflammation of the jejunum
malaise (muh-LAZE)	from Latin *malus* (bad) + *aise* (ease)	overall feeling of discomfort
melena (muh-LEE-nuh)	from the Greek word *melas* (black)	dark-colored, tarry stools due to the presence of blood
pancreatitis (PAN-kree-uh-TYE-tiss)	*pancreat/o* (pancreas); *-itis* (inflammation)	inflammation of the pancreas
pancreatopathy (PAN-kree-uh-TOP-uh-thee)	*pancreat/o* (pancreas); *-pathy* (disease)	any disease of the pancreas
parotiditis (puh-ROT-ih-DYE-tiss)	from the Greek words *para-* (beside) and *otos* (ear); *-itis* (inflammation)	inflammation of the parotid gland
peritonitis (PAIR-ih-toh-NYE-tiss)	from the Greek words *peri-* (around) and *teinein* (to stretch); *-itis* (inflammation)	inflammation of the peritoneal cavity
polyp (PAHL-up)	from the Latin word *polypus* (cuttlefish)	growth protruding from a stalk in the digestive tract

(continues)

Study Table The Digestive System		*(continued)*
Term and Pronunciation	**Analysis**	**Meaning**
Disorders		
sialoadenitis (SIGH-al-oh-ad-eh-NYE-tiss)	*sial/o* (saliva, salivary gland); *aden/o* (gland); *-itis* (inflammation)	inflammation of a salivary gland
sialoangiitis (SIGH-al-oh-an-jee-EYE-tiss)	*sial/o* (saliva, salivary gland); *angi/o* (vessel); *-itis* (inflammation)	inflammation of a salivary duct
sialorrhea (SIGH-al-oh-REE-uh)	*sial/o* (saliva, salivary gland); *-rrhea* (discharge)	excessive production of saliva
sialostenosis (SIGH-al-oh-steh-NO-siss)	*sial/o* (saliva, salivary gland); *-stenosis* (narrowed, blocked)	narrowing of a salivary duct
stomatitis (STOH-muh-tye-tis)	*stomat/o* (mouth); *-itis* (inflammation)	inflammation of the mucous membranes of the mouth
ulcerative colitis (UC) (UL-sur-uh-tiv koh-LYE-tis)	ulcer, from the Latin *ulcus*, related to the Greek word *helkos* (wound, sore) and *col/o* (colon); *-itis* (inflammation)	disorder of unknown origin that causes inflammation and sores (ulcers) on the lining of the large intestine
volvulus (VOL-vyoo-lus)	from the Latin verb *volvere* "to turn, twist"	a twisting of the intestine
Diagnostic Tests, Treatments, and Surgical Procedures		
antacids (ant-ASS-idz)	from *anti-* (against) + acids	medications used to reduce or neutralize acidity
antidiarrheal (an-tee-DYE-uh-REE-ul)	*anti-* (against); from the Greek *dia-* (through) + *-rrhea* (discharge); *-al* (adjective suffix)	drug that relieves diarrhea by absorbing excess water or by decreasing intestinal motility
antiemetic (an-tee-EE-met-ick)	*anti-* (against); *-emesis* (vomit); *-ic* (adjective suffix)	drug used to relieve vomiting
antiflatulence (an-tee-FLAT-yoo-lens)	*anti-* (against); from the Latin word *flatus* (a blowing, a breaking wind)	drug taken to relieve gas or flatus
cholecystectomy (KOH-lee-siss-TEK-toh-mee)	*cholecyst/o* (gallbladder); *-ectomy* (surgical removal)	removal of the gallbladder
cholecystotomy (KOH-lee-siss-TOT-oh-mee)	*cholecyst/o* (gallbladder); *-tomy* (incision)	incision into the gallbladder
colectomy (koh-LEK-toh-mee)	*col/o* (colon); *-ectomy* (surgical removal)	removal of all or part of the colon
colonoscope (koh-LON-oh-skope)	*colon/o* (colon); *-scope* (instrument for viewing)	long, flexible fiber-optic endoscope used in colonoscopy
colonoscopy (koh-lon-OSS-koh-pee)	*colon/o* (colon); *-scopy* (viewing)	visual examination of the colon with a colonoscope
colopexy (KOH-loh-peck-see)	*col/o* (colon); *-pexy* (surgical fixation)	attachment of a portion of the colon to the abdominal wall
colostomy (koh-LOSS-tuh-mee)	*col/o* (colon); *-stomy* (permanent opening)	surgical establishment of an opening into the colon

Term and Pronunciation	Analysis	Meaning
Diagnostic Tests, Treatments, and Surgical Procedures		
colotomy (koh-LOT-uh-mee)	*col/o* (colon); *-tomy* (incision)	incision into the colon
duodenectomy (doo-oh-den-ECK-toh-mee)	*duoden/o* (duodenum); *-ectomy* (surgical removal)	removal of the duodenum
duodenoscopy (doo-oh-den-OS-kuh-pee)	*duoden/o* (duodenum); *-scopy* (viewing)	visual examination of the duodenum with the aid of an endoscope
duodenostomy (doo-oh-den-OS-toh-mee)	*duoden/o* (duodenum); *-stomy* (permanent opening)	surgical establishment of an opening in the duodenum
emetic (ee-MET-ick)	*emesis* (vomit); *-ic* (adjective suffix)	drug that stimulates or induces vomiting; frequently used in poisoning cases
enteroscope (en-TER-oh-skope)	*enter/o* (intestine); *-scope* (instrument for viewing)	lighted instrument for visually examining the intestines
enteroscopy (en-ter-OS-koh-pee)	*enter/o* (intestine); *-scopy* (viewing)	visual examination of the intestines
gastrectomy (gas-TREK-toh-mee)	*gastr/o* (stomach); *-ectomy* (surgical removal)	removal of part of the stomach
gastroscope (GAS-troh-scope)	*gastr/o* (stomach); *-scope* (instrument for viewing)	lighted instrument (endoscope) for visually examining the stomach
gastroscopy (gas-TROS-koh-pee)	*gastr/o* (stomach); *-scopy* (viewing)	visual examination of the stomach with a lighted instrument (endoscope)
gastrostomy (gas-TROS-toh-mee)	from the Greek word *gaster* (stomach) and *-ostomy* (surgical opening)	surgical procedure for making an opening in the stomach
H2 blockers (H 2 BLOCK-urz)	H2 (histamine 2), a common chemical in the body, signals the stomach to make acid; H2 blockers oppose histamine's action and reduce the amount of acid the stomach produces; + blocker, a common English word	drugs that block the release of gastric acid; used to treat gastroesophageal reflux disease, gastritis, and peptic ulcers; also called *H2-receptor antagonists*
H2-receptor antagonists (H 2 ree-SEP-tur an-TAG-uh-nists)	the drugs compete with histamine binding on the H2 receptors, thereby inhibiting binding and histamine action	drugs that work by reducing the amount of stomach acid produced; also called *H2 blockers*
hepatoscopy (hep-uh-TOS-kuh-pee)	*hepat/o* (liver); *-scopy* (viewing)	visual examination of the liver
hepatopexy (HUH-pat-oh-peck-see)	*hepat/o* (liver); *-pexy* (surgical fixation)	anchoring of the liver to the abdominal wall
ileostomy (ill-ee-OS-toh-mee)	from the Latin word *ileum* (variant of ilium) and the Greek word *stoma* (mouth)	surgical opening into the abdomen to create a diversion for the ileum to the body exterior
jejunectomy (jeh-joon-ECK-toh-mee)	*jejun/o* (jejunum); *-ectomy* (surgical removal)	removal of all or part of the jejunum
jejunoplasty (jeh-JOON-oh-plass-tee)	*jejun/o* (jejunum); *-plasty* (surgical repair)	surgical repair of the jejunum
jejunotomy (jeh-joon-OT-oh-mee)	*jejun/o* (jejunum); *-tomy* (incision)	incision into the jejunum

(continues)

Study Table The Digestive System		*(continued)*
Term and Pronunciation	**Analysis**	**Meaning**
Diagnostic Tests, Treatments, and Surgical Procedures		
nasogastric tube (nay-zoh-GAS-trick TOOB)	naso- (nose) + *gastric* (stomach)	a flexible tube passed through the nose and into the stomach to deliver nutrition or to aspirate (suction out) contents
ostomy (OS-toh-mee)	from the Greek word *stoma* (mouth)	surgical opening in the abdomen that allows waste from the intestines to leave the body into an attached sac
pancreatotomy (PAN-kree-uh-TOT-oh-mee)	*pancreat/o* (pancreas); *-tomy* (incision)	incision into the pancreas
sialoadenectomy (SIGH-al-oh-ad-en-ECK-toh-mee)	*sial/o* (saliva, salivary gland); *aden/o* (gland); *-ectomy* (surgical removal)	removal of a salivary gland
sialoadenotomy (SIGH-al-oh-ad-en-OT-oh-mee)	*sial/o* (saliva, salivary gland); *aden/o* (gland); *-tomy* (incision)	incision of a salivary gland
sialography (SIGH-al-OG-ruh-fee)	*sial/o* (saliva, salivary gland); *-graphy* (the process of recording)	radiography (X-rays) of salivary glands and ducts
stool studies (STOOL stuh-DEEZ)	related to Dutch word *stoel* and German word *Stuhl*	laboratory examination of feces (stool culture) to test for fecal occult (hidden) blood, fecal fat, antigens, bacteria, and parasites
total parenteral nutrition (TPN) (TOH-tul puh-REN-ter-ul noo-TRISH-un)	from the Latin *totalis* (whole, entire); *para-* (beside) + from the Greek *enteron* (intestine); from the Latin *nutrition* (to nourish)	nutrition maintained entirely by central intravenous injection or by other non-gastrointestinal route
upper gastrointestinal series (UGIS) (UP-er gas-troh-in-TES-tin-ul sear-EEZ)	from the Middle English *up* + *-er*; *gastrointestinal* (relating to the stomach and intestines); from the Latin *sero* (to join)	radiographic contrast study (X-rays with dye) of the esophagus, stomach, and duodenum
Practice and Practitioners		
gastroenterologist (GAS-troh-en-tur-OL-oh-jist)	*gastr/o* (stomach); *enter/o* (intestine); *-logist* (one who studies a certain field)	a specialist in the diagnosis and treatment of digestive system disorders
gastroenterology (GAS-troh-en-tur-OL-oh-jee)	*gastr/o* (stomach); *enter/o* (intestine); *-logy* (the study of)	the specialty concerned with the digestive system
internal medicine (in-TUR-nul MED-uh-sin)	from the Latin words *internalis* (inward, internal) and *medicus* (physician)	specialty in the diagnosis and nonsurgical treatment of serious and/or chronic illnesses; the phrase is quite commonly used in North America (but not necessarily elsewhere); it also covers subspecialties in specific organs, such as the liver and kidneys
internist (IN-tur-nist)	internal (English adjective meaning "inside"); *-ist* (practitioner)	a specialist in internal medicine
proctologist (prok-TOL-uh-jist)	*proct/o* (anus and rectum); *-logist* (one who studies a certain field)	a specialist in the diagnosis and treatment of rectal and anal disorders
proctology (prok-TOL-uh-jee)	*proct/o* (anus and rectum); *-logy* (study of)	study of the rectum and anus

CASE STUDY WRAP-UP

By morning, Mario still had abdominal pain and was vomiting. He already had an appointment with his physician sched-uled for the late afternoon to get the results of his recent stool studies, blood tests, and colonoscopy. At his appointment, the doctor told him that he likely had Crohn's disease, but since there is no single test for diagnosis, it was a matter of ruling out other causes. However, Mario fit the profile for a typical Crohn's case. Since this was an early probable diagno-sis, the physician explained many treatments possible, ranging from anti-inflammatory drugs and antidiarrheal medica-tions to immune system suppressors and biologics that target immune system proteins. Currently, there is no cure, but medical management has improved the lives of many.

Case Study Application Questions

1. Describe Crohn's disease.
2. Define diarrhea.
3. What is a colonoscopy?
4. Which treatment would decrease inflammation along the intestinal lining?
5. What is the purpose of the stool studies?

END-OF-CHAPTER EXERCISES

Exercise 13.1 Labeling

Using the following list, choose the terms to label the diagram correctly.

anus	large intestine	pharynx
bile duct	liver	salivary gland
esophagus	mouth	small intestine
gallbladder	pancreas	stomach

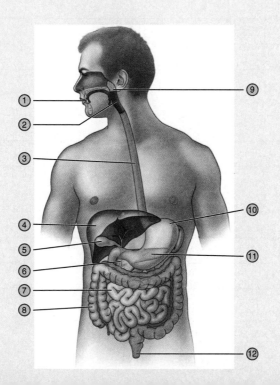

1. _____ 5. _____ 9. _____

2. _____ 6. _____ 10. _____

3. _____ 7. _____ 11. _____

4. _____ 8. _____ 12. _____

Exercise 13.2 Word Parts

Break each of the following terms into its word parts: prefix, root, or suffix. Give the meaning of each word part and then define the term.

1. *cholelithiasis*

   root: _____

   suffix: _____

   suffix: _____

   definition: _____

2. *enterohepatitis*

   root: _____

   root: _____

   suffix: _____

   definition: _____

3. *parotiditis*

   prefix: _____

   root: _____

   suffix: _____

   definition: _____

4. *sialorrhea*

   root: _____

   suffix: _____

   definition: _____

5. *colonoscopy*

   root: _____

   suffix: _____

   definition: _____

6. *gastroenterologist*

   root: _____

   root: _____

   suffix: _____

   definition: _____

7. *colectomy*

   root: _____

   suffix: _____

   definition: _____

8. *jejunotomy*

   root: _____

   suffix: _____

   definition: _____

Exercise 13.3 Word Building

Use the word parts listed to build the terms defined.

-al	enter/o	-ia	phag/o
cholecyst/o	gastr/o	-ic	-pexy
col/o	-genic	-itis	-scope
duoden/o	gingiv/o	jejun/o	sial/o
dys-	hepat/o	-pathy	-stenosis
-ectomy			

1. adjective form of stomach_____

2. any disease of the gallbladder_____

3. inflammation of the gums_____

4. narrowing of a salivary duct_____

5. instrument used to visually examine the intestines_____

6. fixation of the colon_____

7. removal of all or part of the jejunum_____

8. originating in the liver_____

9. difficulty swallowing_____

10. adjective form of duodenum_____

Exercise 13.4 Matching

Match the term with its definition.

1. _____ buccal
2. _____ dentalgia
3. _____ esophagitis
4. _____ duodenum

a. abnormal fluid accumulation in the abdomen

b. cheek

c. narrowing of the esophagus

d. vomiting

5. _____ enteric   e. yellow

6. _____ emesis   f. toothache

7. _____ jaundice   g. first part of small intestine

8. _____ ascites   h. adjective referring to intestine(s)

9. _____ esophagostenosis   i. inflammation of esophagus

10. _____ diarrhea   j. watery discharge from the rectum; liquid stools

Exercise 13.5 Multiple Choice

Choose the correct answer for the following multiple-choice questions.

1. Dysphagia is difficulty with _____.
   a. talking
   b. swallowing
   c. elimination
   d. digestion

2. Anorexia is _____.
   a. difficulty in digestion
   b. hyperemesis
   c. loss of appetite
   d. a small ulcer

3. Gas in the stomach or intestines is _____.
   a. gavage
   b. icterus
   c. flatus
   d. dysentery

4. Diverticulitis is an inflammation of _____.
   a. small pouches in the intestine
   b. the appendix
   c. the pharynx
   d. descending colon

5. Movement of the intestines in which contents are propelled toward the anus is termed _____.
   a. pyloroplasty
   b. volvulus
   c. peristalsis
   d. gastroenteric

6. The buccal mucosa is in the _____.
   a. nostril
   b. stomach and intestines
   c. mouth, inside the cheek
   d. greater curvature of the stomach

7. Belching is called _____.
   a. volvulus
   b. eructation
   c. gastroenteric
   d. halitosis

8. Vomiting blood is called _____.
   a. hematitis
   b. indigestion
   c. mastication
   d. hematemesis

9. Telescoping of the intestines into themselves is called _____.
   a. gastrojejunostomy
   b. intussusception
   c. volvulus
   d. sphincter

10. A colonoscopy is _____.
    a. an endoscopic study of the colon
    b. an upper endoscopy with biopsy
    c. a type of BE
    d. an endoscopic study of the small intestine

Exercise 13.6 Fill in the Blank

Fill in the blank with the correct answer.

1. The sphincter that controls flow from the ileum to the cecum is the _____.
2. The large intestine is divided into the cecum, colon, and _____.
3. Saliva is secreted by the _____.
4. The _____ is responsible for storing, condensing, and delivering bile to the small intestine.
5. A hiatal hernia is a disorder in which the _____ protrudes through the diaphragm.
6. Inflammation of the gallbladder is called _____.
7. Presence of calculi or stones in the gallbladder or bile ducts is called _____.
8. A drug that is used to relieve vomiting is called a(n) _____.
9. The instrument used to view the stomach in a gastroscopy is a(n) _____.
10. Removal of part of the stomach is called a(n) _____.

Exercise 13.7 Abbreviations

Write out the term for the following abbreviations.

1. _____ PO
2. _____ UGIS
3. _____ TPN
4. _____ BM
5. _____ GI
6. _____ GERD
7. _____ IBS
8. _____ LES

Write the abbreviation for the following terms.

9. _____ hydrochloric acid
10. _____ nasogastric
11. _____ barium enema
12. _____ esophagogastro-duodenoscopy
13. _____ nothing by mouth

Exercise 13.8 Spelling

Select the correct spelling of the medical term.

1. The large intestine from the cecum to the rectum is also called the _____.
   a. colon
   b. cologne
   c. collon
   d. colin
2. The GI in GI tract stands for _____.
   a. gastrointestinle
   b. gastrointestinel
   c. gastrointestinal
   d. gastraentestinal
3. A loss of appetite is called _____.
   a. anoresia
   b. anorexia
   c. anarexia
   d. anorexsia
4. _____ is a chronic liver disease characterized by inflammation and degeneration.
   a. Cirosis
   b. Cirrhosis
   c. Cirrosis
   d. Cirhosis
5. A yellowish cast to the skin, scleras, and other mucous membranes caused by bile deposits is called _____.
   a. jandice
   b. juandice
   c. jaundise
   d. jaundice

6. A _____ is a surgical establishment of an opening into the colon.
   a. colostimy
   b. colostamy
   c. colostomy
   d. colostemy
7. Tarry, bloody stool is called _____.
   a. malena
   b. milena
   c. melena
   d. melana
8. A growth protruding from a stalk is a _____.
   a. polyp
   b. polip
   c. pollup
   d. pollyp

9. _____ is an eating disorder characterized by episodes of binge eating followed by self-induced vomiting and misuse of laxatives.
   a. Bullimia
   b. Bullemia
   c. Bulemia
   d. Bulimia
10. A _____ is an enlarged vein in or near the anus that may cause pain or bleeding.
   a. hemoroid
   b. hemorrhoid
   c. hemroid
   d. hemorhoid

Exercise 13.9 Medical Report

Reggie V. is a middle-aged male who began feeling pain in his upper abdomen about a month ago. He described the pain as a burning sensation that at first disappeared after he took over-the-counter antacids. In the last 10 days or so, however, he has noticed that the medication has become less and less helpful.

His pain is not accompanied by SOB, nausea, or chest pains, and his appetite remains normal. His BP was slightly elevated also, and he reported that based on a family history of HTN, his GP had advised him to stop smoking cigarettes and restrict caffeinated drinks to one or two a day.

This patient's WBC count was normal. Endoscopy revealed a 1-cm gastric ulcer.

1. What does the abbreviation SOB stand for? _____
2. What does the abbreviation BP stand for? _____
3. Does the abbreviation HTN have anything to do with the first two abbreviations? Explain how each may relate to the other two. _____
4. What does WBC stand for? _____
5. What word parts make up the word "endoscopy" in the case study? What does the term *endoscopy* mean? _____
6. What is a gastric ulcer? _____

Exercise 13.10 Reflection

1. Bouts of diarrhea are common and any person can get diarrhea. Think about the signs and symptoms you experienced if you had an episode of diarrhea. Do you know what caused the diarrhea?
2. How does the digestive system play a role in your daily activities?
3. What happens to all the food you eat every day?

CHAPTER 14

The Urinary System

LEARNING OUTCOMES

Upon completion of this chapter, you should be able to:

- Name the structures that make up the urinary system.
- Pronounce, spell, and define medical terms related to the urinary system and its disorders.
- Interpret abbreviations associated with the urinary system.
- Apply knowledge gained to case study questions.

CASE STUDY

Skin Frost

J.T. is a 67-year-old male who has type 2 diabetes mellitus. For several days, J.T. had not been feeling well and was very tired. When his daughter came for a routine visit, she found him sleeping in bed. She had great difficulty waking him up. When he finally awakened, his brain was "foggy," and he had trouble talking. He did say that he had not eaten much the past few days, and he could not remember the last time he urinated. When his daughter tried to help him sit up, he was not able to move, and he fell back asleep. Because he was so weak and unresponsive, his daughter called the township emergency medical services.

Introduction

The **urinary system** is composed of the *kidneys, ureters, urinary bladder*, and *urethra* (see **Figure 14.1A**). These organs form, store, and remove urine. These processes start with the **kidneys**, paired structures that remove wastes from the bloodstream, reclaim important electrolytes like sodium and potassium, help regulate blood pressure and fluid balance, and aid in red blood cell production. The kidneys then form **urine**, which is fluid containing water and dissolved substances. The **ureters** are tubular structures that transport urine from the kidneys to the **urinary bladder**, an organ that stores urine. The urine is then eliminated through the **urethra**, a canal leading from the urinary bladder to the exterior. These processes regulate the amount of water in the body and maintain the proper balance of acids and electrolytes, which is necessary for human survival. **Figure 14.1B** shows the processes of urine formation, transport, storage, and elimination.

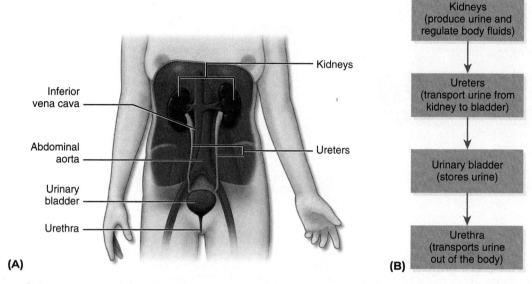

Figure 14.1 Primary organs of the urinary system. **A.** Anterior view of the kidneys, ureters, urinary bladder, and urethra. **B.** The process of urine formation, transport, storage, and elimination, beginning with the kidneys and ending with the urethra.

Word Parts Related to the Urinary System

Nephr/o and ren/o are both root words that mean kidney. The term cyst and the word part cyst/o mean bladder, whereas the word parts ur/o and urin/o mean urine. **Table 14.1** lists word parts used in forming urinary system terms.

What's the difference between the roots nephr/o and ren/o? Both may be used to refer to the kidneys. However, nephr/o is used in the names of most, but not all, kidney disorders and treatments. For example, nephr/o is the root in nephritis, nephralgia, nephrectomy, nephrorrhaphy, nephrotomy, and nephromegaly. In general, the term *nephrology* is also more common than renology, but the adjective renal is far more common than its counterpart, nephric. Renal is more common when naming structures, such as the renal capsule and the renal fascia.

Table 14.1 Word Parts Related to the Urinary System

Word Part	Meaning
cyst/o	bladder
glomerul/o	glomerulus
-iasis	condition, state
lith/o	stone
nephr/o, ren/o	kidney
noct/o	night
olig/o	few, little
poly-	much, many
py/o	pus
pyel/o	pelvis
ur/o, urin/o	urine
ureter/o	ureter
urethr/o	urethra

Word Parts Exercise

After studying Table 14.1, write the meaning of each of the word parts.

1. ur/o, urin/o	1. _____
2. noct/o	2. _____
3. olig/o	3. _____
4. -iasis	4. _____
5. glomerul/o	5. _____
6. nephr/o, ren/o	6. _____
7. urethr/o	7. _____
8. lith/o	8. _____
9. poly-	9. _____
10. py/o	10. _____

Structure and Function

The kidneys are bean-shaped organs (hence the source for the name of the kidney bean) and are about the size of a deck of cards. They lie retroperiotoneally, which is posterior to the peritoneum in the abdominopelvic cavity, along each side of the spinal column. Each kidney is covered by a thin membrane called the *fibrous capsule*. A thicker layer of fatty tissue, called the **perinephric fat** or *pararenal fat body*, surrounds the fibrous capsule and thus provides protection for this vital organ. Finally, a thin layer of connective tissue, called the **renal fascia**, forms each kidney's outer covering. The two regions of the kidney are the outer **renal cortex** and the inner **renal medulla**. The **hilum** is the indented and narrowest part of the kidney, where blood vessels and nerves enter and leave. The flattened funnel-shaped expansion of the upper (superior) end of the ureter where urine collects in the kidney is called the **renal pelvis**. The cup-like structure that drains into the renal pelvis is the **calyx**. **Figure 14.2** shows the anatomy of a kidney.

The kidneys form urine and remove two natural products of metabolism, **urea** and **uric acid**, along with other wastes from the blood. The kidneys also filter, reabsorb, and secrete nonwaste products back into the bloodstream.

Filtration and urine production begin in the **nephrons**, which are the functional units of the kidneys. Each kidney has approximately 1 million nephrons, and each nephron consists of the *renal corpuscle* and *renal tubule*. The **renal corpuscle** is a structure composed of the *glomerulus* and the *glomerular capsule*, also called Bowman's capsule. The **glomerulus** consists of a cluster of capillaries through which blood and wastes are filtered. The **renal tubule** consists of the *proximal convoluted tubule*, *nephron loop* (loop of Henle), and the *distal convoluted tubule* (see **Figure 14.3**). Fluid not returned to the bloodstream becomes urine. It is collected in the *collecting duct* and moves into the renal pelvis before ultimately entering the ureter. The ureters carry the urine to the urinary bladder, where it is stored.

The urinary bladder stores the urine until a sufficient volume causes an increase in pressure and triggers the urge to urinate via the *micturition reflex*. The **micturition reflex** (*urination reflex*) involves contraction of the urinary bladder walls and relaxation of the urethral sphincter in response to the increase in urinary bladder pressure. Micturition is also called *urination*, *uresis*, or *voiding*. Urination is regulated by two sphincters, the circular muscles that surround the urethra. They are the *internal urethral sphincter*, which is located at the entrance to the urethra and

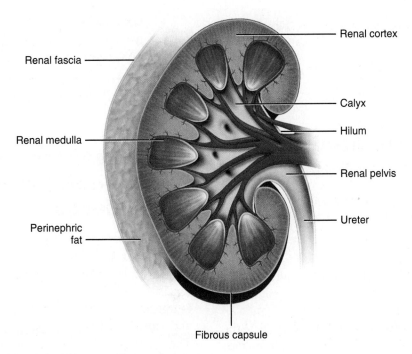

Figure 14.2 Sagittal view of the kidney and internal structures.

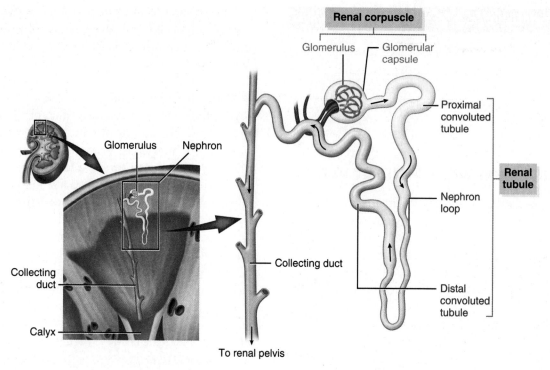

Figure 14.3 Section of the kidney showing a representative nephron.

is involuntarily controlled, and the *external urethral sphincter*, which is located at the distal end of the urethra and is under voluntary control.

QUICK CHECK

Fill in the blanks.

1. Name the primary organs of the urinary system: _____, _____, _____, and _____.

2. The indented part of the kidney, where blood vessels and nerves enter or exit, is called the _____.

3. Name the two urethral sphincters: _____ _____.

Disorders Related to the Urinary System

Disorders of the urinary system can affect any urinary structures. Some of these disorders include the following:

- **Dysuria**: painful, difficult urination
- **Incontinence**: the loss of urinary control
- **Retention**: the inability to completely empty the bladder
- **Urinary tract infection** (UTI): infection of the urinary tract. Examples of urinary tract infections include the following:

- **Cystitis**: inflammation of the urinary bladder, usually caused by infection
- **Glomerulonephritis**: inflammation of the glomerulus, which can involve one or both kidneys, usually caused by infection
- **Nephritis**: inflammation of the kidney(s), usually caused by infection
- **Pyelonephritis**: inflammation of the calyces and renal pelvis, typically due to bacterial infection
- **Urethritis**: inflammation of the urethra, usually caused by infection
- **Renal failure** or *end-stage renal disease* (ESRD) is loss of renal function that results in kidneys ceasing urine production. It can be acute renal failure (ARF) or chronic renal failure (CRF).

Diagnostic Tests, Treatments, and Surgical Procedures

The root cyst/o is used to form terms having to do with the urinary bladder. Examples include **cystalgia** (pain in the urinary bladder), **cystectomy** (excision of the urinary bladder), and **cystopexy** (surgical attachment of the urinary bladder to the abdominal wall or to other supporting structures). These terms come from the Greek word *kystis*, which means bladder.

A test of kidney function is the *glomerular filtration rate* (GFR). This test determines the volume of water filtered out of the blood plasma through the capillary walls into the glomerular capsule per unit of time. An X-ray or computed tomography (CT) scan of the kidneys, ureters, and bladder (KUB) after intravenous injection of a contrast dye is known as an *intravenous pyelogram* (IVP). The contrast dye is injected into a vein and is excreted by the kidneys to show the urinary system. Blood urea nitrogen (BUN) is a blood test that measures kidney function by assessing the levels of nitrogenous waste and urea in the blood.

Practice and Practitioners

A physician who specializes in the diagnosis and treatment of urinary disorders is called a **urologist**, and the specialty practice is **urology**. A physician who treats the kidney and kidney disorders is called a **nephrologist**. This area of specialty is named **nephrology**.

Abbreviation Table The Urinary System

Abbreviation	Meaning
ARF	acute renal failure
BUN	blood urea nitrogen
CAPD	continuous ambulatory peritoneal dialysis
CRF	chronic renal failure
CT	computed tomography
ESRD	end-stage renal disease
GFR	glomerular filtration rate
IVP	intravenous pyelogram
KUB	kidneys, ureter, and bladder
UA	urinalysis
UACR	urine albumin-to-creatinine ratio
UTI	urinary tract infection

Study Table The Urinary System

Term and Pronunciation	Analysis	Meaning
Structure and Function		
calyx (KAY-licks)	from the Greek *kalux* (cup of a flower)	cup-like structure that drains into the renal pelvis
electrolyte (ee-LEK-troh-lyte)	from the Greek words *electron* (able to produce static electricity by friction) and *lytos* (soluble)	an ionizable substance, such as sodium or potassium, in solution within body cells
glomerulus (gloh-MER-yu-lus)	from the Latin word *glomus* (ball of yarn)	capillary network found inside each nephron
hilum (HIGH-lum)	Latin word meaning "a small thing," "a trifle"	narrow part of the kidney where blood vessels and nerves enter and leave
kidney (KID-nee)	originally *kidenere*, perhaps a compound of Old English *cwith* (womb) + *neere* (kidney) in reference to the shape of the organ	organ that excretes urine, removes nitrogenous wastes of metabolism, reclaims electrolytes and water, and contributes to blood pressure and red blood cell production
micturition (mik-chuh-RISH-un)	from the Latin *micturio* (to desire to urinate)	urination; also called *uresis* and *voiding*
micturition reflex (mik-chuh-RISH-un REE-flecks)	from the Latin *micturio* (to desire to urinate) and the Latin word *reflexus* (to bend back)	contraction of the bladder walls and relaxation of the bladder and urethral sphincter in response to an increase in pressure within the bladder
nephron (NEFF-ron)	from the Greek word *nephros* (kidney)	tiny structure within the kidney in which the urine production process begins
pararenal fat (PAIR-uh-ree-nul FAT)	*para-* (beside, next to) + *renal* (kidney)	fatty tissue surrounding the renal capsule; also called *perinephric fat*

(continues)

Study Table The Urinary System		*(continued)*
Term and Pronunciation	**Analysis**	**Meaning**
Structure and Function		
perinephric fat (PAIR-ih-NEF-rick FAT)	*peri-* (around); *nephr-* (kidney) *-ic* (adjective suffix)	fatty tissue surrounding the renal capsule; also called *pararenal fat body*
renal capsule (REE-nul KAP-sul)	*ren/o* (kidney); *-al* (adjective suffix); *capsula*, a Latin word meaning "a small box"	thin membrane covering each kidney, deep to the perinephric fat and renal fascia
renal corpuscle (REE-nul KOR-pus-el)	from the Latin word *renalis* (kidneys) + the Latin word *corpusculum* (body)	the collection of glomerular capillaries and the glomerular (Bowman's) capsule that encloses them
renal cortex (REE-nul KOR-tecks)	from the Latin words *renalis* (kidneys) and *cortex* (bark)	outer region of the kidney
renal fascia (REE-nul FASH-ee-uh)	*ren/o* (kidney); *-al* (adjective suffix); *fascia*, a Latin word meaning band or sash	protective outer covering of the kidney
renal medulla (REE-nul meh-DOO-luh)	from the Latin word *renalis* (kidneys); from the French word *medius* (middle)	inner region of the kidney
renal pelvis (REE-nul PEL-vis)	from the Latin words *renalis* (kidneys) and *pelvis* (basin)	a reservoir in each kidney that collects urine
renal tubule (REE-nul TOOB-yul)	from the Latin words *renalis* (kidneys) and *tubulus* (tube)	small tubes including the proximal convoluted tubule, nephron loop (loop of Henle), and the distal convoluted tubule that convey urine from the glomeruli to the renal pelvis
retroperitoneal (reh-troh-pair-ih-toh-NEE-ul)	*retro-* (backward, behind); from the Greek word *peritenein* (to stretch over)	external or posterior to the peritoneum, which is a serous membrane lining the abdominopelvic cavity
sphincter (SFINK-tur)	from the Greek word *sphincter* (band; anything that binds tight)	circular muscle that surrounds a tube such as the urethra and constricts the tube when it contracts
urea (yu-REE-uh)	from the French word *uree* (urine)	natural waste product of metabolism that is excreted in urine
uresis (yu-REE-sis)	from ancient Greek *ouresis* (urination)	excretion of urine; also called *urination*
ureter (yu-REE-tur; also YUR-eh-tur)	from the Greek word *oureter*, from *ourein* (to urinate)	two tubes that transfer urine from the kidneys to the urinary bladder
urethra (yu-REE-thruh)	from the Greek word *ourethra*, from *ourein* (to urinate)	tube that conducts urine away from the bladder for expulsion
uric acid (YUR-ick ASS-id)	*ur/o* (urine); *-ic* (adjective suffix) + acid from the Latin word *acidus* (sour-tasting)	natural waste product of metabolism that is excreted in urine
urinary bladder (YUR-in-air-ee BLAD-dur)	from the Greek word *ouron* (urine); Anglo-Saxon, *blaedre* (bladder)	temporary storage organ for urine
urinate (YUR-in-ate)	*urin/o* (urine); *-ate* (verb suffix)	passing of urine
urine (YUR-in)	from the Greek word *ouron* (urine)	water and soluble substances excreted by the kidneys

Term and Pronunciation	Analysis	Meaning
Structure and Function		
void (voyd)	from Old French *voide* (empty, hollow, waste)	to urinate
voiding (VOYD-ing)	from Old French *voide* (empty, hollow, waste)	urinating
Disorders		
albuminuria (al-byu-min-YUR-ee-uh)	from the Latin *albumen* (egg white); *ur/o* (urine); *-ia* (condition)	presence of the protein, albumin, in the urine, typically a sign of kidney disease
anuria (an-YUR-ee-uh)	*an-* (without); *ur/o* (urine); *-ia* (condition)	failure of the kidneys to produce urine
azotemia (ay-zoh-TEE-mee-uh)	*-azo* (nitrogen) + *-emia* (substance present in blood); nitrogen is an element in urea	an excess of urea in the blood; also called *uremia*
calculus (KAL-kyu-lus); plural: calculi (KAL-kyu-lye)	a Latin word meaning small pebble	a kidney stone (in the context of this body system)
cystalgia (sis-TAL-jee-uh)	*cyst/o* (bladder); *-algia* (pain)	pain in the urinary bladder
cystitis (sis-TYE-tis)	*cyst/o* (bladder); *-itis* (inflammation)	inflammation of the urinary bladder
cystocele (SIS-toh-seel)	*cyst/o* (bladder); *-cele* (hernia)	hernia of the urinary bladder
cystolith (SIS-toh-lith)	*cyst/o* (bladder); *-lith* (stone)	urinary bladder stone
dysuria (dis-YUR-ee-uh)	*dys-* (difficult); *ur/o* (urine); *-ia* (condition)	difficult or painful urination
enuresis (en-yoo-REE-sis)	from Greek *enourein* (to urinate in)	bedwetting
glomerulonephritis (gloh-mer-yoo-loh-ne-FRY-tis)	*glomerul/o* (glomerulus); *nephr/o* (kidney); *-itis* (inflammation)	inflammation of the kidney glomeruli typically caused by an immune response and not an acute response to kidney infection
glucosuria (GLOO-kohs-YUR-ee-uh)	from French word *glucos* (sugar); *ur/o* (urine); *-ia* (condition)	presence of carbohydrates (sugar) in the urine; also called *glycosuria*
glycosuria (gly-kohs-YUR-ee-uh)	*glycos-* (sugar); *ur/o* (urine); *-ia* (condition)	presence of carbohydrates (sugar) in the urine; also called *glucosuria*
hematuria (hee-muh-CHOO-ree-uh)	*hemat/o* (blood); *ur/o* (urine); *-ia* (adjective suffix)	presence of blood in the urine
incontinence (in-KON-tih-nents)	from the Latin word *incontinentia* (inability to retain)	inability to control urination
nephralgia (nef-RAL-jee-uh)	*nephr/o* (kidney); *-algia* (pain)	pain in the kidneys
nephritis (nef-RYE-tis)	*nephr/o* (kidney); *-itis* (inflammation)	inflammation of the kidney

(continues)

Study Table The Urinary System		*(continued)*
Term and Pronunciation	**Analysis**	**Meaning**
Disorders		
nephrolithiasis (NEF-roh-lih-THY-uh-sis)	*nephr/o* (kidney); *lith/o* (stone); *-iasis* (condition)	the presence of renal calculi
nephromegaly (nef-roh-MEG-uh-lee)	*nephr/o* (kidney); *-megaly* (enlargement)	enlargement of one or both kidneys; also called *renomegaly*
nephropathy (nef-ROP-uh-thee)	*nephr/o* (kidney); *-pathy* (disease)	any disease of the kidney
nephroptosis (nef-ROP-toh-sis)	*nephr/o* (kidney); *-ptosis* (falling downward, prolapse)	prolapse (slipping out of position) of the kidney
nocturia (nok-CHUR-ee-uh)	*noct/o* (night); *ur/o* (urine); *-ia* (condition)	excessive urination at night
oliguria (oh-lig-YUR-ee-uh)	*olig/o* (little); *ur/o* (urine); *-ia* (condition)	diminished urine production
polyuria (pol-ee-YUR-ee-uh)	*poly-* (much, many); *ur/o* (urine); *-ia* (condition)	excessive urine production
pyelonephritis (pye-el-oh-nef-RYE-tis)	*pyel/o* (pelvis); *nephr/o* (kidney); *-itis* (inflammation)	inflammation of the renal calyces and renal pelvis due to local bacterial infection
pyuria (pye-YOUR-ee-uh)	*py/o* (pus); *ur/o* (urine); *-ia* (condition)	pus in the urine
renal calculus (REE-nul KAL-kyu-lus)	*ren/o* (kidney); *calculus*, a Latin word meaning "stone"	a kidney stone
renal failure (REE-nul FAIL-yur)	*ren/o* (kidney); *-al* (adjective suffix); from the French word *failer* (failure)	impairment of renal function, either acute or chronic, with retention of urea, creatinine (compound produced by the metabolism of creatinine), and other wastes
renomegaly (REN-oh-meg-uh-lee)	*reno-* (kidney) + *-megaly* (enlargement)	enlargement of one or both kidneys; also called *nephromegaly*
renal hypoplasia (REE-nul HIGH-poh-PLAY-zee-uh)	*ren/o* (kidney); *hypo-* (below normal); *-plasia* (formation, development)	an underdeveloped kidney
retention (ree-TEN-shun)	from the Latin word *retentio* (a retaining, a holding back)	the inability to empty the bladder
uremia (yu-REE-mee-uh)	*ur/o* (urine); *-emia* (blood condition)	an excess of urea in the blood; also called *azotemia*
uremic frost (yu-REE-mick FROST)	from Greek words *ouron* (urine) and *haima* (blood) + German word *Frost* (freeze)	manifestation of azotemia (excess urea in the blood) in which small, yellow-white urea crystals deposit on the skin as sweat evaporates
ureteritis (yu-ree-tur-EYE-tis)	*ureter/o* (ureter); *-itis* (inflammation)	inflammation of a ureter
urethralgia (yu-ree-THRAL-jee-uh)	*urethr/o* (urethra); *-algia* (pain)	pain in the urethra; *urethrodynia*

Term and Pronunciation	Analysis	Meaning
Disorders		
urethritis (yu-ree-THRIGH-tis)	*urethr/o* (urethra); *-itis* (inflammation)	inflammation of the urethra
urethrostenosis (yu-REE-throh-sten-OH-sis)	*urethr/o* (urethra); *sten/o* (narrow); *-sis* (condition)	narrowing of the urethra
urinary tract infection (yur-in-AIR-ee TRAKT in-FEK-shun)	*urin/o* (urine); *-ary* (adjective suffix)	microbial infection of any part of the urinary tract
Diagnostic Tests, Treatments, and Surgical Procedures		
antibiotic (an-tee-BYE-ot-ick)	from *anti-* (against) + the Greek word *biotikos* (fit for life)	medicine that inhibits the growth of bacteria
blood urea nitrogen (BUN) (BLUD yoo-REE-uh nigh-TROH-jen)	term related to German *Blut* (blood) + from Greek *ouron* (urine) + from French *nitrogene* (chemical element, nitrogen)	test that measures the amount of urea nitrogen in the blood; the liver produces urea as a waste product of protein metabolism; the test is an indicator of kidney function; increased amounts indicate high protein diet or decreased glomerular filtration rate (GFR)
catheter (CATH-eh-tur)	from the Greek word *kathienai* (to let down, thrust in)	a flexible tube that enables passage of fluid from or into a body cavity
continuous ambulatory peritoneal dialysis (CAPD) (KUN-tin-yu-us pair-ih-TOH-nee-ul- dye-AL-ih-sis)	from Latin words *continuus* (unbroken) and *ambulatorius* (to walk) + Greek words *peritonaion* (stretched round) and *dialusis* (to separate)	filtration to remove colloidal particles from a fluid; a method of artificial kidney function; fluid flows through a catheter (tube) in the abdomen where the peritoneum acts as the filter to remove wastes
cystectomy (sis-TEK-toh-mee)	*cyst/o* (bladder); *-ectomy* (excision)	excision of the urinary bladder
cystopexy (SIS-toh-peks-ee)	*cyst/o* (bladder); *-pexy* (fixation)	surgical attachment (fixation) of the urinary bladder to the abdominal wall or other supporting structures
cystoscopy (sis-TOS-koh-pee)	*cyst/o* (bladder); *-scopy* (use of an instrument for viewing)	visual inspection of the urinary bladder by means of an instrument called a cystoscope
dialysis (dye-AL-ih-sis)	a Greek word meaning "dissolution," "separation"	filtration to remove colloidal particles from a fluid; a method of artificial kidney function; types include continuous ambulatory peritoneal dialysis (CAPD) and extracorporeal dialysis
diuretic (dye-yu-RET-ick)	from the Greek words *dia-* (through) and *ourein* (urine)	drug that promotes urination
extracorporeal dialysis (EKS-truh-kor-POR-ee-ul dye-AL-ih-sis)	from the Latin words *extra* (outside) and *corpus* (body) and from Greek word, *dialusis* (to separate)	filtering blood through a semipermeable membrane outside the body
glomerular filtration rate (GFR) (glow-MER-you-lur fill-TRAY-shun RATE)	from the Latin words *glomus* (ball of thread) and *filtrum* (felt used as a filter)	test that indicates kidney function by measuring the flow of filtered fluid through the kidney

(continues)

Study Table The Urinary System		*(continued)*
Term and Pronunciation	**Analysis**	**Meaning**
Diagnostic Tests, Treatments, and Surgical Procedures		
hemodialysis (HEE-moh-dye-AL-ih-sis)	*hemo-* (blood); *dialysis*, a Greek word meaning "dissolution," "separation"	removal of unwanted substances from the blood by passage through a semipermeable membrane; also called *kidney dialysis*
kidney transplant (KID-nee TRANS-plant)	originally *kidenere*, perhaps a compound of Old English *cwith* (womb) + *neere* (kidney) in reference to the shape of the organ; from the late Latin *transplantare* (something moved to a new place)	operation in which a donor kidney is placed into a recipient
lithotripsy (LITH-oh-trip-see)	*lith/o* (stone); *-tripsy* (crushing)	treatment in which a stone in the kidney, urethra, or urinary bladder is broken up into small particles
nephrectomy (nef-REK-toh-mee)	*nephr/o* (kidney); *-ectomy* (removal)	removal of a kidney
nephrolithotomy (NEF-roh-lith-OT-oh-mee)	*nephr/o* (kidney); *lith/o* (stone); *-tomy* (incision into)	incision into the kidney to remove a kidney stone
nephropexy (NEF-roh-pek-see)	*nephr/o* (kidney) + the Greek work *pexis* (fixation)	operative fixation of a floating or mobile kidney
ureteroplasty (yu-REE-tur-oh-plass-tee)	*ureter/o* (ureter); *-plasty* (surgical repair)	surgical repair of a ureter
ureterorrhaphy (yu-ree-tur-OR-uh-fee)	*ureter/o* (ureter); *-rrhaphy* (surgical suturing)	suturing a ureter
ureteroscope (yu-REE-tur-oh-skope)	*ureter/o* (ureter); *-scope* (instrument for viewing)	instrument used to visually examine the ureter
urinalysis (UA) (yur-in-AL-ih-sis)	*urin/o* (urine); *-alysis* from the English word analysis	analysis of urine by physical, chemical, and microscopic means to test for the presence of substances or disease
Practice and Practitioners		
nephrologist (nef-ROL-oh-jist)	*nephr/o* (kidney); *-logist* (one who studies a special field)	a medical specialist who diagnoses and treats disorders of the kidney
nephrology (nef-ROL-oh-jee)	*nephr/o* (kidney); *-logy* (study of)	medical specialty dealing with the kidneys
urologist (yur-OL-oh-jist)	*ur/o* (urine); *-logist* (one who studies a special field)	a medical specialist who diagnoses and treats disorders of the urinary system
urology (yur-OL-oh-jee)	*ur/o* (urine); *-logy* (study of)	the medical specialty dealing with the urinary system

CASE STUDY WRAP-UP

J.T. was transported to the local hospital where the emergency department staff began a series of tests. J.T.'s skin also had a frosted appearance, a condition known as uremic frost. Given J.T.'s history of diabetes and his presumed failure to urinate, a glomerular filtration test and a urine test for albumin were ordered. The results follow:

GFR Results	Normal	Kidney Disease	Kidney Failure
30	60 or greater	15–60	0–15
Urine albumin-to-creatinine ratio (UACR) Results		Normal	Kidney Disease
35 mg/g		30 mg/g or less	30 mg/g or more

Case Study Application Questions

1. Identify J.T.'s underlying medical condition.
2. Define GFR, and explain what it measures.
3. What do the test results indicate?
4. Give the term for albumin in the urine.
5. What is the term for excess urea in the blood?

END-OF-CHAPTER EXERCISES

Exercise 14.1 Labeling

Using the following word list, choose the terms to label the diagram correctly.

abdominal aorta   kidneys   urethra

inferior vena cava   ureters   urinary bladder

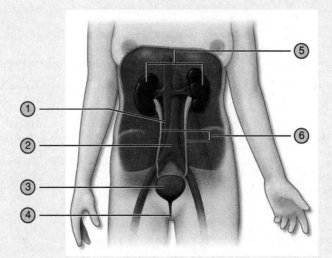

1. _____   3. _____   5. _____

2. _____   4. _____   6. _____

Exercise 14.2 Word Parts

Break each of the following terms into its word parts: root, prefix, or suffix. Give the meaning of each word part and then define each term.

1. *anuria*

   prefix: _____

   root: _____

   suffix: _____

   definition: _____

2. *cystalgia*

   root: _____

   suffix: _____

   definition: _____

3. *nephrolithiasis*

   root: _____

   root: _____

   suffix: _____

   definition: _____

4. *hematuria*

   root: _____

   root: _____

   suffix: _____

   definition: _____

5. *glomerulonephritis*

   root: _____

   root: _____

   suffix: _____

   definition: _____

6. *nephrologist*

   root: _____

   suffix: _____

   definition: _____

7. *urology*

   root: _____

   suffix: _____

   definition: _____

8. *nephrectomy*

   root: _____

   suffix: _____

   definition: _____

Exercise 14.3 Word Building

Use the word parts listed to build the terms defined.

albumen	urethro	-tripsy	cyst/o
-ur/o	-stenosis	ur/o	-ectomy
-ia	ur/o	-logist	-scope
nephro	-emia	nephr/o	urter/o
-aliga	lith/o	-logy	-rrhaphy

1. presence of protein in urine _____

2. pain in the kidneys _____

3. narrowing of the urethra _____

4. an excess of urea in the blood _____

5. treatment in which a stone is broken into smaller particles _____

6. one who studies the urinary system _____

7. study of the kidney _____

8. excision of the bladder _____

9. instrument used to examine the bladder _____

10. suture of a ureter _____

Exercise 14.4 Matching

Match the term with its definition.

1. _____ nephron
2. _____ urethra
3. _____ renal calculus
4. _____ glomerulus
5. _____ micturition
6. _____ uric acid
7. _____ ureters
8. _____ hilum
9. _____ electrolyte
10. _____ UA
11. _____ nephralgia
12. _____ nephritis
13. _____ urethrostenosis
14. _____ nephrolithotomy
15. _____ nephroureterocystectomy
16. _____ ureterography
17. _____ cystalgia
18. _____ nephropathy

a. capillary network found inside each nephron
b. urination
c. pain in the bladder
d. tube that conducts urine away from the bladder for excretion
e. an ionizable substance in solution within body cells
f. narrow part of the kidney where blood vessels and nerves enter and exit
g. functional unit of the kidney
h. two tubes that transfer urine from the kidneys to the urinary bladder
i. X-ray of the ureter
j. natural waste product of metabolism excreted in the urine
k. a kidney stone
l. excision of a kidney, ureter, and at least part of the urinary bladder
m. inflammation of the kidney
n. narrowing of the urethra
o. any disease of the kidney
p. pain in the kidneys
q. incision into the kidney to remove a calculus (kidney stone)
r. urinalysis

Exercise 14.5 Multiple Choice

Choose the correct answer for the following multiple-choice questions.

1. The _____ carry the urine from the renal pelvis to the urinary bladder.
   a. urethra
   b. meatus
   c. cortex
   d. ureters
2. The inability to hold urine is called _____.
   a. polyuria
   b. incontinence
   c. hematuria
   d. enuresis
3. Excretion of urine from the bladder is properly termed as _____.
   a. voiding
   b. micturition
   c. urination
   d. all the above
4. The functioning unit of the kidney is the _____.
   a. nephron
   b. cortex of the kidney
   c. glomeruli
   d. pelvis of the kidney

5. What does anuria mean?
   a. failure to produce urine
   b. no urine from the kidney
   c. painful urination
   d. pus in the urine
6. What term means destruction of kidney tissue?
   a. nephrolithiasis
   b. neurolysis
   c. nephrolysis
   d. resection
7. What is the correct plural form of the word calculus?
   a. calcula
   b. calculuses
   c. calculi
   d. calculae

8. What is the term for surgical repair of a ureter?
   a. ureterectomy
   b. ureteroplasty
   c. ureterectasia
   d. ureterolysis
9. A hernia of the urinary bladder is called a _____.
   a. cystitis
   b. cystocele
   c. cystalgia
   d. cystolith
10. Which of the following is NOT a correct match between a word part and its definition?
   a. cyst/o; bladder
   b. py/o; pus
   c. pyel/o; pelvis
   d. urethr/o; ureter

Exercise 14.6 Fill in the Blank

1. Tom suffered from CRF. His sister donated one of her normal kidneys to him and he had a(n) _____.
2. Cindy had a floating kidney that required surgical fixation. Her urologist performed a surgical procedure known as a(n) _____.
3. The surgeons operated on Robert to remove a kidney stone (calculus) from his kidney. The name of this surgery is _____.
4. Gabbi had to have one of her ureters repaired because of a stricture. This procedure is called _____.
5. The physician had to examine Joshua's bladder for blood. They used a special instrument. This procedure is called a(n) _____.
6. _____ are medications that promote urination.
7. The two tubes that transfer urine from the kidneys to the urinary bladder are the _____.
8. Natural waste products of metabolism that are excreted in urine include _____.
9. Filtration to remove colloidal particles from a fluid is called _____.
10. The word part *-logist* in urologist means _____.

Exercise 14.7 Abbreviations

Write out the term for the following abbreviations.

1. _____ UTI
2. _____ GFR
3. _____ ESRD
4. _____ BUN
5. _____ CRF

Write the abbreviation for the following terms.

6. _____ urinalysis
7. _____ kidney, ureter, and bladder
8. _____ acute renal failure
9. _____ intravenous pyelogram
10. _____ continuous ambulatory peritoneal dialysis

Exercise 14.8 Spelling

Select the correct spelling of the medical term.

1. The _____ is a tiny structure within the kidney in which the urine production process begins.
   a. nephron
   b. nephran
   c. nephren
   d. nefron

2. An _____ is an ionizable substance in solution.
   a. electrolyte
   b. electralyte
   c. electrolite
   d. electrelyte

3. A circular muscle that surrounds a tube and constricts the tube when it contracts is called a _____.
   a. spincter
   b. sphincter
   c. sphicter
   d. sphinter

4. The presence of protein in the urine is _____.
   a. albumineria
   b. albumineralia
   c. albumineuria
   d. albuminuria

5. A _____ is a drug that promotes the excretion of urine.
   a. diretic
   b. diuritic
   c. diuretic
   d. duiretic

6. Excessive urination at night is known as _____.
   a. nocturia
   b. nocturnia
   c. nocteria
   d. nockturia

7. A _____ is a flexible tube that enables passage of fluid from or into a body cavity.
   a. cathater
   b. cathiter
   c. catheter
   d. cathuter

8. Difficult or painful urination is called _____.
   a. dysurea
   b. disuria
   c. disurea
   d. dysuria

9. A treatment in which a stone in the kidney, urethra, or urinary bladder is broken up into small particles is called _____.
   a. lithutripsy
   b. lithetripsy
   c. lithotripsy
   d. lithotripsee

10. The purpose of a _____ is to detect and manage a wide range of disorders, which can include diabetes, kidney disease, or UTIs.
    a. urinalasis
    b. urinealysis
    c. urinlasis
    d. urinalysis

Exercise 14.9 Medical Report

Read the following case study. There are 11 phrases that can be reworded with a medical term that was introduced in this chapter. Determine what the term is, and write your answers in the space provided.

Heather is a 40-year-old female who saw a (1) specialist who treats disorders of the urinary system for complaints of urinary frequency, (2) painful urination, (3) blood in her urine, and lower abdominal pain. She was also experiencing a low-grade fever and general fatigue. The doctor ordered a (4) laboratory reading of her urine and an (5) X-ray of her kidneys, ureters, and bladder. The laboratory results showed red blood cells in the urine, and the urine was cloudy with an odor. Tests indicated multiple (6) small, round, calcified objects in the (7) urine reservoir. Heather was diagnosed with a (8) condition of having bacteria in the urinary tract and (9) stones in her bladder. The doctor ordered a(n) (10) drug used to kill bacteria, and he told Heather that she needed to have a(n) (11) procedure in which a scope is inserted into the bladder to remove the stones. Heather's signs and symptoms improved, and she returned to have the procedure. Her recovery was uneventful.

1. _____
2. _____
3. _____
4. _____
5. _____
6. _____
7. _____
8. _____
9. _____
10. _____

Exercise 14.10 Reflection

1. Describe something that you found particularly interesting in this chapter.
2. Think about what would happen to all the liquid a person ingests in a day if the kidneys were not producing urine.

CHAPTER 15

The Reproductive System

LEARNING OUTCOMES

Upon completion of this chapter, you should be able to:

- Label diagrams of the male and female reproductive systems.
- Name the structures that make up the reproductive system.
- Understand medical terms related to pregnancy.
- Pronounce, spell, and define medical terms related to the reproductive system and its disorders.
- Interpret abbreviations associated with the reproductive system.
- Apply knowledge gained to case study questions.

CASE STUDY

Paige's Problematic Pregnancy

Paige is a 36-year-old active, healthy female with two children and a demanding career. She is also 23 weeks pregnant. Her pregnancy has been unremarkable except for fatigue, which she considered normal because she was tired during her last two pregnancies. That morning, while walking up a flight of stairs at home, she felt blood trickle down her leg. She rushed to the bathroom to see what was happening. Paige discovered that she was having vaginal bleeding, so she phoned her OB/GYN, who told her to come to the office immediately. Paige then texted her husband, who drove her to the healthcare provider's office.

Introduction

The primary function of the reproductive system is to perpetuate life. The reproductive process begins with fertilization, which occurs when sex cells called **gametes** fuse. Male gametes are known as **sperm**, and female gametes are known as **oocytes**. The name for the organ that produces a gamete is **gonad**. Male gonads are *testes*, whereas female gonads are *ovaries*.

The single cell formed at **fertilization** (the fusion of a sperm with an oocyte) is called a **zygote**. A zygote contains more than a trillion molecules, despite its diameter of only 0.1 mm (0.0039 in.).

These trillion or so molecules all communicate and work together with the eventual goal of forming a human organism.

Word Parts Related to the Reproductive System

The reproductive system is the one body system where both structure and function vary greatly between the sexes. For this reason, different word parts are used to describe the male and the female reproductive systems. Word parts that refer to the testes, prostate, sperm, and penis typically apply to the male system, whereas word parts that refer to the breasts, vagina, ovaries, uterine tubes, and uterus typically apply to the female system.

Anatomists and clinicians use the singular term *testis* or the plural term *testes* to refer to the male gonad(s), but *testicle* and *testicles* are also commonly used. The Latin word for "testis" is *testis*, but the Latin word for "testicle" is *testiculus*, which is a diminutive form of *testis*. The Greek word for testicle is *orkheos*, which is where the roots orch/o, orchi/o, and orchid/o originate. The roots for sperm are spermat/o and sperm/o, which comes from the late Latin word *sperma*, meaning seed or to sow.

The word roots for vagina are colp/o and vagin/o. The root colp/o comes from the Greek word *kolpos* (womb) but refers to the vagina and not the uterus. *Vagina* is a Latin word meaning "sheath" or "covering."

The word roots for uterus are metr/o, hyster/o, and uter/o. *Uterus* is a Latin word, meaning womb. Hyster/o comes from the Greek word *hystera*, which also translates to womb. **Table 15.1** shows common word parts related to the reproductive system.

Table 15.1 Word Parts Related to the Reproductive System

Word Part	Meaning
amni/o	amnion
balan/o	glans penis
cervic/o	cervix, neck
circum/o	around
colp/o	vagina
gonad/o	gonads, sex glands
gynec/o	woman, female
hyster/o	uterus
lact/o	milk
mamm/o	breast
mast/o	breast
men/o	menses, menstruation
metr/o	uterus
nat/o	birth
oophor/o	ovary, egg-bearing
orch/o, orchi/o, orchid/o	testes
ovari/o	ovary, egg-bearing
prostat/o	prostate gland

Word Part	Meaning
salping/o	tube, uterine tube
sperm/o, spermat/o	sperm
uter/o	uterus
vagin/o	vagina
vas/o	vessel, vas deferens
vulv/o	vulva

Word Parts Exercise

After studying Table 15.1, write the meaning of each of the word parts.

Word Part	Meaning
1. mast/o, mamm/o	1._____
2. spermat/o, sperm/o	2._____
3. salping/o	3._____
4. vas/o	4._____
5. circum/o	5._____
6. ovari/o	6._____
7. colp/o	7._____
8. prostat/o	8._____
9. amni/o	9._____
10. nat/o	10._____
11. hyster/o	11._____
12. vulv/o	12._____
13. orchid/o	13._____
14. cervic/o	14._____
15. balan/o	15._____
16. gonad/o	16._____
17. gynec/o	17._____
18. lact/o	18._____
19. men/o	19._____
20. oophor/o	20._____

Structure and Function

This section describes the male reproductive system and then the female reproductive system. Functions of the male reproductive system include synthesizing the hormone testosterone; producing, storing, and transporting sperm; and making and releasing fluid from glands that support the sperm. This male reproductive fluid is called **semen**. Main functions of the female reproductive system are producing the hormones estrogen and progesterone; propagating life by producing oocytes; transporting oocytes to sites where they can be fertilized by sperm; supporting and nurturing a developing human organism; and providing an infant's first source of nutrition and protective antibodies through breast milk. Note that in males, the urethra is part of both the urinary and reproductive systems. In females, the urethra does not play a role in reproduction, but the opening to the exterior is enclosed by the **vulva**, the term for the external genitalia.

The Male Reproductive System

The male reproductive system is divided into internal *genitalia* (reproductive organs) and external genitalia. Internal genitalia include the testes, epididymis, ductus deferens (vas deferens), seminal glands (seminal vesicles), prostate (prostate gland), and bulbourethral glands. **Testes** are two oval-shaped gonads, located in a sac known as the *scrotum*, that produce sperm and testosterone. The **seminal glands**, also called

the **seminal vesicles**, are two glands located at the base of the urinary bladder that produce seminal fluid, which becomes a component of semen. The gland that surrounds the beginning of the urethra (inferior to the bladder) that secretes a fluid that becomes part of the semen is the **prostate**. The **bulbourethral glands** (*Cowper's glands*) are two glands inferior to the prostate that secrete a sticky fluid that also becomes a component of semen. External genitalia include the penis and scrotum. The **penis** is the external male organ used in urination and sexual intercourse, whereas the **scrotum** is a pouch that is suspended on each side of and behind the penis that encloses the testes. The rounded head of the penis forms a structure called the **glans penis**. A free fold of skin covers the glans penis and is known as the **foreskin** or **prepuce**. **Figure 15.1** shows the structures of the male reproductive system.

An important function of the male reproductive system is to produce sperm. The process, called **spermatogenesis**, involves stem cells dividing and differentiating into sperm. *Differentiating* means that a cell matures and develops into a cell with specific structures and functions. Spermatogenesis involves cell division known as **meiosis**, which reduces the number of chromosomes from 46 to 23.

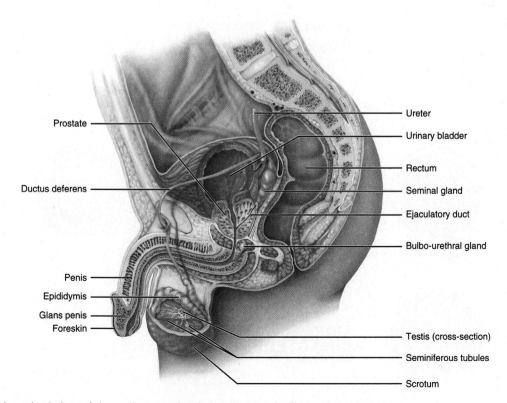

Figure 15.1 A sagittal view of the male reproductive system and adjacent structures.

Meiosis is a type of cell division that occurs in sex cells to reduce the number of chromosomes. Mitosis is a different type of cell division that occurs in cells to produce two daughter cells that both have the same number of chromosomes as the original cell. *Meiosis* is a Greek word meaning "a lessening." Mitosis comes from the Greek word *mitos* meaning "thread" and reflects what the process of mitosis looks like when the thread-like chromosomes bend and twist as they replicate.

Spermatogenesis begins in the *seminiferous tubules* of the testes and is initiated by the secretion of **androgens**, which are a group of hormones. The most significant androgen is **testosterone**. After spermatogenesis is complete, the sperm migrate from the seminiferous tubules to the **epididymis**, a coil-shaped tube at the upper part of each testis where the sperm mature as they are stored. Sperm are released during ejaculation, which begins with erection. When stimulated, the tissues in the penis become filled with blood, causing an *erection*. During erection, mature sperm leave the epididymis and enter the muscular tube of the **ductus deferens**, which leads to the *ejaculatory duct* that passes through the prostate. Fluid from the seminal glands is secreted into the ejaculatory duct. This fluid nourishes the sperm and forms much of the semen volume. The ductus deferens and the duct of the seminal gland unite to form the **ejaculatory duct**. The sperm and the fluid are now propelled through the ejaculatory duct toward the urethra. As the urethra passes through the prostate, milky secretions are added, forming semen. During ejaculation, the semen is expelled from the urethra at the tip of the penis. **Figure 15.2** shows the pathway of sperm, beginning with production in the testes.

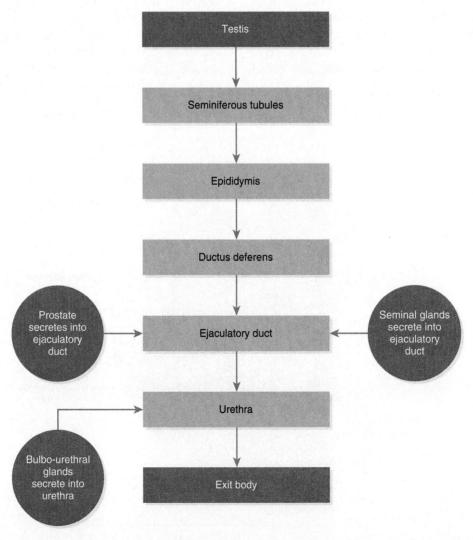

Figure 15.2 Pathway of sperm. The secretions from the glands that contribute to seminal fluid are shown in circles.

The Female Reproductive System

Like the male reproductive system, the female reproductive system is also divided into internal and external genitalia. The internal reproductive organs are the *uterus*, two *ovaries*, two *uterine tubes*, and the *vagina*. Female external genitalia include the *clitoris*, *labium majus*, and *labium minus* (see **Figure 15.3**). Breasts are technically part of the integumentary system because their tissue contains modified sweat glands. We will discuss them here because breasts are the female organs of milk secretion.

The **uterus** is a pear-shaped organ that has a dome-shaped top portion called the **fundus** and a lower, narrow portion referred to as the **cervix**, which extends into the vagina. The uterus is composed of three layers of tissues: the **perimetrium**, which is the outer surrounding layer; the **myometrium**, which is the middle muscular layer; and the **endometrium**, which is the inner layer. The endometrium reacts to hormonal changes every month, and the result is **menstruation**, which involves a shedding of the endometrial lining.

Two **ovaries** lie on each side of the uterus in the pelvic cavity. The ovaries produce oocytes, the female gametes (sex cells). When an oocyte is fertilized by a sperm, it develops into an **ovum** (egg) and can develop into a new individual.

The **uterine tubes** (*fallopian tubes*) extend from the ovaries to the uterus. They provide the path by which an oocyte travels from the ovary to the uterus. Fertilization takes place in the uterine tube.

The vagina is a muscular tube that extends from the cervix to the body's exterior. The vagina has the following functions:

- Allows for passage of the monthly menstrual flow of blood to the exterior
- Is the organ for sexual intercourse
- Serves as the birth canal during a vaginal birth

The external genitalia, commonly known as the **vulva**, include organs that enable sperm to enter the body, protect the internal genital organs from infectious organisms, and provide sexual pleasure. The **clitoris** is a small mass of erectile tissue that responds to sexual stimulation. *Labia* are two sets of skin folds that cover the female external genitalia and tissues. The **labium majus** (plural, *labium majora*) is one of two rounded external folds, and the **labium minus** (plural, *labium minora*) is one of two inner folds that surround the openings to the vagina and urethra (see Figure 15.3).

Breasts are protruding organs that have a *nipple* and an *areola*. The **nipple** is a projection on the breast surface through which *lactiferous* (milk) *ducts* open onto the body surface. The **areola** is the dark-pigmented area around the nipple.

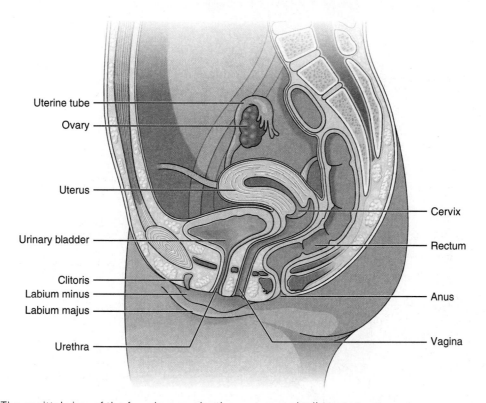

Figure 15.3 The sagittal view of the female reproductive system and adjacent structures.

Each breast contains a **mammary gland**, the modified sweat gland that produces milk. The subdivisions of the mammary gland are called *lobules* (see **Figure 15.4**). Breast milk provides nourishment for the newborn. **Lactation** is the term given to the production of milk.

Like the male reproductive system, the female reproductive system provides gametes for fertilization, but its function in the process continues by providing an environment for a fertilized egg to develop into to a fully formed baby.

The preparation for the process is accommodated by the **menstrual cycle** (also called the **uterine cycle**), a recurrent periodic change in the ovaries and uterus that occurs approximately every 28 days. The first time this cycle occurs in a female, around age 11 or 12, it is called **menarche**. When this monthly cycle stops occurring for the final time, around age 45 to 55, it is called **menopause**. Hormones control the menstrual cycle, which has three phases: **menstrual phase** (days 0 to 7; destruction and shedding of the endometrium), **proliferative phase** (days 7 to 14; repair and regeneration of the endometrium and preparation of the endometrial lining for implantation if fertilization occurs after ovulation on day 14), and the **secretory phase** (days 14 to 28; secretion of hormones). If male sperm are present during **ovulation** (the release of an oocyte), the possibility of fertilization exists.

Pregnancy

Pregnancy, or **gestation**, is the condition of having a developing embryo or fetus in the uterus. When a secondary oocyte is fertilized by sperm, it forms a *zygote*, which travels through the uterine tube and implants into the uterus. Once implanted, the zygote is called an **embryo** during the first 8 weeks of gestation. Between the end of the 8th week and birth, which under normal circumstances occurs between weeks 38 and 40, the term **fetus** is used. The fetus receives nourishment from the uterine wall through the *umbilical cord* and the *placenta*. The **umbilical cord** is the structure that contains blood vessels and connects the embryo or fetus to the placenta, whereas the **placenta** is a temporary organ formed during pregnancy that is implanted in the uterus. The **amnion** (*amniotic sac*) is the inner layer of the membrane that surrounds the fetus and contains *amniotic fluid*. **Amniotic fluid** encases the fetus and provides a cushion for the fetus as the pregnant person moves (see **Figure 15.5**).

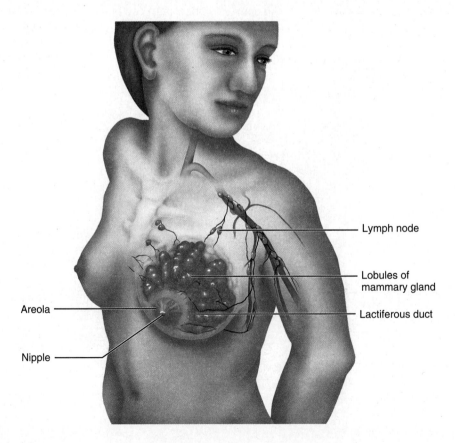

Figure 15.4 Frontal view of the breasts.

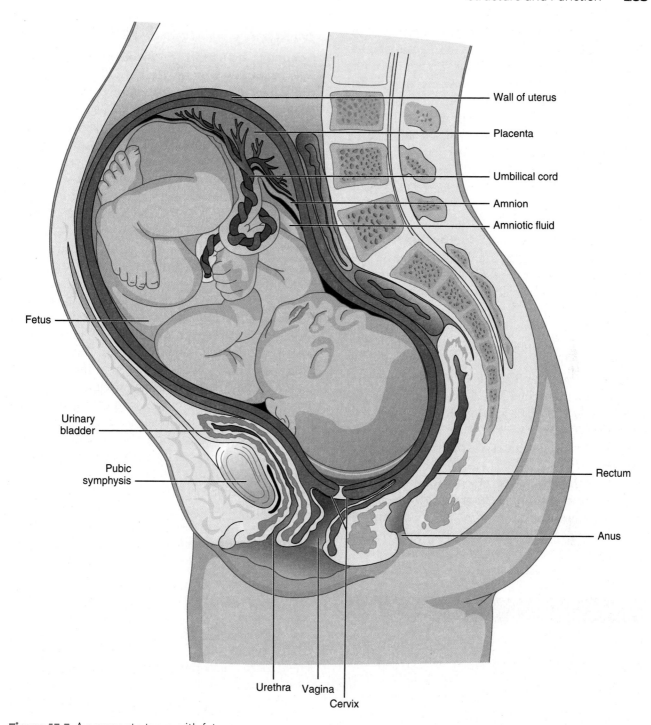

Wall of uterus

Placenta

Umbilical cord

Amnion

Amniotic fluid

Fetus

Urinary
bladder

Pubic
symphysis

Rectum

Anus

Urethra Vagina

Cervix

Figure 15.5 A pregnant uterus with fetus.

Terms Associated with Pregnancy

Gravida, para, and abortus are shorthand notations for a female's pregnancy history. The term **gravida** (G), derived from the Latin word *gravidus* (heavy), means a pregnant person. Gravida is usually followed by a numeral (Roman or Arabic) and indicates the number of pregnancies. For example, gravida I, GI, and G1 all refer to a female in her first pregnancy and gravida II, GII, and G2 refer to a female in her second pregnancy. The term can also be preceded by the Latin prefix primi- for first and secundi- for second, as in primigravida (first pregnancy) and secundigravida (second pregnancy). The number following gravida indicates the number of times a patient has been pregnant regardless of whether these pregnancies were carried to term. A current pregnancy, if any, is included in this count. The term **para** (P), derived from the Latin word *pario* (to bring forth), refers to a female who has given birth to one or more infants. Like gravida, it is followed by a numeral (Roman or Arabic) or preceded by a Latin prefix. For example, para I, primipara, PI, and P1 refer to a female who has given birth for the first time, whereas para II, secundipara, PII, and P2 refer to a female who has given birth for a second time to one or more infants. Para indicates the number of births that occurred after 20 weeks, including viable and nonviable (stillbirths). Pregnancies consisting of multiples, such as twins or triplets, count as one birth for the purpose of this notation. **Abortus** (A) is the Latin word for "miscarriage" and indicates the number of pregnancies that were lost for any reason, including induced abortions or miscarriages. Stillbirths are not included.

In the United States, Arabic numerals are typically used. Therefore, the obstetric history of a female who has had two pregnancies (both of which resulted in live births) would be noted as G2P2. The obstetrical history of a female who has had four pregnancies, one of which was a miscarriage before 20 weeks, would be noted as G4P3A1. That of a female who has had one pregnancy of twins with successful outcomes would be noted as G1P1.

The **estimated date of confinement** (EDC) or **estimated date of delivery** (EDD) is the date an infant is expected to be born and is calculated by counting forward 280 days (40 weeks) from the first day of the pregnant person's last menstrual period (LMP). It is also called the *due date*.

QUICK CHECK

Fill in the blanks.

1. List functions of the male reproductive system.
   _____
   _____
2. The term for milk production is _____
   _____.
3. A synonym for pregnancy is _____
   _____.

Disorders Related to the Reproductive System

Disorders of the reproductive system are briefly described under the following sections: sexually transmitted diseases (STDs), inflammation, structural abnormalities, and tumors. Additional conditions affecting females and males, respectively, are included at the end of this section.

Sexually Transmitted Diseases

Sexually transmitted diseases (STDs), also called **sexually transmitted infections** (STIs), are contagious diseases acquired during sexual contact. Examples include human immunodeficiency virus, herpes simplex virus, gonorrhea, chlamydia, pelvic inflammatory disease, syphilis, and human papillomavirus infection.

Human immunodeficiency virus (HIV) attacks the immune system after it is transmitted through blood or other infected body fluids. **Herpes simplex virus** (HSV) includes a variety of infections caused by herpesvirus types 1 and 2 that produce cold sores, genital inflammation, and conjunctivitis. Gonorrhea (GC) is a highly contagious disease caused by *Neisseria gonorrhoeae* bacteria that may also be transmitted to a child from an infected pregnant person during birth. **Chlamydia** is another common infection spread through sexual contact and is caused by a very small parasitic bacterium from the *Chlamydia* genus. **Pelvic inflammatory disease** (PID), an infection of the uterus, ovaries, and uterine tubes, can prevent fertilization. If a female has PID and an oocyte does become fertilized, the zygote may implant outside the uterus, which is known as an **ectopic pregnancy**. An ectopic pregnancy can be life threatening. **Syphilis** is a highly contagious disease caused by the *Treponema pallidum* bacterium. A developing fetus can contract the disease through an infected mother. **Human papilloma virus** (HPV) is a sexually transmitted virus that can lead to cervical cancer.

Why is GC sometimes used as an abbreviation for gonorrhea? The abbreviation, GC, stands for gonococcal. Gonorrhea is an infection caused by the *Neisseria gonorrhoeae* bacterium, which is also known as gonococcus, a species of Gram-negative diplococci bacteria first isolated in 1879 by Albert Neisser. The abbreviation GC for gonococcus is derived from the first letter G for gono and C for coccus. Coccus refers to any spherical-shaped bacterium.

Inflammation

Infections of the female reproductive system may result from exposure to bacteria, fungi, or viruses. Many of the conditions are marked by inflammation, the terms for which are indicated by the suffix *-itis*.

Female reproductive system inflammation disorders include **mastitis** (breast inflammation), **oophoritis** (ovary inflammation), **salpingitis** (uterine tube inflammation), **cervicitis** (inflammation of the uterine cervix), and **vaginitis** (inflammation of the vagina). Salpingitis can lead to a closing of the uterine tubes, thereby causing infertility.

Male reproductive system inflammation conditions include **epididymitis** (inflammation of the epididymis), **prostatitis** (inflammation of the prostate), **balanitis** (inflammation of the glans penis), and **orchitis** (inflammation of a testis). Balanitis occurs in uncircumcised males who still have an intact glans penis.

Female Structural Abnormalities

In adult females, the uterus may be out of position, or it may have a bend in its main body. **Anteflexion** (forward bending) is the normal position of the uterus (see **Figure 15.6A**). **Anteversion** (forward turning) is the tilting of the uterus in which it is angled slightly posteriorly toward the cervix (see **Figure 15.6B**). **Retroflexion** (backward bending) is an abnormal tipping with the body of the uterus bent back on itself, forming an angle with the cervix (see **Figure 15.6C**). **Retroversion** (backward turning) is an abnormal tipping of the entire uterus backward (see **Figure 15.6D**). A **prolapsed uterus** involves the descent of the uterus or cervix into the vaginal canal. Two other conditions involving structural abnormalities of the female reproductive system are a **cystocele**, which is a protrusion of the urinary bladder into the anterior wall of the vagina, and a **rectocele**, which is a protrusion of the rectum into the posterior wall of the vagina.

Tumors

Benign tumors of the uterus are called *fibroleiomyomas* or **fibroids**. Cysts, which may also be considered benign tumors, are usually caused by hormonal disturbances.

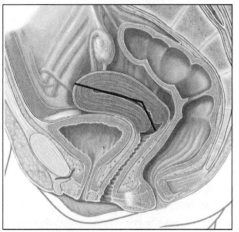

(A) Anteflexion

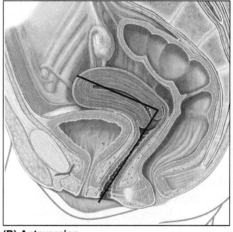

(B) Anteversion

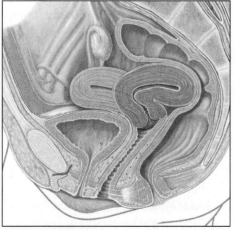

(C) Retroflexion

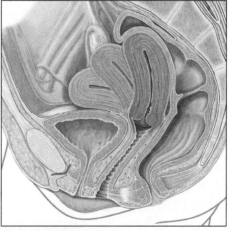

(D) Retroversion

Figure 15.6 Variants of uterine position within the pelvis. The pink-shaded organ is the uterus.

Cancer of the endometrium is the most common type of cancer in the female reproductive system. A **hysterectomy** (removal of the uterus) is a common treatment. **Endometriosis** is a condition in which endometrial tissue grows outside the uterus, frequently forming cysts, and causing pelvic pain.

Menstrual Cycle Disorders

Menstruation, commonly called a *period* or a *menstrual period*, generally occurs once per month. However, menstrual cycle disorders are common. **Amenorrhea** is the absence of menstruation. **Dysmenorrhea** is painful menstruation. **Menorrhagia** is an increased amount and duration of blood flow. **Oligomenorrhea** is infrequent menstrual period (fewer than six to eight per year) and is accompanied by reduced blood flow.

Disorders That Affect Males

Any disease that affects the testes is called **orchiopathy**. This includes **azoospermia** (absence of living sperm in the semen), **oligospermia** (low sperm count), **orchialiga** (pain in the testes), **anorchism** (absence of one or both testes; may be congenital or acquired), and **cryptorchidism** (failure of one testis or both testes to descend into the scrotum). Other disorders that affect the male reproductive system include the following:

- **Benign prostatic hyperplasia** (BPH): an enlarged, noncancerous prostate
- **Hydrocele**: fluid accumulation in the scrotum
- **Phimosis**: narrowing of the opening of the foreskin so it cannot be retracted (pulled back) to expose the glans penis
- **Varicocele**: enlargement of veins in the spermatic cord (bundle of nerves and blood vessels connecting the testes to the abdominal cavity)

Diagnostic Tests, Treatments, and Surgical Procedures

Some diagnostic tests, surgical treatments, and procedures of the female reproductive system are as follows:

- **Amniocentesis**: amniotic fluid is tested for fetal abnormalities; can also help determine fetal lung maturity, age, and sex (see **Figure 15.7**)

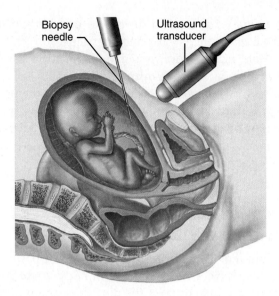

Figure 15.7 Amniocentesis. A biopsy needle is inserted through the abdominal wall into the uterus, and a sample of amniotic fluid is removed from the amniotic sac using guided ultrasound.

- **Colposcopy**: visual examination of the tissues of the cervix and vagina using a surgical instrument called a colposcope
- **Papanicolaou test (Pap smear)**: scraping of the cervical tissues to diagnose cervical cancer or other conditions of the cervix and surrounding tissues
- **Dilation and curettage** (D&C): dilation (widening) of the cervix and scraping the lining of the uterus with a surgical instrument called a curette, which has a loop, ring, or scoop with sharpened edges attached to a handle
- **Cone biopsy**: surgical removal of a cone-shaped section of the cervix
- **Laparoscopy**: visual examination of the interior of the abdomen by means of a surgical instrument called a laparoscope
- **Oophorectomy**: removal of one ovary
- **Bilateral oophorectomy**: removal of both ovaries
- **Salpingo-oophorectomy**: removal of an ovary and a uterine tube
- **Bilateral salpingo-oophorectomy**: removal of both ovaries and uterine tubes
- **Hysterosalpingography**: a radiographic examination of the uterus and uterine tubes
- **Hysterectomy**: surgical removal of the uterus
- **Mammography**: radiographic examination of the breast
- **Mastectomy**: removal of a breast
- **Tubal ligation**: surgical procedure that involves severing and tying the uterine tubes to prevent future fertilization (conception)

Some diagnostic tests, treatments, and surgical procedures of the male reproductive system are as follows:

- **Circumcision**: a surgical procedure to remove the foreskin of the penis
- **Orchiectomy**: removal of one testis or both testes
- **Orchioplasty**: surgical repair of a testis
- **Transurethral resection of the prostate** (TURP): the removal of part or all the prostate through the urethra
- **Varicocelectomy**: the removal of a portion of an enlarged vein to remove a varicocele
- **Vasovasostomy**: procedure to restore fertility to a vasectomized male by reconnecting the ductus (vas) deferens

Practice and Practitioners

Obstetrics (OB) is the medical specialty concerned with the medical care of females during pregnancy and childbirth, and **obstetricians** (from *obstetrix*, the Latin word for midwife) are the specialists who provide medical care to pregnant person and who deliver babies. **Gynecology** (GYN) is the study of the female reproductive system, and **gynecologists** diagnose and treat disorders of the female reproductive system. **Urologists** diagnose and treat disorders of the urinary system; urologists also diagnose and treat male reproductive system disorders. **Neonatology** is the medical specialty dealing with newborns, and **pediatrics** is the medical specialty dealing with children. Specialists in these fields are **neonatologists**, who specialize in newborns, and **pediatricians**, who specialize in the diagnosis and treatment of childhood disorders.

Abbreviation Table	The Reproductive System
Abbreviation	**Meaning**
A	abortus
BPH	benign prostatic hyperplasia
CS	cesarean section
C-section	cesarean section
D&C	dilation and curettage
EDC	estimated date of confinement (due date)
EDD	estimated date of delivery (due date)
G	gravida
GC	gonorrhea
GYN	gynecology
HIV	human immunodeficiency virus
HPV	human papillomavirus
HSV	herpes simplex virus
LMP	last menstrual period
OB	obstetrics
P	para
Pap smear	Papanicolaou smear
PID	pelvic inflammatory disease
STD	sexually transmitted disease
STI	sexually transmitted infection
TURP	transurethral resection of the prostate

Study Table	The Reproductive System	
Term and Pronunciation	**Analysis**	**Meaning**
Structure and Function		
abortus (uh-BOR-tus)	from the Latin word *abortus* (miscarriage)	any product of a miscarriage
amniotic fluid (am-nee-OT-ik FLOO-id)	*amni/o* (amnion); *-ic* (suffix meaning pertaining to); fluid (from the Latin word for fluid, *fluidus*)	the fluid within the amnion (amniotic sac) that surrounds the embryo/fetus and helps to protect it from physical injury
amnion (AM-nee-on)	from the Greek word, *amnion* (membrane around the fetus) and diminutive of *amnos* (lamb)	innermost membrane enveloping the embryo/fetus in the uterus; *amniotic sac*
amniotic sac (am-nee-OT-ik SAK)	*amni/o* (amnion); *-ic* (suffix meaning pertaining to); sac (from the Latin word for bag, *saccus*)	innermost membrane enveloping the embryo/fetus in the uterus; *amnion*

(continues)

Study Table The Reproductive System		*(continued)*
Term and Pronunciation	**Analysis**	**Meaning**
Structure and Function		
androgens (AN-droh-jenz)	from the Greek words *andros* (male, man) and *genein* (to produce)	hormones that stimulate the activity of accessory sex hormones; testosterone is an androgen
areola (uh-REE-oh-luh)	diminutive of *area*, Latin word for "small area"	circular pigmented area surrounding the nipple
bulbo-urethral gland (bul-boh-yoo-REE-thrul GLAND)	from the Latin word *bulbus* (bulb); from the Greek word *ourethra* (passage for urine) + French *glande* (gland)	one of a pair of small glands at the base of the penile urethra that secretes fluid that becomes a component of seminal fluid; also called *Cowper's gland*
cervix (SER-viks)	Latin word for "neck" (as in the neck of the uterus)	common term for the neck of the uterus that projects into the vagina
chromosome (KROH-moh-sohm)	from the Greek word *khroma* (color) and *soma* (body), so called because the structures contain a substance that stains readily with basic dyes	a gene-bearing bundle of DNA found in the nucleus of cells
clitoris (KLIT-or-is)	from the Greek word *kleitoris* (small, sensitive, erectile part)	small (less than 2 cm) mass of erectile tissue in females that responds to sexual stimulation
Cowper's gland (COW-perz GLAND)	named after English anatomist, William Cowper (1666–1709)	one of a pair of small glands at the base of the penile urethra that secretes fluid that becomes a component of seminal fluid; also called *bulbourethral gland*
ductus deferens (DUCK-tus DEF-ur-enz)	from words *ductus* (leading) and *deferens* (carrying down)	duct leading out of the epididymis; also called *vas deferens*
embryo (EM-bree-oh)	from the Greek word *embryon* (young animal, literally, "that which grows")	name change from zygote after the first cell division until the 8th week of pregnancy
endometrium (en-doh-MEE-tree-um)	endo- (within); from the Greek *metra* (uterus)	membrane forming the inner layer of the uterine wall
epididymis (ep-ih-DID-ih-mus)	from the Greek words *epi-* (on) + *didymos* (testicle)	organ in which the sperm become functional
estimated date of confinement (ESS-tih-may-ted DATE UV kun-FINE-munt)	from the Latin words *aestimat-* (determined, appraised) and *daktulos* (finger)	the day that spontaneous (not induced) labor is expected to occur during pregnancy, typically lasting between 38 and 42 weeks; also called *estimated date of delivery*
estimated date of delivery (EDD) (ESS-tih-may-ted DATE UV dih-LIV-uh-ree)	from the Latin word *aestimat-* (determined, appraised) and French word *delivree* (to deliver)	the day that spontaneous (not induced) labor is expected to occur during pregnancy, typically lasting between 38 and 42 weeks; also called *estimated date of confinement*
fallopian tubes (fuh-LOH- pee-un TOOBZ)	named after Gabriello Fallopio (1523–1562), an Italian anatomist who first described them	tubular structures between the ovaries and the uterus; also called *uterine tubes*
fertilization (fer-til-ih-ZAY-shun)	from the Latin word *fertilis* (fruitful)	the joining of the male and female gametes (in the context of the human reproductive system)

Term and Pronunciation	Analysis	Meaning
Structure and Function		
fetus (FEE-tus)	Latin word meaning "the bearing," "bringing forth," or "hatching of young"	name change from embryo after the 8th week of pregnancy to birth
fundus (FUN-dus)	Latin word for "bottom"	the upper rounded portion of the uterus above (superior to) the openings of the uterine tubes
gamete (GAH-meet)	Greek word meaning "a wife"; also, *gametes* (a husband), from *gamein* (to take a wife, to marry)	term given to both the sex cells; female oocyte and male sperm
gestation (jes-TAY-shun)	from the Latin word *gestare* (to bear, carry, gestate)	period of development that occurs between the formation of the zygote and birth of the fetus; also called *pregnancy*
gonad (GOH-nad)	from the Greek word *gone* (generation, seed)	gamete-generating organ (ovary or testis)
gravida (GRAV-ih-duh)	from the Latin word *gravis* (heavy, profound, important)	a pregnant person
labor (LAY-bur)	from the Latin word *labor* (toil, trouble)	process of childbirth
lactation (lak-TAY-shun)	from the Latin words *lactare* (to suckle) and *lac* (milk)	milk production
labium majus (LAY-bee-um MAY-jus)	from the Latin words *labium* (lip) + *magnus* (great)	part of the labia that covers and protects the female external genital organs
labium minus (LAY-bee-um MYE-nus)	from the Latin words *labium* (lip) + *minor* (smaller)	inner folds of the labia that surround the openings to the vagina and urethra
mammary gland (MAM-uh-ree GLAND)	from the Latin word *mamma* (breast)	modified sweat gland that produces milk
meiosis (migh-OH-sis)	Greek word meaning "a lessening"	cell division comprising two nuclear divisions in rapid succession that results in four gametocytes (a cell that divides to form gametes)
menarche (meh-NAR-kee)	from the Greek words *men* (month) and *arkhe* (beginning)	beginning of menstruation (menses)
menopause (MEN-oh-pawz)	from the Latin words *mensis* (month) and *pausis* (a cessation, a pause)	normal stopping of the monthly menstrual cycle (periods)
menses (MEN-seez)	plural form of the Latin word *mensis* (month)	periodic bleeding occurring at intervals of about 4 weeks in which the endometrial lining is shed; also called *menstruation*
menstruation (men-stroo-AYE-shun)	from the Latin word *menstruus* (monthly); *-atio* (process)	cyclic endometrial shedding and discharge of a bloody fluid from the uterus; also called *menses*
menstrual (MEN-stroo-ul)	from the Latin word *mensis* (month)	relating to the menses (menstruation)
menstrual cycle (MEN-stroo-ul SIGH-kul)	from the Latin words *mensis* (month) and *cyclus* (cycle)	part of the reproductive system process in females, comprising three phases: menstrual, proliferative, and secretory; also called *uterine cycle*

(continues)

Study Table The Reproductive System		*(continued)*
Term and Pronunciation	**Analysis**	**Meaning**
Structure and Function		
mitosis (my-TOH-shs)	from the Greek word *mitos* (wrap, thread); *-osis* (process)	process of cell division by which one cell becomes two, both of which contain the maternal and paternal chromosomes
myometrium (my-oh-MEE-tree-um)	*myo-* (muscle); from the Greek *metra* (uterus)	the muscular wall of the uterus
ovary (OH-vah-ree)	from the Latin word *ovum* (egg)	small almond-shaped organ located on each side of the uterus that produces hormones and releases oocytes
ovulation (OV-yoo-lay-shun)	from the Latin word *ovum* (egg); *-atio* (process)	release of an oocyte from the ovary
ovum (OH-vuhm) plural, ova (OH-vuh)	Latin word meaning "egg"	fertilized oocyte before implantation
para (PAR-uh)	from the Latin verb *pario* (to bring forth, produce, create)	a female who has given birth to a viable fetus
penis (PEE-nis)	from the Latin *penis* (tail)	external male sex organ used in urination and sexual intercourse that transports the male sperm into the female vagina
placenta (pluh-SEN-tuh)	from the Greek word *plakous* (flat cake)	a spongy organ that attaches the fetus to the pregnant person and provides nourishment to the developing fetus
pregnancy (PREG-nun-see)	*pre-* (before); from the Latin word *gnascor* (to be born)	time when the embryo/fetus grows inside the uterus; also called *gestation*
proliferative phase (pro-LIF-er-uh-tiv FAZE)	from the Latin words *proles* (offspring) and *ferre* (to carry, to bear)	menstrual phase (days 7–14) controlled by estrogen secreted by ovarian follicles (cell aggregations in the ovary that contains an oocyte), simultaneous with their development
prostate (PROS-tate)	from the Greek word *prostates* (one standing in front)	male gland that produces and stores prostatic fluid, a fluid medium that is part of semen; also called *prostate gland*
prostate gland (PROS-tate GLAND)	from the Greek word *prostates* (one standing in front) + a variant of Scots *glam* (clamp)	male gland that produces and stores prostatic fluid, a fluid medium that is part of semen; also called *prostate*
scrotum (SKROH-tum)	from the Latin word *scrotum* cognate with Old English *scrud* (garment, source of shroud)	the sac that encloses and protects the testes
secretory phase (SEE-kruh-tor-ee FAZE)	from the Latin verb *secretionem* (to separate)	menstrual phase (days 14–28) controlled by the hormone progesterone that coincides with the formation of the corpus luteum (a hormone-secreting structure that develops in the ovary after the oocyte has been released, but degenerates after a few days unless fertilization occurs)

Term and Pronunciation	Analysis	Meaning
Structure and Function		
semen (SEE-men)	a Latin word meaning "seed"	combination of sperm, their associated glandular secretions, and prostatic fluid
seminal gland (SEM-in-ul GLAND)	from the Latin word *semen* (seed); -al (adjective suffix) + variant of Scots *glam* (clamp)	gland at the base of the urinary bladder that secretes a thick substance that nourishes sperm; also called *seminal vesicle*
seminal vesicle (SEM-in-ul VES-ih-kul)	from the Latin words *semen* (seed) and *vesica* (bladder, balloon)	gland at the base of the urinary bladder that secretes a thick substance that nourishes sperm; also called *seminal gland*
sperm (SPURM)	from the Greek words *sperma* (seed)	mature, motile male gamete; sperm is singular or plural; also called *spermatozoon* and *spermatozoa*
spermatic cord (spur-MAT-ick KORD)	*spermat/o* (sperm); + suffix -*ic* + Old French *corde* (string of a musical instrument)	bundle of nerves, ducts, and blood vessels that connect the testes to the abdominal cavity
spermatocyte (SPUR-mat-oh-SITE)	from the Greek words *sperma* (seed) + *cyte* (cell)	cell produced at the second stage of spermatogenesis in the formation of spermatozoa
spermatogenesis (SPUR-mat-toh-JEN-ih-sis)	*spermat/o* (sperm); + *genesis* (production)	production of sperm
spermatozoon (spur-mat-oh-ZOH-un) plural, spermatozoa (SPUR-mat-oh-zoh-uh)	*spermat/o* (sperm); + *zoion* (animal)	mature, motile male gamete; also called *sperm*
testicle (TES-tih-kul)	from Latin word *testiculus* (a witness to virility)	the organ that produces and stores the male gametes (sperm); also called *testis*
testis (TES-tis) plural, testes (TES-teez)	from the Latin word *testiculus* diminutive of *testis* (witness) (the organ being evidence of virility)	the organ that produces and stores the male gametes (sperm); also called *testicle*
testosterone (tes-TOS-ter-ohn)	from the Latin word *testis* (witness) + -*sterone* (steroid hormone)	hormone (androgen) prominent in male gamete production
umbilical cord (um-BILL-ih-kul KORD)	from the Latin words *umbilicus* (navel) + *chorda* (string)	connecting stalk between the embryo/fetus and the placenta that contains two arteries and one vein
urethra (yoo-REETH-ruh)	from the Greek word *ourethra* (passage for urine)	canal leading from the bladder to the exterior; male ductwork that acts as a part of both the male urinary system and male reproductive system
uterine cervix (YOO-ter-in SUR-viks)	*uter/o* (uterus); -*ine* (adjective suffix) + *cervix*, Latin word for neck	the "neck" located at the lower end of the uterus
uterine cycle (YOO-ter-in SIGH-kul)	from the Latin words *uterinus* (born of the same mother) and *cyclus* (cycle)	part of the reproductive system process in females, comprising three phases: menstrual, proliferative, and secretory; also called *menstrual cycle*

(continues)

Study Table The Reproductive System		*(continued)*
Term and Pronunciation	**Analysis**	**Meaning**
Structure and Function		
uterine tubes (YOO-ter-in TOOBZ)	*uter/o* (uterus); *-ine* (adjective suffix); from the Latin word *tubus* (tube)	tubular structures between the ovaries and the uterus; also called *fallopian tubes*
uterus (YOO-ter-us)	Latin word meaning "womb" or "belly"	reproductive organ in which the fertilized oocyte is implanted and in which the embryo/fetus develops
vagina (vuh-JYE-nuh)	Latin word for sheath	the female genital canal extending between the cervix of the uterus and the body exterior
vas deferens (VAS DEF-ur-enz)	from the Latin words *vas* (vessel) and *deferens* (carrying down)	duct leading out of the epididymis; also called *ductus deferens*
vulva (VUL-vuh)	from the Latin word *vulva* (wrapper or covering)	female external genital organs
zygote (ZYE-goat)	from the Greek word *zygotos* (yoked)	single cell formed at fertilization from the union of the oocyte with the sperm
Disorders		
amenorrhea (ah-MEN-oh-REE-uh)	*a-* (without); *men/o* (menses); *-rrhea* (flowing, discharge)	absence of menstruation
anorchism (an-ORK-izm)	*an-* (without); *orch/o* (testes); *-ism* (condition)	congenital absence of one testis or both testes
anteflexion (an-tee-FLEX-shun)	*ante-* (something positioned in front of); from the Latin word *flectere* (to bend)	forward bend of the uterus
anteversion (an-tee-VER-zhun)	*ante-* (something positioned in front of); from the Latin word *versio* (turning)	turning forward of the entire uterus
azoospermia (aye-ZOH-oh-SPER-mee-uh)	*a-* (without); from the Greek word *azoos* (lifeless); *sperm/o* (sperm)	absence of living sperm in the semen
balanitis (bal-an-EYE-tiss)	*balan/o* (glans penis); *-itis* (inflammation)	inflammation of the glans penis
benign prostatic hyperplasia (BPH) (bee-NINE pros-TAT-ik high-per-PLAY-zhee-uh)	benign (common English word) + *prostat/o* (prostate) + *-ic* (adjective suffix); *hyper-* (above normal); *-plasia* (development, growth)	an enlarged, noncancerous prostate
cervicitis (sur-vih-SIGH-tiss)	*cervic/o* (cervix); *-itis* (inflammation)	inflammation of the uterine cervix
cryptorchidism (kript-OR-kid-iz-um)	from the Greek word *kryptos* (hidden); *orch/o* (testes); *-ism* (condition)	undescended testes or when one testis or both testes fail to descend into the scrotum
cystocele (SIS-toh-seel)	*cyst/o* (bladder); *-cele* (hernia)	protrusion of the bladder into the anterior wall of the vagina
dysmenorrhea (dis-MEN-oh-REE-uh)	*dys-* (bad, difficult); *men/o* (menses); *-rrhea* (flowing, discharge)	painful menstruation
ectopic pregnancy (ek-TOP-ik PREG-nun-see)	from the Greek word *ektopos* (out of place) + from the Latin prefix *praegnant-* (be born)	out of place; a pregnancy occurring elsewhere than in the uterus

Term and Pronunciation	Analysis	Meaning
Disorders		
endometriosis (EN-doh-MEE-tree-OH-sis)	from the Greek words *endon* (within) and *metra* (womb) + *-osis* (condition)	presence of endometrial tissue outside the uterus
epididymitis (ep-ih-did-ih-MY-tiss)	from the Greek words *epi* (on) and *didymos* (testicle); *-itis* (inflammation)	inflammation of the epididymis
gonorrhea (GC) (gon-oh-REE-uh)	from the Greek *gonos* (offspring); *-rrhea* (discharge, flowing)	highly contagious sexually transmitted disease (infection) caused by *Neisseria gonorrhoeae* bacteria
herpes simplex virus (HSV) (HUR-peez SIM-pleks VYE-rus)	from the Latin words *herpes* (spreading skin eruption), *simplex* (simple), and *virus* (poison)	infections caused by herpesvirus types 1 and 2; signs include groups of vesicles and lesions on the genitalia
human immunodeficiency virus (HIV) (HYOO-mun IM-yoo-noh-dee-fish-en-see VYE-rus)	from the Latin words *immunis* (exempt), *deficientem* (deficient), and *virus* (poison)	virus that attacks the immune system; can be sexually transmitted
human papillomavirus (HPV) (HYOO-mun pap-ih-LOH-muh VYE-rus)	from the Latin words *papilla* (nipple), *oma* (tumor), and *virus* (poison)	most common sexually transmitted disease (infection); causes certain types of genital warts
hydrocele (HIGH-droh-seel)	*hydro-* (water); *-cele* (hernia)	swelling in the scrotum caused by fluid accumulation in the testes
hysteralgia (HIS-ter-AL-jee-uh)	*hyster/o* (womb, uterus); *-algia* (pain)	pain in the uterus; also called *hysterodynia*
hysterodynia (HIS-ter-oh-DIN-ee-uh)	*hyster/o* (womb, uterus); *-dynia* (pain)	pain in the uterus; also called *hysteralgia*
hysteropathy (hiss-ter-OP-uh-thee)	*hyster/o* (womb, uterus); *-pathy* (disease)	any disease of the uterus
leiomyoma (LYE-oh-my-oh-muh)	from the Greek *leio-* (smooth) + *myo-* (muscle) + *oma* (tumor)	benign tumor originating in the smooth muscle lining the myometrium (middle layer of uterus); also called *uterine fibroid*
mastitis (mast-EYE-tiss)	*mast/o* (breast); *-itis* (inflammation)	inflammation of the breast
menorrhagia (MEN-oh-RAJ-ee-uh)	*men/o* (menses); *-rrhagia* (rapid flow of blood)	increased amount and duration of menstrual flow
oligomenorrhea (oh-LIG-oh-MEN-oh-REE-uh)	*olig/o* (having little); *men/o* (menses); *-rrhea* (discharge, flowing)	infrequent, irregular menstrual periods
oligospermia (oh-LIG-oh-SPER-mee-uh)	*olig/o* (having little); *-sperm/o* (sperm); *-ia* (condition)	low sperm count
oophoritis (oh-oh-for-EYE-tiss)	*oophor/o* (ovary); *-itis* (inflammation)	inflammation of an ovary; also called *ovaritis*
orchialgia (or-kee-AL-jee-uh)	*orchi/o* (testes); *-algia* (pain)	pain in the testes
orchitis (or-KIGH-tiss)	*orchi/o* (testes); *-itis* (inflammation)	inflammation of a testis
ovarialgia (oh-vahr-ee-AL-jee-uh)	*ovari/o* (ovary); *-algia* (pain)	pain in an ovary

(continues)

Study Table The Reproductive System		(continued)
Term and Pronunciation	**Analysis**	**Meaning**
Disorders		
ovaritis (oh-var-EYE-tiss)	*ovari/o* (ovary); *-itis* (inflammation)	inflammation of an ovary; also called *oophoritis*
pelvic inflammatory disease (PID) (PEL-vik in-FLAM-uh- tor-ee dih-ZEEZ)	*pelvic* (relating to the pelvis); Latin word *inflammare* (flame) + Old French *desaise* (lack of ease)	acute or chronic suppurative inflammation of female pelvic structures (endometrium, uterine tubes, pelvic peritoneum) due to infection by *Neisseria gonorrhoeae*, *Chlamydia trachomatis*, or other organisms
phimosis (figh-MOH-sis)	from the Greek word *phimoo* (to muzzle); *-osis* (condition)	narrowing of the foreskin opening so it cannot be retracted or pulled back to expose the glans penis
placenta previa (pluh-SEN-tuh PREV-ee-uh)	from the Greek word *plakous* (flat cake) and the Latin word *praevia* (going before)	condition of pregnancy in which the placenta partially or completely blocks the cervix (neck of uterus), interfering with normal delivery
prolapsed uterus (proh-LAPSED YOO-ter-us)	from the Latin words *prolapsus* (displacement) and *uterus* (womb)	descent of the uterus or cervix into the vagina
prostatitis (PROS-tuh-TYE-tiss)	*prostat/o* (prostate); + *-itis* (inflammation)	inflammation of the prostate
rectocele (REK-toh-seel)	*rect/o* (rectum); *-cele* (hernia)	protrusion of the rectum into the posterior wall of the vagina
retroflexion (re-troh-FLEX-shun)	*retro-* (backward) + flexion, from the Latin word *flectere* (to bend)	abnormal tipping with the body of the uterus bent back on itself
retroversion (re-troh-VER-zhun)	*retro-* (backward); from the Latin word *versio* (to turn)	an abnormal tipping of the entire uterus backward
salpingitis (sal-pin-JYE-tis)	*salping/o* (tube, uterine tube); *-itis* (inflammation)	inflammation of the uterine tube
sexually transmitted disease (STD) (SEK-shoo-uh-lee trans-MIT-ted dih-ZEEZ)	from late Latin words *sexualis* (sex) and *transmittere* (across) + Old French *desaise* (lack of ease)	disease such as HIV, syphilis, and chlamydia that are transmitted through sexual intercourse or sexual contact; also called *sexually transmitted infection* (STI)
sexually transmitted infection (STI) (SEK-shoo-uh-lee trans-MIT-ted in-FECK-shun	from late Latin words *sexualis* (sex), *transmittere* (across), and *infection* (dip in, taint)	infection such as HIV, syphilis, and chlamydia that are transmitted through sexual intercourse or sexual contact; also called *sexually transmitted disease* (STD)
syphilis (SIF-ih-lis)	from the title of a 1530 poem *Syphilis sive Morbus Gallicus* by Fracastorius, *Syphilus* being the title character who supposedly had the disease	a highly contagious sexually transmitted disease/infection that is caused by the spirochete bacterium, *Treponema pallidum*
uterine fibroid (YOO-ter-in FIGH-broid)	*uter/o* (uterus); *-ine* (adjective suffix); from the Latin word *fibra* (a fiber, filament); *-oid* (resembling)	benign tumor originating in the smooth muscle lining the myometrium (middle layer of uterus); also called *leiomyoma*
vaginitis (VAJ-ih-NIGH-tiss)	*vagin/o* (vagina); *-itis* (inflammation)	inflammation of the vaginal tissues that may be infectious or due to several other causes
varicocele (VAIR-ih-koh-seel)	*varic/o* (varix, varicose, varicosity); *-cele* (hernia)	mass of varicose veins within the spermatic cord

Term and Pronunciation	Analysis	Meaning
Diagnostic Tests, Treatments, and Surgical Procedures		
amniocentesis (am-nee-oh-sen-TEE-siss)	*amni/o* (amnion); *-centesis* (surgical puncture for aspiration)	extraction and diagnostic examination of amniotic fluid from the amniotic sac
bilateral oophorectomy (bye-LAT-er-ul oh-oh-for-EK-tuh-mee)	*bi-* (two); lateral (side); *oophor/o* (ovary); *-ectomy* (excision)	removal of both ovaries
bilateral salpingo-oophorectomy (bye-LAT-er-ul sal-ping-oh-oh-for-EK-tuh-mee	*bi-* (two); lateral (side); *salping/o* (tube, fallopian tube); *oophor/o* (ovary); + *ectomy* (excision)	removal of both sets of ovaries and uterine tubes
cervicectomy (surv-ih-SEK-toh-mee)	*cervic/o* (cervix); + *ectomy* (excision)	excision of the uterine cervix; also called *trachelectomy*
cervicoplasty (SUR-vih-koh-plass-tee)	*cervic/o* (cervix); + *plasty* (surgical repair)	surgical repair of the uterine cervix
cervicotomy (sur-vih-KOT-oh-mee)	*cervic/o* (cervix); + *-tomy* (incision into)	incision into the uterine cervix
cesarean section (CS or C-section) (seh-SAIR-ee-un SEK-shun)	perhaps from the story that Roman general and statesman Julius Caesar (100–44 BCE) was delivered by this method; other spellings are caesarean and caesarian	surgical operation through the abdominal wall and uterus for delivery of the baby
circumcision (SER-kum SIZH-un)	*circum/o* (around); from the Latin word *caedo* (cut)	a surgical procedure to remove the foreskin (prepuce) of the penis
colposcope (kol-POH-skope)	*colp/o* (vagina); *-scope* (instrument used to view)	endoscopic instrument used to magnify and examine the tissues of the vagina and cervix
colposcopy (kol-POSS-koh-pee)	*colp/o* (vagina); *-scopy* (use of an instrument for viewing)	using an endoscopic instrument to examine the vagina and cervix
dilation and curettage (D&C) (dye-LAY-shun AND KYOO-ruh-tahzh)	from the Latin word *dilatare* (to make wider, enlarge); from the French word *curette* (scoop)	dilation of the cervix and scraping of the lining of the uterus (curettage)
hysterectomy (his-ter-EK-tuh-mee)	*hyster/o* (uterus); *-ectomy* (excision)	surgical removal of the uterus
hysteropexy (his-ter-oh-PEK-see)	*hyster/o* (uterus); *-pexy* (fixation)	surgical lifting and holding of the uterus back into its normal position; also called *uteropexy*
hysteroplasty (his-ter-oh-PLAS-tee)	*hyster/o* (uterus); *-plasty* (surgical repair)	surgical repair of the uterus; also called *uteroplasty*
hysterosalpingography (HISS-ter-roh-sal-ping-goh-gruh-fee)	*hyster/o* (uterus); *salping/o* (tube, fallopian tube); *-graphy* (process of recording)	radiography of the uterus and uterine tubes
hysterotomy (his-ter-OT-oh-mee)	*hyster/o* (uterus); *-tomy* (incision into)	incision of the uterus; also called *uterotomy*
laparoscopy (lap-pair-OS-kuh-pee)	*lapar/o* (of or pertaining to the abdominal wall, flank); *-scopy* (use of an instrument for viewing)	direct visualization of the abdomen interior using a laparoscope

(continues)

Study Table The Reproductive System		*(continued)*
Term and Pronunciation	**Analysis**	**Meaning**
Diagnostic Tests, Treatments, and Surgical Procedures		
mammography (mah-MOG-ruh-fee)	*mamm/o* (breast); *-graphy* (process of recording)	examination of the breast by means of an imaging technique, such as radiography
mastectomy (mas-TEK-toh-mee)	*mast/o* (breast); *-ectomy* (excision)	removal of a breast
oophorectomy (oh-oh-for-EK-tuh-mee)	*oophor/o* (ovary); *-ectomy* (excision)	excision of an ovary; also called *ovariectomy*
oophoroplasty (oh-oh-for-oh PLAS-tee)	*oophor/o* (ovary); *-plasty* (surgical repair)	surgical repair of an ovary
oophorotomy (oh-oh-for-OT-uh-mee)	*oophor/o* (ovary); *-tomy* (incision into)	incision into an ovary
orchidectomy (or-kid-EK-toh-mee)	*orchi/o* (testes); *-ectomy* (excision)	removal of one testis or both testes; also called *orchiectomy*
orchiectomy (or-kee-EK-toh-mee)	*orchi/o* (testes); *-ectomy* (excision)	removal of one testis or both testes; also called *orchidectomy*
orchioplasty (OR-kee-oh-plass-tee)	*orchi/o* (testes); *-plasty* (surgical repair)	surgical repair of a testis
orchiotomy (or-kee-OT-uh-mee)	*orchi/o* (testes); *-tomy* (incision into)	incision into a testis
ovariectomy (oh-vair-ee-EK-toh-mee)	*ovari/o* (ovary); *-ectomy* (excision)	excision of one ovary or both ovaries
ovariotomy (oh-vair-ee-OT-oh-mee)	*ovari/o* (ovary); *-tomy* (incision into)	incision of an ovary
Pap smear (PAP SMEER)	named after George Papanicolaou, who developed the technique	exfoliative biopsy or a scraping of the cervix to diagnose conditions of the cervix and surrounding tissues
salpingo-oophorectomy (sahl-ping-goh oh-oh-fuh-REK-tuh-mee)	*salping/o* (tube, uterine tube); *oophor/o* (ovary); *-ectomy* (excision)	removal of an ovary and uterine tube
trachelectomy (tray-kuh-LEK-tuh-mee)	from the Greek word *trachelos* (neck) + *-ectomy* (removal)	surgery to remove the cervix (neck of the uterus); also called *cervicectomy*
transurethral resection of the prostate (TURP) (TRANS-yoo-ree-thrul ree-SEK-shun UV THE PROS-tate)	from the Latin *trans* (across); from the Greek word *ourethra* (urethra); + re- (again), and from the Latin word *secare* (to cut)	the removal of part or all the prostate through the urethra
tubal ligation (TOO-bul lye-GAY-shun)	from the Latin word *tubus* (tube) + *-al* (adjective suffix); ligation, from the Latin word *ligare* (to bind)	surgical procedure performed for female sterilization where each fallopian tube is tied off or "ligated" to prevent the oocyte from reaching the uterus
uteropexy (yoo-tur-oh-PEK-see)	*uter/o* (uterus); *-pexy* (fixation)	surgical fixation (holding in place) of the uterus; also called *hysteropexy*
uteroplasty (yoo-tur-oh-PLAS-tee)	*uter/o* (uterus); *-plasty* (surgical repair)	surgical repair of the uterus; also called *hysteroplasty*
uterotomy (yoo-tur-OT-uh-mee)	*uter/o* (uterus); *-tomy* (incision into)	incision of the uterus; also called *hysterotomy*

Term and Pronunciation	Analysis	Meaning
Diagnostic Tests, Treatments, and Surgical Procedures		
varicocelectomy (VAIR-ih- koh-seh-LEK-tuh-mee)	*varic/o* (varix, varicose, varicosity); *-cele* (hernia); *-ectomy* (excision)	the removal of a portion of an enlarged vein to remove a varicocele
vasovasostomy (vay-soh-vay-ZOS-toh-mee)	*vas/o* (vessel, vas deferens); *-stomy* (creation of an opening)	procedure to restore fertility to a vasectomized male; reconnect the ductus (vas) deferens
Practice and Practitioners		
gynecologist (guy-nuh-KOL-oh-jist)	*gynec/o* (woman, female); *-logist* (one who studies a certain field)	physician who specializes in female reproductive health
gynecology (guy-neh-KOL-oh-jee)	*gynec/o* (woman, female); *-logy* (study of)	the study of the female reproductive system
neonatology (NEE-oh-nay-TOL-oh-jee)	*neo-* (new); *nat/o* (birth); *-logy* (study of)	the medical specialty dealing with newborns
neonatologist (NEE-oh-nay-TOL-oh-jist)	*neo-* (new); *nat/o* (birth); *-logist* (one who studies a certain field)	physician who specializes in caring for newborns.
obstetrician (OB-stuh-trish-un)	from the Latin word *obstetricis* (midwife), derived from the Latin word *obstare* (to stand opposite to)	a physician who specializes in the medical care of females during pregnancy and childbirth
obstetrics (OB) (ob-STET-riks)	from the Latin word *obstetricis* (midwife), derived from the Latin word *obstare* (to stand opposite to)	medical specialty concerned with the medical care of females during pregnancy and childbirth
pediatrician (pee-dee-uh-TRISH-un)	from *paedo-* (of children) +*-iatr/o* (pertaining to medicine)	physician who specializes in treating children and their diseases
pediatrics (pee-dee-AT-riks)	from the Greek *paid-*, stem of *pais* (child); *-iatr/o* (pertaining to medicine)	medical specialty dealing with children
urologist (yoo-ROL-uh-jist)	*uro-* (urinary) + *logos* (study)	physician who diagnoses and treats disorders of the urinary system and male reproductive system

CASE STUDY WRAP-UP

Upon arrival, Paige was taken to an exam room where her physician performed a transvaginal ultrasound. Carefully positioning the wand, her physician took great care not to disrupt the placenta. Within minutes, Paige was diagnosed with placenta previa and admitted to the hospital's labor and delivery unit, where she and the fetus could be carefully monitored. Her doctor explained that there was a good chance that the bleeding would stop. Paige and her husband hoped this would be the case, but her OB/GYN stressed that she would need to limit standing for long amounts of time, she would need to avoid heavy lifting, and that the baby might have to be delivered by C-section.

Case Study Application Questions

1. What is an OB/GYN?
2. Describe placenta previa.
3. Which test diagnosed placenta previa?
4. What is a C-section, and why may Paige need one?

END-OF-CHAPTER EXERCISES

Exercise 15.1 Labeling

Using the following list, choose the terms to label the diagrams correctly.

Label the figure of the male reproductive system.

ductus deferens or vas deferens   glans penis   scrotum

epididymis   penis   seminal gland

foreskin   prostate   testis

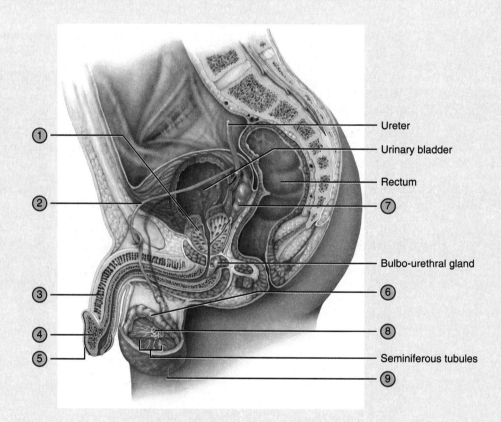

1. _____   4. _____   7. _____

2. _____   5. _____   8. _____

3. _____   6. _____   9. _____

Label the figure of the female reproductive system.

anus   labium minus   urinary bladder

cervix   ovary   uterine tube

clitoris   rectum   uterus

labium majus   urethra   vagina

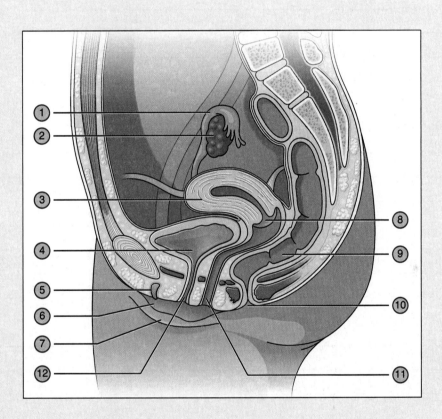

1. _____   5. _____   9. _____

2. _____   6. _____   10. _____

3. _____   7. _____   11. _____

4. _____   8. _____   12. _____

Exercise 15.2 Word Parts

Break each of the following terms into its word parts: prefix, root, or suffix. Give the meaning of each word part and then define the term.

1. *amenorrhea*

   prefix: _____

   root: _____

   suffix: _____

   definition: _____

2. *azoospermia*

   prefix: _____

   prefix: _____

   root: _____

   suffix: _____

   definition: _____

3. *dysmenorrhea*

   prefix: _____

   root: _____

   suffix: _____

   definition: _____

4. *menorrhagia*

   root: _____

   suffix: _____

   definition: _____

5. *prostatitis*

   root: _____

   suffix: _____

   definition: _____

6. *hysterotomy*

   root: _____

   suffix: _____

   definition: _____

7. *mastectomy*

   root: _____

   suffix: _____

   definition: _____

8. *neonatology*

   prefix: _____

   root: _____

   suffix: _____

   definition: _____

Exercise 15.3 Word Building

Use the word parts listed to build the terms defined.

-algia	-graphy	-logist	-pexy
amni/o	gynec/o	mamm/o	-pathy
-cele	hyster/o	mast/o	-scopy
-centesis	-itis	oophor/o	-tomy
cyst/o	lapar/o	orchi/o	uter/o

1. protrusion of the bladder into the anterior wall of the vagina _____

2. pain in the uterus _____

3. inflammation of the breast _____

4. any disease of the testes _____

5. extraction and diagnostic examination of amniotic fluid from the amniotic sac _____

6. examination of the breast by means of an imaging technique, such as radiography _____

7. direct visualization of the interior of the abdomen with the use of a laparoscope _____

8. incision into an ovary _____

9. surgical fixation of the uterus _____

10. medical specialist of the female reproductive system _____

Exercise 15.4 Matching

Match the term with its definition.

1. _____ vas deferens

2. _____ prostate

3. _____ spermatogenesis

4. _____ epididymis

5. _____ semen

6. _____ orchialgia

7. _____ testes

8. _____ hysterectomy and bilateral oophorectomy

9. _____ ovarialgia

10. _____ hysteropexy

11. _____ period of gestation

12. _____ oophoritis

13. _____ ovulation

a. combination of sperm and associated liquids that nourish the sperm

b. pain in the ovary

c. organs that produce and store male gametes

d. duct leading out of the epididymis

e. production of sperm

f. inflammation of an ovary

g. pain in the testes

h. release of the female gamete from the ovary

i. organ in which the male sperm become functional; lies on top of the testes

j. excision of the uterine cervix

k. surgical fixation of the uterus

l. the female gamete

m. surgical removal of the uterus and right and left ovaries

14. _____ oocyte

15. _____ cervicectomy

n. time lapse between zygote formation and birth

o. gland that surrounds the urethra; secretes alkaline fluid that assists in sperm motility

Exercise 15.5 Multiple Choice

Choose the correct answer for the following multiple-choice questions.

1. The surgical removal of testes is called _____.
    a. orchiectomy
    b. vasectomy
    c. circumcision
    d. cauterization
2. A prolapsed uterus means that the uterus is _____.
    a. bent backward on itself
    b. descended into the vagina
    c. tipped forward
    d. tipped backward
3. Menarche is _____.
    a. the beginning of menstruation
    b. the end of menopause
    c. part of the first trimester
    d. another name for gestation
4. Cryptorchidism is _____.
    a. underdeveloped testes
    b. small ovaries
    c. ruptured ovaries
    d. undescended testes
5. Removal of fluid from the area around the fetus to analyze it is called _____.
    a. cervicentesis
    b. amniocentesis
    c. intrauterine analysis
    d. uterocentesis

6. The surgical procedure that removes the prostate is called a _____.
    a. vasectomy
    b. prostatectomy
    c. vasoligation
    d. circumcision
7. A Papanicolaou test is done to detect _____.
    a. fibroids
    b. metritis
    c. cancer of the cervix
    d. ovarian cancer
8. A difficult or painful monthly blood flow is termed _____.
    a. dysmenorrhea
    b. menorrhea
    c. dysmetrorrhagia
    d. menometrorrhagia
9. A colposcope is used to visualize the _____.
    a. testis
    b. epididymis
    c. breast
    d. vagina

Exercise 15.6 Fill in the Blank

Fill in the blank with the correct answer.

1. A male gamete is also called a(n) _____.
2. A female gamete is also called a(n) _____.
3. Spermatogenesis is initiated by the secretion of the androgen _____.
4. The male glands located at the base of the urinary bladder that produce a fluid that nourishes the sperm are the _____.
5. The inner layer of the uterus is the _____.
6. A fertilized egg is called a(n) _____ during the first 8 weeks of gestation.
7. A fertilized egg that implants outside the uterus is called a(n) _____ pregnancy.
8. A Pap smear uses tissue from the _____.
9. The plural of ovum is _____.
10. The plural of ovary is _____.

Exercise 15.7 Abbreviations

Write out the term for the following abbreviations.

1. BPH _____
2. G _____
3. HIV _____
4. EDD _____
5. CS _____
6. OB _____
7. EDC _____
8. STD _____
9. GYN _____
10. PID _____
11. HSV _____

Write the abbreviation for the following terms.

12. abortus _____
13. sexually transmitted infection

   _____
14. transurethral resection of the prostate

   _____
15. gonorrhea _____
16. last menstrual period _____
17. dilation and curettage _____
18. para _____
19. human papillomavirus _____

Exercise 15.8 Spelling

Select the correct spelling of the medical term.

1. The Latin word for neck is
    _____, which is a common
    term for a structure found in the uterus.
    a. cirvix
    b. cervics
    c. cerviks
    d. cervix
2. The term for a female oocyte and a male sperm
    is _____.
    a. gameat
    b. gameet
    c. gamete
    d. gemete
3. The beginning of menses is called
    _____.
    a. menarche
    b. menarch
    c. menerch
    d. mennarche
4. The plural of testis is _____.
    a. testeas
    b. testes
    c. testies
    d. testees
5. A gene-bearing bundle of DNA found in the
    nucleus of all cells is a _____.
    a. cromosome
    b. chromasome
    c. chromosome
    d. chromosone

6. The absence of menstruation is called
    _____.
    a. amenorrhea
    b. amenorhea
    c. amenorea
    d. amenoria
7. A low sperm count is known as
    _____.
    a. oligaspermia
    b. oligospermia
    c. oligospermea
    d. oliguspermiea
8. The STD caused by the bacterium *Treponema
    pallidum* is _____.
    a. sipilis
    b. siphilis
    c. siphylis
    d. syphilis
9. A _____ is a practitioner who
    specializes in the female reproductive system.
    a. gynacologist
    b. gynecologist
    c. gynicologist
    d. gynocologist
10. The extraction and diagnostic examination of
    amniotic fluid from the amniotic sac is called
    _____.
    a. amiocentesis
    b. aminocentesis
    c. amniocentesis
    d. amnoicentesis

Exercise 15.9 Medical Report

The patient is a 27-year-old gravida II, para I female without significant medical history. Blood work was normal before delivery of a stillborn 1-pound, 11-ounce infant during week 21. Although ultrasound studies during week 14 and amniocentesis during week 15 were unremarkable, intrauterine fetal demise had occurred during week 18.

1. What does gravida II para I mean? _____
2. What is amniocentesis? _____
3. Using your knowledge of word parts, define intrauterine _____

Exercise 15.10 Reflection

1. What were you thinking might be wrong with Paige, the person in the chapter-opening case study?
2. Who might benefit from reading this chapter in your medical terminology book?
3. Why is it important for every person to know most of the terms in this chapter?

Appendix A

Answers to In-Text Questions

Chapter 1

QUICK CHECK

prefix = intra-
root = cran/i
suffix = -al

CASE STUDY APPLICATION ANSWERS

1. A geriatrician is a physician specializing in the care of older and aging adults.
2. Arthralgia is joint pain; it is derived from the word parts arthr- meaning joint and -algia meaning pain.
3. Osteoarthritis is a degenerative joint disease with inflammation of the bone; it is derived from the word parts osteo- meaning bone, arthr- meaning joint, and -itis meaning inflammation.
4. Greta was referred to an orthopedic surgeon because this is the medical specialty that deals with bone and joint issues.
5. The word root in the term neuroscience is neuro.

End-of-Chapter Exercises

Exercise 1.1 Defining Terms

1. cardiology
2. gerontology
3. hematology
4. dermatology
5. neurology
6. psychology

Exercise 1.2 Analyzing Terms

Term	Root	Suffix	Definition
1. neuropathy	neuro	-pathy	disease of the nerves
2. psychology	psycho	-logy	the study and science of the mind and behavior
3. pathogenic	patho	-genic	causing disease
4. neuralgia	neur	-algia	nerve pain
5. systemic	system	-ic	relating to a body system or systems
6. psychiatrist	psychiatr	-ist	a physician who specializes in the diagnosis and treatment of mental and emotional disorders
7. pediatrician	pediatr	-ician	a physician who specializes in treating children
8. iatrogenic	iatro	-genic	refers to ailments caused by a physician or other medical personnel
9. cardialgia	cardi	-algia	pain in the heart (or stomach)
10. neuritis	neur	-itis	inflammation of a nerve or nerves

Exercise 1.3 Fill in the Blank

1. around
2. study of
3. skin
4. osteo- and arthr- are roots; -itis is a suffix
5. logos, word

Chapter 2

QUICK CHECK		
anti-	definition: against	refers to: negation
hyper-	definition: above	refers to: position
tachy-	definition: rapid	refers to: speed

CASE STUDY APPLICATION ANSWERS

1. Dehydration is a condition characterized by severe water loss in the body. The body has lost more fluids than are taken in. The word part de- means "without," and the root word hydr- means "water."
2. The prefix hypo- means low. Hypotension is "low blood pressure."
3. Oliguria is very little urinary output; Bear wasn't urinating much. The word part olig- means "a little," and uria refers to "urine."
4. Ringer's lactate solution is a physiological saline solution containing sodium chloride, potassium, and calcium dissolved in water.

End-of-Chapter Exercises

Exercise 2.1 Adding Prefixes of Time and Speed

1. anteroom; outer room that leads into another room
2. neoclassic; new classic work
3. postglacial; following the glacial period
4. predominant; important
5. tachometer; instrument used to compute speed

Exercise 2.2 Adding Prefixes of Direction

1. abnormal; adjective meaning "away from normal"
2. adjoining; adjective meaning "next to"
3. concentric; having the same center
4. contralateral; the other side
5. diagram; illustration that gives an overall view
6. sympathetic; sharing emotions with another person
7. synthesis; assembling parts into a whole

6. inflammation, tendon
7. before
8. Pain, -dynia
9. -itis
10. psychology

Reflection answers will vary.

Exercise 2.3 Adding Prefixes of Position

1. eccentric; outside the center; unusual
2. ectomorph; slightly built person
3. enslave; to make a slave of
4. endocardial; adjective meaning "inside the heart"
5. epidemic; great number of occurrences of a particular disease
6. exchange; give something in return for another
7. exosphere; the far reaches of the atmosphere
8. extraterrestrial; beyond the earth
9. hypersensitive; highly sensitive
10. hypothesis; a possible explanation underlying the facts
11. infrastructure; the internal framework of a system or an organization
12. intercollegiate; participation involving at least two colleges
13. intramural; inside the walls; often applied to sports teams within a school
14. mesosphere; the middle part of the earth's atmosphere
15. metaphysics; beyond physics
16. panorama; a wide expansive view of everything
17. paralegal; a trained assistant to a lawyer

Exercise 2.4 Adding Prefixes of Size and Number

1. biannual; occurring twice a year
2. hemisphere; half of a sphere
3. macrocosm; the whole of something as in the whole world or universe
4. microscope; an instrument for viewing objects invisible to the human eye
5. monorail; a railway system on which the vehicle travels on one rail
6. oligarchy; rule by a small group of people
7. quadrilateral; having four sides
8. semiannual; twice a year
9. triangle; three-sided geometric shape
10. unicycle; a vehicle having one wheel

Exercise 2.5 Combining Roots and Suffixes That Denote Medical Conditions

1. card/i/o
   a. cardiocele; herniation of the heart
   b. cardiodynia; heart pain
   c. cardiectasia; dilation of the heart
   d. carditis; inflammation of the heart
   e. cardiomalacia; softening of the heart
   f. cardiomegaly; enlargement of the heart
   g. cardioptosis; drooping of the heart
   h. cardioplegia; paralysis of the heart
   i. cardiorrhexis; rupture of the heart wall
   j. cardiospasm; spasm of the heart
2. dermat/o
   a. dermatitis; inflammation of the skin
   b. dermatoma; tumor of the skin
   c. dermatomegaly; enlargement of the skin (congenital condition in which the skin hangs in folds)
   d. dermatosis; abnormal condition of the skin
3. hem/o, hemat/o
   a. hemolysis; destruction of the blood cells
   b. hematogenesis; produced by the blood
   c. hematoma; localized mass of blood
4. neur/o
   a. neuralgia; nerve pain
   b. neurectasis; dilation (stretching) of a nerve
   c. neuritis; inflammation of a nerve
   d. neuroma; tumor of a nerve
5. oste/o
   a. osteodynia; bone pain
   b. osteoma; bone tumor
   c. osteomalacia; softening of the bone
   d. osteopenia; reduction of bone density
   e. osteoporosis; porous bone, condition resulting in decreased bone mass
   f. osteitis; inflammation of the bone
6. psych/o
   a. psychosis; severe mental and behavioral disorder

Exercise 2.6 Combining Roots and Suffixes That Denote Diagnostic Terms, Tests, and Surgical Procedures

1. card/i/o
   a. cardiogenic; originating in the heart
   b. cardiogram; graphic record of the heart
   c. cardiograph; machine that produces a cardiogram
   d. cardiography; process of electrically measuring heart function
   e. cardiopathy; heart disease
   f. cardiorrhaphy; suture of the wall of the heart
2. dermat/o
   a. dermatoplasty; surgical repair of the skin
3. hemat/o
   a. hematogenesis; originating with or in the blood
   b. hematometry; examination of blood
4. neur/o
   a. neurectomy; removal of a nerve or part of a nerve
   b. neurogenic; adjectival form of neurogenesis; originating in the nervous system
   c. neurogenesis; originating in the nervous system
5. oste/o
   a. osteorrhaphy; suturing broken bone together
   b. osteoplasty; surgical repair of the bone
   c. osteogenesis; formation of bone
   d. ostectomy; excision of bone
   e. osteotomy; cutting of bone
6. path/o
   a. pathogen; a disease-causing agent
   b. pathogenic; adjectival form of pathogen; disease causing
   c. pathogenesis; development of a disease
7. psych/o
   a. psychogenic; adjectival form of psychogenesis; of brain origin
   b. psychogenesis; mental development
   c. psychometry; mental testing
   d. psychopathy; mental illness or disorder

Exercise 2.7 Combining Roots and Suffixes Associated with Medical Practices and Practitioners

1. card/i/o
   a. cardiology; medical specialty that diagnoses and treats heart diseases
   b. cardiologist; heart specialist
2. derm/o, dermat/o
   a. dermatology; medical specialty that diagnoses and treats skin disorders
   b. dermatologist; skin specialist
3. ger/o/nt/o
   a. geriatrics; medical specialty that diagnoses and treats the aged
   b. gerontology; the study of the process and results of aging
   c. gerontologist; specialist in gerontology
4. hem/o, hemat/o
   a. hematology; medical specialty that diagnoses and treats blood disorders

b. hematologist; a specialist who treats blood disorders

5. neur/o
   a. neurology; medical specialty that diagnoses and treats the nervous system
   b. neurologist; specialist who treats the nervous system

6. oste/o
   a. osteology; medical specialty that diagnoses and treats disorders of the skeletal system
   b. osteologist; a bone specialist

7. path/o
   a. pathology; study of disease
   b. pathologist; a medical specialist who studies pathology

8. psych/o
   a. psychology; study of the mind
   b. psychiatry; the medical specialty that diagnoses and treats mind disorders
   c. psychiatrist; a medical specialist in psychiatry

Exercise 2.8 Combining Roots and Suffixes That Denote Adjectives

1. card/i/o
   a. cardiac; refers to the heart
2. hem/o, hemat/o
   a. hemotoxic; destructive of red blood cells
3. derm/o, dermat/o
   a. dermal; adjective denoting skin
   b. dermatic; adjective denoting skin
4. ger/o, geront/o
   a. geriatric; adjective meaning "pertaining to the elderly or aging"
   b. gerontal; adjective meaning "old-age related"
5. neur/o
   a. neural; adjective meaning "related to the nervous system"
   b. neurotic; adjective meaning "pertaining to neurosis"
6. spin/o
   a. spinal; adjective referring to spinal column
   b. spinous; adjective meaning "having spines"
7. oste/o
   a. osteal; adjective meaning "bone"
   b. osteoid; adjective meaning "resembling bone"

Exercise 2.9 Matching Suffixes with Meanings

1. g
2. i
3. b
4. m
5. j
6. d
7. c
8. h
9. f
10. e
11. a
12. o
13. n
14. k
15. l

Exercise 2.10 Fill in the Blank

1. -algia, -dynia
2. angiectasis
3. adjective
4. suture of a blood vessel
5. -graphy
6. tumor of the blood vessel
7. surgical repair
8. dermatologist
9. old patients
10. gerontology is the study of old age; geriatrics is the branch of medicine dealing with the care of older people
11. ad-
12. ante-
13. abnormally slow heartbeat
14. beyond
15. hyper-
16. medicine to prevent coagulation (clotting)
17. three
18. The instrument will make objects visible that are too small to be seen with the unaided eye.
19. endocarditis; inflammation of the inside of the heart
20. Tachypnea is rapid breathing; dyspnea is difficulty or painful breathing.

Reflection answers will vary.

Chapter 3
Word Parts Exercise

1. across
2. back
3. near
4. cartilage
5. front, anterior
6. muscle
7. superior
8. neck
9. groin
10. spinal cord

> **QUICK CHECK**
>
> distal: proximal
> inferior: superior
> anterior: posterior
> dorsal: ventral

CASE STUDY APPLICATION ANSWERS

1. The trainer and the medical personnel stated that the injury was to the left leg. This means that in the anatomical position, the left leg is the patient's left. So, no matter the position of the medical team, to avoid wrong-site X-rays or surgeries, everyone must consider the anatomical position.
2. Supine means that Trayvon is lying face upward.
3. Anteroposterior means front to back; lateral means toward the side.
4. A proximal break of the tibia means that it is closer to the knee.

End-of-Chapter Exercises
Exercise 3.1 Matching
A Planes of the Body

1. c
2. b
3. a

B Directional Terms

1. f
2. g
3. h

4. j
5. i
6. e
7. a
8. d
9. c
10. b

Exercise 3.2 Fill in the Blank

1. distal
2. proximal
3. anterior, ventral
4. medial
5. superior
6. lateral
7. posterior, dorsal
8. inferior

Exercise 3.3 Word Building

1. hypo-, -ic; hypogastric
2. -al; dorsal
3. -itis; chondritis
4. trans-, -ic; transthoracic
5. -itis; neuritis
6. epi-, -al; epicardial

Exercise 3.4 Short Answer

1. lateral
2. toward the back
3. proximal
4. anterior or forward
5. ventral

Exercise 3.5 True or False

1. False
2. True
3. False
4. True
5. True
6. False
7. True
8. False
9. False
10. True

Reflection answers will vary.

Chapter 4
Word Parts Exercise

1. skin
2. fungus
3. cell
4. sweat
5. red
6. dry
7. to carry
8. below
9. sebum (oil; fat)
10. upon
11. white
12. blue
13. dry, scaly (fishlike)
14. skin
15. horn
16. skin
17. nail
18. black
19. hair
20. hardening
21. yellow

QUICK CHECK	
Suffix	**Term**
-ous	subcutaneous
-cyte	melanocyte
-aceous	sebaceous

CASE STUDY APPLICATION ANSWERS

1. Folliculitis is inflammation of the hair follicles.
2. The folliculitis was caused by *Pseudomonas aeuriginosa*.
3. Pruritis is the medical term for itching.
4. *Pseudomonas aeruginosa* is a bacterium. The nurse practitioner recommended an antibacterial topical cream. Antibacterials are medicines that kill bacteria. If it were a viral infection, an antiviral medicine would have been recommended.

End-of-Chapter Exercises

Exercise 4.1 Labeling the Skin

1. hair
2. epidermis
3. dermis
4. hypodermis (subcutaneous) layer
5. nerve
6. artery
7. vein
8. adipose tissue
9. sudoriferous (sweat) gland
10. hair follicle
11. arrector pili muscle
12. sebaceous (oil) gland
13. pore (opening of sweat gland)

Exercise 4.2 Word Parts

1. *avascular*
   prefix: a-, without
   root: vascular, small vessels
   definition: without blood vessels
2. *epidermis*
   prefix: epi-, upon
   root: dermis, skin
   definition: outer layer of the skin
3. *melanocyte*
   root: melano
   suffix: -cyte, cell
   definition: cell that produces melanin
4. *scabicide*
   root: scabies, infection caused by mites
   suffix: -icide, destruction
   definition: agent lethal to mites
5. *dermatomycosis*
   root: dermato, skin
   root: myc, fungus
   suffix: -osis, abnormal condition
   definition: fungal infection of the skin
6. *onychectomy*
   root: onych, nail
   suffix: -ectomy, excision
   definition: surgical removal of a nail
7. *ecchymosis*
   prefix: ec-, out
   root: chymos, juice
   suffix: -osis, abnormal condition
   definition: a purple patch more than 3 mm in diameter caused by blood under the skin
8. *antiseptic*
   prefix: anti-, against
   root: septic, poison
   definition: agent that inhibits the growth of infectious agents

Exercise 4.3 Word Building

1. dermatoplasty
2. hemangioma
3. dermatitis
4. subcutaneous
5. onchotomy
6. dermatology
7. onchyomalacia
8. paronchia
9. ichthyosis
10. hyperhidrosis

Exercise 4.4 Matching

1. d
2. e
3. i
4. f
5. b
6. c
7. g
8. j
9. h
10. a
11. l
12. k

Exercise 4.5 Multiple Choice

1. b
2. b
3. b
4. d
5. b
6. c
7. b
8. b
9. d
10. d
11. d
12. b
13. b
14. a
15. c

Exercise 4.6 Fill in the Blank

1. keloid
2. fissure
3. Cyanosis
4. scleroderma

5. alopecia
6. albinism
7. vitiligo
8. Urticaria
9. biopsy
10. polyp

Exercise 4.7 Abbreviations

1. body surface area
2. incision and drainage
3. SLE
4. UV

Exercise 4.8 Spelling

1. d.
2. d
3. c
4. a
5. d
6. c
7. b
8. d
9. a
10. a

Exercise 4.9 Medical Report

1. antibiotic; medication used to kill bacteria or treat an infection
2. impetigo; contagious superficial skin infection that presents with vesicles
3. dermatologist; medical specialist who diagnoses and treats disorders of the skin
4. dermatitis; inflammation of the skin
5. erythematous; redness of the skin
6. pustules; small, elevated areas of skin that contains pus
7. edema; swelling in the tissues
8. antipruritic medication; medication used to reduce or stop itching
9. pruritus; itching
10. One reason the dermatologist may have been asking about pets is that allergies to pets may cause some of the signs and symptoms of an allergic reaction. Another possible reason to ask about children and pets is that they can carry diseases that are uncommon in adult populations, but more common in children and animals.

Reflection answers will vary.

Chapter 5
Word Parts Exercise

1. swayback, curve
2. joined (yoked) together
3. wrist
4. foot, child
5. bone
6. bones of fingers and toes
7. pain
8. cranium
9. joined together
10. inflammation
11. muscle
12. to visually examine
13. movement
14. correct, straight
15. femur, thighbone
16. softening
17. surgical repair
18. joint
19. pelvis
20. growth
21. arm
22. finger, toe
23. rib
24. bone marrow
25. electricity
26. thorax, chest
27. humerus, upper arm bone
28. porous
29. stiff, fused, closed
30. vertebrae
31. written record of something
32. movement
33. both sides
34. calcaneus, heel bone
35. hump
36. neck
37. study of
38. cartilage
39. lower back
40. removal of, excision of
41. tumor

QUICK CHECK

1. osteocytes
2. synovial
3. mandible

CASE STUDY APPLICATION ANSWERS

1. The femur is the broken bone.
2. The femur attaches to the hip at the acetabulum.
3. Osteoporosis is a bone disorder characterized by loss of bone mass and density.
4. THR stands for total hip replacement.

End-of-Chapter Exercises
Exercise 5.1 Labeling: Skeleton

1. cranium
2. facial bones
3. mandible
4. sternum
5. costal cartilage
6. vertebral column
7. ilium
8. pubis
9. sacrum
10. calcaneus
11. metatarsals
12. phalanges
13. tarsal bones
14. tibia
15. fibula
16. patella
17. femur
18. clavicle
19. scapula
20. humerus
21. ribs
22. radius
23. ulna
24. carpal bones
25. metacarpals
26. phalanges

Exercise 5.2 Labeling: Long Bone

1. proximal epiphysis
2. diaphysis
3. distal epiphysis
4. spongy bone
5. epiphyseal plate

6. periosteum
7. compact bone
8. medullary cavity
9. endosteum

Exercise 5.3 Word Parts

1. *osteorraphy*
   root: oste/o = bone
   suffix: -rrhaphy = surgical suturing
   definition: suturing together the fragments of a broken bone
2. *arthrocentesis*
   root: arthr/o = joint
   suffix: -centesis = surgical puncture for aspiration
   definition: aspiration of fluid from a joint by needle puncture
3. *brachialgia*
   root: brachi/o = arm
   suffix: -algia (pain)
   definition: pain in the arm
4. *osteochondritis*
   root: oste/o = bone
   root: chondr/o = cartilage
   suffix: -itis = inflammation
   definition: inflammation of bone and its overlying cartilage
5. *carpectomy*
   root: carp/o = wrist
   suffix: -ectomy = surgical removal
   definition: excision of a portion or all the wrist
6. *chondrosarcoma*
   root: chondr/o = cartilage
   root: sarc/o = flesh
   suffix: -oma = tumor
   definition: malignant tumor originating from cartilage
7. *dactylomegaly*
   root: dactyl/o = finger, toe
   suffix: - megaly = enlargement
   definition: enlargement of one or more fingers or toes

Exercise 5.4 Word Building

1. osteomyelitis
2. arthroscopy
3. chondromalacia
4. arthrogram
5. arthralgia
6. kinesiology
7. chondroplasty
8. intercostal
9. osteitis

10. osteosarcoma
11. arthroplasty
12. myelogram
13. chondritis
14. osteoporosis
15. costalgia

Exercise 5.5 Matching

1. e
2. d
3. b
4. c
5. a
6. f
7. g

Exercise 5.6 Multiple Choice

1. d
2. a
3. d
4. a
5. c
6. b
7. c
8. d
9. a
10. a
11. d
12. b
13. a
14. a
15. b

Exercise 5.7 Fill in the Blank

1. arthritis
2. arthrocentesis
3. orthopedic surgeon
4. compound
5. medullary
6. ligament
7. herniated disc

Exercise 5.8 Abbreviations

1. anterior cruciate ligament
2. computed tomography
3. cervical vertebra 1
4. total knee arthroplasty
5. lumbar vertebra 5
6. rheumatoid arthritis
7. nonsteroidal anti-inflammatory drug

8. magnetic resonance imaging
9. THR
10. Fx
11. Tx
12. ROM
13. T12
14. TKR
15. MRI

Spelling

1. a
2. b
3. b
4. d
5. c
6. d
7. a

Chapter 6
Word Parts Exercise

1. ligament
2. tendon
3. tone
4. paralysis
5. muscle
6. movement
7. partial or incomplete paralysis
8. strength
9. muscle
10. four
11. fibrous membrane
12. fiber
13. half
14. alongside, near

QUICK CHECK

Muscle Tissue Type Location

1.	skeletal	voluntary, striated muscle tissue found throughout the body attached to bones
2.	smooth	involuntary muscle tissue lining blood vessels, hollow organs, and respiratory passageways
3.	cardiac	involuntary, striated muscle tissue making up the heart wall

---

8. c
9. a
10. b

Exercise 5.9 Medical Report

1. a physician who treats and diagnoses skeletal disorders
2. ROM = range of motion; her limited ROM in her right wrist indicates that she is unable to flex or move her wrist much.
3. A wrist bone was broken in several places.
4. Her left hip bone, which is formed by the fusion of the ilium, ischium, and pubis, was broken, and it pressed into another part of the bone.
5. realignment
6. a treatment using elastics or pulley and weights

Reflection answers will vary.

CASE STUDY APPLICATION ANSWERS

1. A rheumatologist is a physician who specializes in infectious and inflammatory diseases of the musculoskeletal system.
2. Dysphagia is difficulty swallowing.
3. Nushi has polymyositis.
4. Myopathy is a disease of muscle tissue.
5. Bilateral asthenia and atrophy mean that Nushi is experiencing muscle weakness (asthenia) and muscle wasting (atrophy) on both sides of her body (bilateral).

End-of-Chapter Exercises
Exercise 6.1 Word Parts

1. *fibromyalgia*
   root: fibro, fiber
   root: my/o, muscle
   suffix: -algia, pain
   definition: a chronic disorder characterized by widespread aching and stiffness of muscles and soft tissues
2. *periostitis*
   prefix: peri-, around
   root: osteo, bone
   suffix: -itis, inflammation

definition: inflammation of the periosteum, which is the covering that surrounds the bone

3. *tendinoplasty*
   root: tendo, tendon
   suffix: -plasty, restoring function to a part
   definition: surgical procedure to restore function to the tendon

4. *myology*
   root: my/o, muscle
   suffix: -ology, study of
   definition: study of muscles

5. *electromyography*
   root: electro, electricity
   root: myo, muscle
   suffix: -graphy, process of writing
   definition: diagnostic technique that records the strength of muscle contractions by means of electrical stimulation

6. *epicondylitis*
   prefix: epi-, around
   root: condyl, rounded end surface of bone
   suffix: -itis, inflammation
   definition: inflammation of the tissues around the elbow

7. *hemiplegia*
   prefix: hemi-, half
   root: plegia, paralysis
   definition: total paralysis of one side of the body

8. *paralysis*
   prefix: para-, not normal
   suffix: -lysis, loosening
   definition: loss of sensation and voluntary muscle movements caused by an injury or disease

Exercise 6.2 Word Building

1. tenotomy
2. neurologist
3. paraplegia
4. myocele
5. hemiparesis
6. fasciitis
7. kinesialgia
8. fibromyalgia
9. myopathy; musculopathy
10. myositis

Exercise 6.3 Matching

1. d
2. i
3. f
4. b

5. c
6. e
7. a
8. g
9. k
10. h
11. l
12. j

Exercise 6.4 Multiple Choice

1. c
2. c
3. b
4. d
5. a
6. a
7. c
8. a
9. d
10. a

Exercise 6.5 Fill in the Blank

1. Epicondylitis
2. ligament
3. plantar flexion
4. Asthenia
5. myocele
6. Plantar fasciitis
7. electromyography (EMG)
8. tendinoplasty
9. Myology
10. myalgia

Exercise 6.6 Abbreviations

1. muscular dystrophy
2. rest, ice, compression, elevation
3. cumulative trauma disorder
4. myasthenia gravis
5. EMG
6. ALS
7. IM
8. Fx
9. MD

Exercise 6.7 Spelling

1. c
2. a
3. b
4. d
5. d

6. c
7. c
8. b
9. a
10. a

Exercise 6.8 Medical Report

1. flexion (closing the angle of a joint); extension (opening the angle of a joint); rotation (turning a body part on its own axis); abduction (movement away from midline)
2. inflammation of a tendon
3. Range of motion is the amount of movement that is possible at the joint.
4. nonsteroidal anti-inflammatory drug

Reflection answers will vary.

Chapter 7

Word Parts Exercise

1. slight paralysis
2. outer layer or covering
3. referring to the mind
4. paralysis
5. memory
6. physician; to treat
7. fear
8. brain
9. the cerebrum; also, the brain in general
10. water
11. a membrane
12. ganglia (ganglion, singular)
13. suffix meaning mental abnormality or obsession
14. in connection with the nervous system, refers to the spinal cord and medulla oblongata
15. nerve, nerve tissue
16. spider
17. to split
18. head
19. mind
20. resembling
21. the cerebellum
22. spine
23. speech
24. glue

QUICK CHECK

1. brain and spinal cord
2. homeostasis
3. brainstem

CASE STUDY APPLICATION ANSWERS

1. Amyotrophic lateral sclerosis (ALS) is a fatal, progressive, degenerative disease of motor neurons leading to muscle atrophy (wasting) and loss of function.
2. Upper motor neurons originate in the brain and lower motor neurons originate in the spinal cord.
3. Signs that Pierce has motor neuron issues include those associated with voluntary muscle movement including slurred speech; hand weakness; foot slapping while walking; and difficulty buttoning his shirt, opening a juice container, and playing guitar.
4. Electromyography (EMG) is a test that evaluates electrical activity of muscles during contraction and relaxation.
5. The nerve conduction study was ordered to measure the speed at which the nerves are transmitting impulses to different body areas. This test determines nerve damage or nerve diseases.

End-of-Chapter Exercises

Exercise 7.1 Labeling

1. dendrites
2. nucleus
3. cell body
4. myelin
5. axon

Exercise 7.2 Word Parts

1. *psychosis*
   root: psycho, of or pertaining to the mind
   suffix: -sis, condition of
   definition: a serious disorder involving a marked distortion of, or sharp break from, reality
2. *electroencephalography*
   root: electro, electic
   root: encephalo, brain
   suffix: -graphy, process of recording
   definition: record of the electrical potential of the brain
3. *astrocytoma*
   root: astro, star
   root: cyt, cell
   suffix: -oma, tumor
   definition: star-shaped tumor that usually develops in the cerebrum
4. *cerebrovascular*
   root: cerebro, brain
   root: vascul
   suffix: -ar, adjective suffix
   definition: of or relating to the brain and its blood vessels
5. *encephalitis*
   root: encephal, of or pertaining to the brain
   suffix: -itis, inflammation
   definition: inflammation of the brain
6. *epidural*
   prefix: epi-, above
   root: dura, relating to the dura mater
   suffix: -al, adjective suffix
   definition: on or around the dura mater
7. *psychiatrist*
   root: psych, of or pertaining to the mind
   root: iatr, of or pertaining to medicine or a physician
   suffix: -ist, one who specializes in
   definition: a medical doctor who specializes in the diagnosis and treatment of psychological disorders
8. *meningioma*
   root: mening, membrane
   suffix: -oma, tumor
   definition: benign tumor of the meninges

Exercise 7.3 Word Building

1. encephalitis
2. glioma
3. hemiparesis
4. lobotomy
5. neuroglia

6. parasympathetic
7. paranoia
8. neuroplasty
9. diencephalon
10. paresthesia

Exercise 7.4 Matching

1. k
2. f
3. c
4. n
5. h
6. j
7. e
8. b
9. m
10. g
11. d
12. a
13. l
14. i

Exercise 7.5 Multiple Choice

1. d
2. c
3. a
4. b
5. a
6. b
7. c
8. c
9. d
10. c
11. b
12. d
13. b
14. b
15. d

Exercise 7.6 Fill in the Blank

1. hyperesthesia
2. poliomyelitis
3. dementia
4. multiple sclerosis
5. myelomeningocele
6. cerebral thrombosis
7. Ataxia
8. epilepsy
9. Syncope
10. neuralgia

Exercise 7.7 Abbreviations

1. intracranial pressure
2. cerebral spinal fluid
3. lumbar puncture
4. electroencephalography
5. multiple sclerosis
6. obsessive–compulsive disorder
7. Parkinson's disease
8. peripheral nervous system
9. cerebrovascular accident
10. dopamine
11. PTSD
12. PNS
13. CVA
14. MRI
15. TIA

Exercise 7.8 Spelling

1. a
2. c

3. c
4. d
5. a
6. b
7. d
8. b
9. c
10. a

Exercise 7.9 Medical Report

1. transient ischemic attack; sometimes called a ministroke
2. cerebrovascular accident
3. dys- means "difficult"; -phasia means "speak"
4. partial or incomplete paralysis
5. Hemiparesis means "partially paralyzed on half the body"; hemiplegia means "complete paralysis on half the body."
6. Hemi- means "half"; -plegia means "paralysis."

Reflection answers will vary.

Chapter 8
Word Parts Exercise

1. retina
2. hard, cornea
3. tear, lacrimal apparatus
4. light, eye, vision
5. eye
6. denoting the pigmented middle eye layer
7. two, double
8. tears, lacrimal sac, or lacrimal duct
9. iris
10. eye
11. lens
12. old age
13. eyelid
14. conjunctiva (plural: conjunctivae)
15. pupil
16. horny
17. relating to the sclera; hard

QUICK CHECK

1. fibrous, vascular, inner
2. choroid
3. pupil

Word Parts Exercise

1. sound
2. ear
3. hearing
4. tympanic membrane (eardrum)
5. eardrum
6. ear
7. stapes
8. ear

QUICK CHECK

1. malleus, incus, and stapes
2. conductive hearing loss, sensorineural hearing loss, presbycusis, and anacusis
3. cochlea

CASE STUDY APPLICATION ANSWERS

1. Floaters are flashes of specks or spots that dart about the field of vision. The eye "sees" them, but they are not caused by external light events, such as camera flashes or light flashes.

2. Thad saw an ophthalmologist because he needed a specialist in eye disorders and eye treatments. Family physicians are generalists and do not have the training that ophthalmologists do regarding eye diseases, diagnoses, and treatments.
3. Thad was diagnosed with retinal detachment (the retina has separated from the posterior eyeball) and vitreous hemorrhage (bleeding into the vitreous humor).
4. Thad needed a vitrectomy, an eye surgery that removes the vitreous humor and replaces it with a gel-like substance similar to vitreous humor. This surgery will treat his eye problem by also putting pressure on the retina and holding it in place against the posterior eye.

End-of-Chapter Exercises

Exercise 8.1 Labeling: The Eye

1. conjunctiva
2. cornea
3. iris
4. pupil
5. lens
6. anterior chamber (containing aqueous humor)
7. posterior chamber (containing vitreous humor)
8. sclera
9. choroid
10. retina
11. optic nerve

Exercise 8.2 Word Parts

1. *extraocular*
   prefix: extra-, outside
   root: ocul, eye
   suffix: -ar, adjective suffix
   definition: situated outside the eye
2. *xerophthalmia*
   root: xero, dry
   root: ophthalm, eye
   suffix: -ia, condition
   definition: dry eyes
3. *scleroiritis*
   root: sclera, sclera
   root: ir/o, iris
   suffix: -itis, inflammation
   definition: inflammation of the sclera and iris
4. *blepharoconjunctivitis*
   root: blephar, eyelid
   root: conjunctiv, mucous membrane covering the anterior surface of the eyeball and inner eyelid
   suffix: -itis, inflammation

   definition: inflammation of the palpebral conjunctiva, the inner lining of the eyelids
5. *audiometry*
   root: audio, hearing
   suffix: -metry, process of measuring
   definition: measuring hearing with an audiometer
6. *otosclerosis*
   root: oto, ear
   root: sclero, hardening
   suffix: -osis, abnormal condition
   definition: formation of spongy bone in the inner ear producing hearing loss
7. *mastoidectomy*
   root: mastoid, mastoid process
   suffix: -ectomy, excision
   definition: surgical removal of the mastoid process
8. *otorhinolaryngologist*
   root: oto, ear
   root: rhino, nose
   root: laryngo, throat
   suffix: -logist, one who studies a certain field
   definition: physician who specializes in the diagnosis and treatment of ear, nose, and throat disorders

Exercise 8.3 Word Building

1. dacryolith
2. phacolysis
3. dacryocystotomy
4. retinopexy
5. iridomalacia
6. tympanocentesis
7. otodynia
8. myringotomy
9. otorrhea
10. otitis

Exercise 8.4 Matching: The Eye

1. j
2. g
3. e
4. d
5. h
6. a
7. f
8. i
9. c
10. b

Exercise 8.5 Matching: The Ear

1. c
2. g

3. d
4. i
5. b
6. j
7. e
8. a
9. h
10. f

Exercise 8.6 Multiple Choice

1. b
2. a
3. d
4. c
5. a
6. d
7. b
8. c
9. a
10. d

Exercise 8.7 Fill in the Blank

1. cataract
2. presbycusis
3. diplopia
4. vertigo
5. Tinnitus
6. auricle
7. hordeolum
8. Otalgia
9. astigmatism
10. keratitis
11. cochlea
12. semicircular
13. auditory tube
14. Blepharoptosis
15. conductive

Chapter 9

Word Parts Exercise

1. secreting internally
2. pituitary gland
3. adrenal glands
4. suffix used in the formation of names of chemical substances
5. suffix meaning nourishment or stimulation
6. tumor
7. pancreas
8. extremities
9. gland

Exercise 8.8 Abbreviations

1. right ear
2. otitis media
3. right eye
4. left ear
5. both eyes
6. left eye
7. laser-assisted in situ keratomileusis
8. AU
9. EOM
10. AD
11. IOP
12. OS
13. OD or O.D.

Exercise 8.9 Spelling

1. a
2. c
3. b
4. b
5. d
6. d
7. a
8. b
9. c
10. a

Exercise 8.10 Medical Report

1. middle ear infection or inflammation
2. incision into the tympanic membrane
3. earwax
4. passageway leading inward from the auricle to the tympanic membrane (eardrum)

Reflection answers will vary.

10. thyroid gland
11. enlargement
12. sugar, glucose, glycogen
13. to separate or secrete
14. parathyroid gland
15. calcium

QUICK CHECK

1. hypophysis
2. suprarenal gland
3. Endocrine

CASE STUDY APPLICATION ANSWERS

1. Felicity was constantly hungry (polyphagia), constantly thirsty (polydipsia), and she had to urinate frequently (polyuria).
2. A fasting blood sugar test is a blood test taken after a person has not eaten (fasted) overnight. The results indicate normal, prediabetes, or diabetes.
3. The HbA1c test is a blood test that measures blood glucose levels over the past 3 months and is a good indicator of blood sugar levels over an extended time.

End-of-Chapter Exercises

Exercise 9.1 Labeling

1. pineal gland
2. thyroid
3. adrenal glands
4. testes
5. pituitary gland
6. parathyroid glands
7. thymus
8. pancreas
9. ovaries

Exercise 9.2 Word Parts

1. *adenogenous*
   root: aden/o (gland)
   suffix: -genous (originating)
   definition: originating in a gland
2. *epinephrine*
   prefix: epi- (upon)
   root: nephr/o (kidney)
   suffix: -ine (chemical substance)
   definition: hormone secreted from the adrenal medulla, which is the central region of the adrenal gland located on the superior border of each kidney
3. *suprarenal*
   prefix: supra- (above)
   root: ren/o (kidney)
   suffix: -al (pertaining to)
   definition: above the kidney
4. *adrenomegaly*
   root: adren/o (adrenal gland)
   suffix: -megaly (enlargement)
   definition: enlargement of the adrenal gland
5. *hyperglycemia*
   prefix: hyper- (above normal)
   root: glyc/o (glucose; sugar)
   suffix: -ia (condition)
   definition: excessive glucose (sugar) in the blood

6. *adenotomy*
   root: aden/o (gland)
   suffix: -tomy (cutting operation)
   definition: incision of a gland
7. *thyroparathyroidectomy*
   root: thryr/o (thyroid gland)
   root: parathyr/o (parathyroid gland)
   suffix: -ectomy (excision)
   definition: excision of the thyroid and parathyroid glands
8. *endocrinology*
   root: endocrin/o (endocrine)
   suffix: -ology (study of)
   definition: medical specialty of the endocrine system

Exercise 9.3 Word Building

1. adrenomegaly
2. adrenalectomy
3. adrenopathy
4. hypothyroidism
5. throiditis
6. throidotomy
7. thyromegaly
8. pancreatoma
9. pancreatitis
10. pancreatogenic

Exercise 9.4 Matching

1. d
2. k
3. g
4. i
5. a
6. e
7. f
8. m
9. j
10. b
11. c
12. l
13. h

Exercise 9.5 Multiple Choice

1. a
2. b
3. b
4. c
5. b
6. a
7. d
8. a
9. d

Exercise 9.6 Fill in the Blank

1. thyromegaly
2. diabetes mellitus
3. hyperglycemia
4. polyuria
5. glycosuria
6. glucagon
7. acromegaly
8. Homeostasis

Exercise 9.7 Abbreviations

1. glucose tolerance test
2. parathyroid hormone
3. thyroxine or tetraiodothyronine
4. fasting blood sugar
5. antidiuretic hormone
6. hemogloboin A$_{1c}$
7. growth hormone
8. parathyroid hormone
9. ACTH
10. FSH
11. DM
12. CT
13. MSH
14. T$_3$
15. PRL
16. TSH
17. LH

Exercise 9.8 Spelling

1. d
2. c
3. b
4. a
5. a
6. c
7. d
8. b
9. b
10. d

Exercise 9.9 Medical Report

1. difficulty speaking
2. goiter, thyromegaly
3. thyroid stimulating hormone

Reflection answers will vary.

Chapter 10

Word Parts Exercise

1. ven/o or phlebo
2. cardi/o
3. angi/o or vas/o
4. endo-
5. tachy-
6. thromb/o
7. peri-
8. ather/o
9. atri/o
10. -gram
11. -emia
12. my/o
13. -stenosis
14. hem/o, hemat/o
15. arteri/o
16. phleb/o or ven/o
17. valv/o, valvul/o
18. aort/o
19. brady-
20. varic/o
21. coron/o
22. -ectasis
23. vas/o or angi/o
24. electr/o
25. ventricul/o
26. isch

QUICK CHECK

1. arterioles
2. Veins
3. red blood cell

CASE STUDY APPLICATION ANSWERS

1. A physician is a person qualified to practice medicine who has a medical degree (doctor of medicine, MD or doctor of osteopathic medicine, DO) from an accredited institution, has completed the required internships and residencies, and passed medical boards. A physician assistant (PA) is similar to a physician in that they are both medical professionals who diagnose, treat, prescribe medications, and manage patients, but PA's have not gone to medical school. Physician assistants do go through specialized medical training programs associated with medical schools, and they do have considerable clinical experience, but their licensing requirements and medical boards are different and their scope of practice is not as broad.
2. A deep vein thrombosis (DVT) is a blood clot in a blood vessel that is below the skin surface (deep). It typically develops in the legs where blood can pool, especially from inactivity.
3. Lovenox and warfarin are blood thinners used to prevent blood clot formation.
4. An embolism is a blood clot, air bubble, or fatty fragment that breaks loose and travels throughout the bloodstream to a distant site where it can lodge in another vessel, creating an obstruction. If it travels to the lungs, it is known as a pulmonary embolism.

End-of-Chapter Exercises

Exercise 10.1 Labeling

1. superior and inferior vena cava
2. right atrium
3. right atrioventricular valve; also called tricuspid valve
4. right ventricle
5. pulmonary valve
6. pulmonary arteries
7. pulmonary veins
8. left atrium
9. left atrioventricular valve; also called mitral valve
10. left ventricle
11. aortic valve
12. aorta

Exercise 10.2 Word Parts

1. *erythrocyte*
   root: erythr/o (red)
   suffix: -cyte (cell)
   definition: red blood cell

2. *atherosclerosis*
   root: ather/o (fatty)
   root: scler/o (hardening)
   suffix: -osis (abnormal condition)
   definition: hardening and narrowing of the arteries
3. *cardiomyopathy*
   root: cardi/o (heart)
   root: my/o (muscle)
   suffix: -pathy (disease)
   definition: disease of the heart muscle
4. *endocarditis*
   prefix: endo- (within)
   root: cardi/o (heart)
   suffix: -itis (inflammation)
   definition: inflammation of the endocardium
5. *thrombocytopenia*
   root: thromb/o (blood clot)
   root: cyt/o (cell)
   suffix: -penia (deficiency)
   definition: abnormal decrease in the number of thrombocytes
6. *angiogram*
   root: angi/o (blood vessel)
   suffix: -gram (record or picture)
   definition: printed record of a blood vessel
7. *hematology*
   root: hemat/o (blood)
   suffix: -logy (study of)
   definition: medical specialty dealing with blood
8. *pericardiotomy*
   prefix: peri- (surrounding)
   root: cardi/o (heart)
   suffix: -tomy (cutting operation)
   definition: incision into the pericardium

Exercise 10.3 Word Building

1. cardiogenic
2. atriotomy
3. erythrocyte
4. hemophilia
5. vasospasm
6. thrombectomy
7. vasodilation
8. cardiomegaly
9. arteriostenosis
10. atheroma
11. leukocyte
12. valvectomy
13. cardiac
14. hemolysis, erythrolysis
15. interventricular
16. anemia

17. myocardium
18. atherectomy
19. arrhythmia

Exercise 10.4 Matching

1. g
2. i
3. b
4. a
5. f
6. h
7. j
8. c
9. e
10. d

Exercise 10.5 Multiple Choice

1. b
2. a
3. b
4. b
5. a
6. a
7. b
8. d
9. d
10. d

Exercise 10.6 Fill in the Blank

1. hypotension
2. tachycardia
3. hematologist
4. pulmonary
5. O, AB
6. cardiology
7. phlebotomy
8. hyperlipidemia
9. bicuspid
10. superior vena cava, inferior vena cava

Exercise 10.7 Abbreviations

1. blood pressure
2. atrial fibrillation
3. low-density lipoprotein
4. shortness of breath
5. white blood cell
6. atrioventricular
7. coronary artery disease
8. congestive heart failure
9. heart rate
10. hemoglobin
11. myocardial infarction
12. transient ischemic attack
13. Hb
14. A-fib
15. RBC
16. SA
17. CHF
18. ECG or EKG
19. CABG
20. HTN
21. DIC
22. HDL
23. PTCA

Exercise 10.8 Spelling

1. b
2. a
3. c
4. d
5. a
6. b
7. d
8. b
9. c
10. a

Exercise 10.9 Medical Report

1. pain in the chest due to ischemia
2. shortness of breath
3. high blood pressure
4. electrocardiogram; record of the heart's electrical activity
5. aspirin—anticoagulant effect; antiarrhythmics—decrease abnormal atrial heart beats; diuretics—decrease fluid volume by increasing urination; vasodilators—increase diameter of blood vessels to decrease blood pressure and increase blood flow
6. myocardial infarction or heart attack; lack of blood supply (infarction) to the heart muscle; my/o means "muscle" and cardi/o means "heart"
7. irregular atrial contractions; frequently a rapid irregular rhythm

Reflection answers will vary.

Chapter 11
Word Parts Exercise

1. immune system
2. ingest or engulf
3. protection
4. enlargement
5. tonsil
6. spleen
7. without
8. lymph nodes
9. lymph vessels
10. lymph or lymphatic system
11. thymus
12. resembling
13. disease

QUICK CHECK

1. fluid; fats
2. tonsils, lymph nodes, thymus, spleen, appendix, lymphoid nodules of the small intestine (Peyer's patches)
3. antigen

CASE STUDY APPLICATION QUESTIONS

1. Ibuprofen is an over-the-counter medication that is used as an analgesic (pain reliever) and an anti-inflammatory (swelling reducer). Petra had both pain and swelling, which could be alleviated with this medication.
2. A C-reactive protein (CRP) test is a blood test that measures levels of C-reactive protein, a marker of inflammation. It can be used to aid in diagnosing inflammatory diseases such as rheumatoid arthritis (RA) or lupus.
3. Rheumatoid arthritis is a chronic inflammatory autoimmune disorder characterized by joint swelling, pain, and joint distortion. As an autoimmune disorder, the body mistakenly attacks the joint lining, resulting in bone erosion and joint deformity.
4. A rheumatologist is a physician who specializes in the treatment of inflammatory conditions of the musculoskeletal system, particularly the joints.

End-of-Chapter Exercises
Exercise 11.1 Labeling

1. cervical lymph nodes
2. axillary lymph nodes
3. thymus
4. mediastinal lymph nodes
5. spleen
6. superficial lymphatics of lower limb

Exercise 11.2 Word Parts

1. *lymphocyte*
   root: lymph/o (lymph)
   suffix: -cyte (cell)
   definition: white blood cell in the lymphatic system
2. *phagocytosis*
   root: phag/o (ingest or engulf)
   root: cyt/o (cell)
   suffix: -osis (condition of)
   definition: process carried out by white blood cells to ingest and digest solid substances
3. *anaphylaxis*
   prefix: ana- (without)
   root: phylaxis (protection)
   definition: life-threatening reaction to a foreign substance
4. *hemolysis*
   root: hem/o (blood)
   suffix: -lysis (destruction)
   definition: destruction of red blood cells
5. *lymphoma*
   root: lymph/o (lymph)
   suffix: -oma (tumor)
   definition: tumor of lymph tissue
6. *splenectomy*
   root: splen/o (spleen)
   suffix: -ectomy (excision)
   definition: excision (removal) of the spleen
7. *thymectomy*
   root: thym/o (thymus)
   suffix: -ectomy (excision)
   definition: excision (removal) of the thymus
8. *immunology*
   root: immun/o (immune system)
   suffix: -logy (study of)
   definition: study of the immune system

Exercise 11.3 Word Building

1. lymphadenitis
2. lymphoma
3. thymomegaly
4. lymphangitis
5. lymphadenopathy
6. immunologist
7. lymphography
8. phagocytosis

Exercise 11.4 Matching

1. e
2. f
3. g
4. i
5. a
6. j
7. b
8. d
9. h
10. c

Exercise 11.5 Multiple Choice

1. b
2. c
3. c
4. a
5. d
6. b
7. c
8. b
9. c
10. d

Exercise 11.6 Fill in the Blank

1. lymphocytes
2. maintain fluid balance

3. lymph nodes
4. Innate
5. tonsils
6. lymphedema
7. splenectomy
8. allergist
9. thymus
10. immunodeficiency

Exercise 11.7 Abbreviations

1. systemic lupus erythematosus
2. rheumatoid arthritis
3. Epstein–Barr virus
4. AIDS
5. HIV

Exercise 11.8 Spelling

1. a
2. c
3. c
4. a
5. d
6. b
7. d
8. c
9. b
10. a

Exercise 11.9 Medical Report

1. disease of the lymph nodes
2. splenomegaly
3. an infectious disease caused by the Epstein–Barr virus (EBV)

Reflection answers will vary.

Chapter 12

Word Parts Exercise

1. voice
2. trachea
3. thorax, chest
4. bronchus
5. breathing
6. larynx
7. sinus cavity
8. rib, side, pleura
9. lungs, air
10. nose
11. oxygen
12. pharynx
13. diaphragm
14. lung
15. mouth, opening

CASE STUDY APPLICATION ANSWERS

1. Wheezing is a whistling breath sound that indicates excessive secretions or partially obstructed airways.
2. Cystic fibrosis (CF) is a genetic disorder in which the lungs become clogged with excessive amounts of abnormally thick mucus.
3. A pulmonologist is a physician who specializes in the respiratory system.
4. Mucolytics thin mucous secretions, and bronchodilators expand the bronchial tree to ease air passage.

End-of-Chapter Exercises

Exercise 12.1 Labeling

1. paranasal sinuses
2. lungs
3. trachea
4. bronchi
5. alveoli

Exercise 12.2 Word Parts

1. *nasopharynx*
   root: nas/o (nose)
   root: pharyng/o (pharynx)
   definition: upper portion of the pharynx
2. *pulmonary*
   root: pulmon/o (lung)
   suffix: -ary (related to)
   definition: adjective meaning related to the lungs
3. *dysphonia*
   prefix: dys- (painful)
   root: phon/o (sound)
   suffix: -ia (condition)
   definition: condition of painful speech
4. *hemoptysis*
   root: hem/o (blood)
   suffix: -ptysis (spitting)
   definition: spitting or coughing up blood

5. *laryngostenosis*
   root: laryng/o (larynx)
   root: sten/o (narrowing)
   suffix: -osis (abnormal condition)
   definition: condition of a narrowing of the larynx
6. *antipyretic*
   prefix: anti- (against)
   root: pyretos (fever)
   suffix: -ic (adjective)
   definition: drug used to reduce fever
7. *rhinoplasty*
   root: rhin/o (nose)
   suffix: -plasty (surgical repair)
   definition: surgical repair of the nose
8. *otolaryngologist*
   root: ot/o (ear)
   root: laryng/o (larynx)
   suffix: -logist (one who studies)
   definition: physician who specializes in ear, nose, and throat diseases

Exercise 12.3 Word Building

1. bronchitis
2. bronchiectasis
3. laryngitis
4. sinusitis
5. epiglottitis
6. tachypnea
7. bradypnea
8. dyspnea
9. orthopnea

Exercise 12.4 Matching

1. e
2. d
3. c
4. f
5. a
6. g
7. b
8. j
9. k
10. l
11. r
12. n
13. o
14. h
15. m
16. q
17. i
18. p

Exercise 12.5 Multiple Choice

1. c
2. c
3. b
4. d
5. b
6. b
7. c
8. b
9. b
10. c

Exercise 12.6 Fill in the Blank

1. hemoptysis
2. bradypnea
3. pneumocentesis
4. inflammation of the pleura (membrane that surrounds the lungs and lines the walls of the thoracic cavity)
5. pleura
6. orthopnea
7. bronchiectasis
8. rhinorrhea
9. Cheyne–Stokes respirations

Exercise 12.7 Abbreviations

1. chronic obstructive pulmonary disease
2. arterial blood gas

3. total lung capacity
4. cystic fibrosis
5. tonsillectomy and adenoidectomy
6. upper respiratory infection
7. TB
8. O_2
9. CO_2
10. PFT
11. RV
12. SOB

Exercise 12.8 Spelling

1. d
2. b
3. c
4. a
5. a
6. b
7. d
8. c
9. b
10. a

Exercise 12.9 Medical Report

1. a
2. b

Reflection answers will vary.

Chapter 13

Word Parts Exercise

1. eat or swallow
2. common bile duct
3. mouth
4. sigmoid colon
5. abdomen
6. intestine
7. abdomen
8. rectum
9. stone
10. salivary glands
11. liver
12. pylorus
13. bile, gall
14. bile duct
15. esophagus
16. vomit
17. instrument used for viewing
18. tongue
19. jejunum
20. stomach
21. lip
22. ileum
23. pancreas
24. cheek
25. gallbladder
26. digestion
27. colon
28. teeth
29. eating, swallowing
30. duodenum
31. anus and rectum
32. gums
33. visual examination
34. nutrition

1. bolus
2. The stomach also secretes acid and enzymes to help break down proteins, fats, and carbohydrates.
3. duodendum, jejunum, ileum

CASE STUDY APPLICATION ANSWERS

1. Crohn's disease is a type of inflammatory bowel disease characterized by abdominal pain, diarrhea, and immune-mediated inflammation.
2. Diarrhea is loose, watery, and frequent bowel movements.
3. Colonoscopy is a medical procedure in which a colonoscope is inserted through the anus to visually inspect the colon.
4. Anti-inflammatory drugs decrease inflammation.
5. Stool studies are used to test for hidden (occult) blood, bacteria, parasites, antigens, and fat in a fecal (stool) sample.

End-of-Chapter Exercises
Exercise 13.1 Labeling

1. mouth
2. pharynx
3. esophagus
4. liver
5. gallbladder
6. bile duct
7. small intestine
8. large intestine
9. salivary gland
10. stomach
11. pancreas
12. anus

Exercise 13.2 Word Parts

1. *cholelithiasis*
   root: chol/e (bile, gall)
   suffix: -lith (stone)
   suffix: -iasis (condition of)
   definition: formation or presence of stones in the gallbladder or common bile duct
2. *enterohepatitis*
   root: enter/o (intestine)
   root: hepat/o (liver)
   suffix: -itis (inflammation)
   definition: inflammation of the intestine and liver

3. *parotiditis*
   prefix: para- (beside)
   root: ot/o (ear)
   suffix: -itis (inflammation)
   definition: inflammation of the parotid salivary gland
4. *sialorrhea*
   root: sial/o (saliva, salivary gland)
   suffix: -rrhea (discharge)
   definition: excessive production of saliva
5. *colonoscopy*
   root: colon/o (colon)
   suffix: -scopy (viewing)
   definition: visual examination of the colon
6. *gastroenterologist*
   root: gastr/o (stomach)
   root: enter/o (intestine)
   suffix: -logist (one who studies)
   definition: a specialist in the diagnosis and treatment of digestive system disorders
7. *colectomy*
   root: col/o (colon)
   suffix: -ectomy (surgical removal)
   definition: excision of all or part of the colon
8. *jejunotomy*
   root: jejun/o (jejunum)
   suffix: -tomy (incision)
   definition: incision into the jejunum

Exercise 13.3 Word Building

1. gastric
2. cholecystopathy
3. gingivitis
4. sialostenosis
5. enteroscope
6. colopexy
7. jejunectomy
8. hepatogenic
9. dysphagia
10. duodenal

Exercise 13.4 Matching

1. b
2. f
3. i
4. g
5. h
6. d
7. e
8. a
9. c
10. j

Exercise 13.5 Multiple Choice

1. b
2. c
3. c
4. a
5. c
6. c
7. b
8. d
9. b
10. a

Exercise 13.6 Fill in the Blank

1. ileocecal sphincter
2. rectum
3. salivary glands
4. gallbladder
5. stomach
6. cholecystitis
7. cholelithiasis
8. antiemetic
9. gastroscope
10. gastrectomy

Exercise 13.7 Abbreviations

1. *per os* or nothing by mouth
2. upper gastrointestinal series
3. total parenteral nutrition
4. bowel movement
5. gastrointestinal
6. gastroesophageal reflux disease
7. irritable bowel syndrome
8. lower esophageal sphincter

9. HCl
10. NG
11. BE
12. EGD
13. NPO

Exercise 13.8 Spelling

1. a
2. c
3. b
4. b
5. d
6. c
7. c
8. a
9. d
10. b

Exercise 13.9 Medical Report

1. shortness of breath
2. blood pressure
3. HTN stands for hypertension, which is high blood pressure. Hypertension and shortness of breath may accompany each other. Smoking and excessive caffeine intake may be related to both conditions.
4. white blood cell
5. Endo- means within; -scopy means "look" or "see." Endoscopy may be defined as looking inside, by means of an instrument called an endoscope.
6. A gastric ulcer is a sore on the lining (mucous membrane) of the stomach.

Reflection answers will vary.

Chapter 14

Word Parts Exercise

1. urine
2. night
3. little, few
4. condition, state
5. glomerulus
6. kidney
7. urethra
8. stone
9. much, many
10. pus

11. pelvis
12. ureter
13. bladder

QUICK CHECK

1. kidneys, ureters, urinary bladder, and urethra
2. hilum
3. internal urethral sphincter and external urethral sphincter

CASE STUDY APPLICATION ANSWERS

1. J.T.'s underlying medical condition is type 2 diabetes mellitus.
2. GFR stands for glomerular filtration rate and is a measure of how well the kidneys are filtering the blood.
3. Both the GFR and UACR test results indicate kidney disease.
4. Albuminuria is the term for albumin in the blood.
5. Azotemia, also called uremia, is a term for excess urea in the blood.

End-of-Chapter Exercises
Exercise 14.1 Labeling

1. inferior vena cava
2. abdominal aorta
3. urinary bladder
4. urethra
5. kidneys
6. ureters

Exercise 14.2 Word Parts

1. *anuria*
   prefix: an-, without
   root: ur/o, urine
   suffix: -ia, condition
   definition: absence of urine formation
2. *cystalgia*
   root: cyst/o, bladder
   suffix: -algia, pain
   definition: pain in the bladder
3. *nephrolithiasis*
   root: nephr/o, kidney
   root: lith/o, stone
   suffix: -iasis, condition
   definition: presence of a kidney stone
4. *hematuria*
   root: hemat/o, blood
   root: ur/o, urine
   suffix: -ia, condition
   definition: blood in the urine
5. *glomerulonephritis*
   root: glomerul/o, glomerulus
   root: nephr/o, kidney
   suffix: -itis, inflammation
   definition: renal disease characterized by inflammation of the glomeruli

6. *nephrologist*
   root: nephr/o, kidney
   suffix: -logist, one who studies
   definition: a specialist who treats kidney disorders
7. *urology*
   root: ur/o, urine
   suffix: -logy, study of
   definition: study of the urinary system
8. *nephrectomy*
   root: nephr/o, kidney
   suffix: -ectomy, removal
   definition: removal of a kidney

Exercise 14.3 Word Building

1. albuminuria
2. nephralgia
3. urethrostenosis
4. uremia
5. lithotripsy
6. urologist
7. nephrology
8. cystectomy
9. cystoscope
10. ureterorrhaphy

Exercise 14.4 Matching

1. g
2. d
3. k
4. a
5. b
6. j
7. h
8. f
9. e
10. r
11. p
12. m
13. n
14. q
15. l
16. i
17. c
18. o

Exercise 14.5 Multiple Choice

1. d
2. b
3. d
4. a
5. a

6. c
7. c
8. b
9. b
10. d

Exercise 14.6 Fill in the Blank

1. kidney transplant
2. nephropexy
3. nephrolithotomy
4. ureteroplasty
5. cystoscopy
6. Diuretics
7. ureters
8. urea and uric acid
9. dialysis
10. one who studies

Exercise 14.7 Abbreviations

1. urinary tract infection
2. glomerular filtration rate
3. end-stage renal disease
4. blood urea nitrogen
5. chronic renal failure
6. UA
7. KUB
8. ARF
9. IVP
10. CAPD

Exercise 14.8 Spelling

1. a
2. a
3. b
4. d
5. c
6. a
7. c
8. d
9. c
10. d

Exercise 14.9 Medical Report

1. urologist
2. dysuria
3. hematuria
4. urinalysis (UA)
5. intravenous pyelogram (IVP)
6. calculi
7. urinary bladder
8. urinary tract infection (UTI)
9. calculi
10. antibiotic
11. cystoscopy

Reflection answers will vary.

Chapter 15

Word Parts Exercise

1. breast
2. sperm
3. uterine tube
4. vessel, vas deferens
5. around
6. ovary, egg-bearing
7. vagina
8. prostate gland
9. amnion
10. birth
11. uterus
12. vulva
13. testes
14. cervix, neck
15. glans penis
16. gonads, sex glands
17. woman, female
18. milk
19. menses, menstruation
20. ovary, egg-bearing

QUICK CHECK

1. synthesizing testosterone, producing and storing sperm, and making and releasing fluid from glands that support the sperm
2. lactation
3. gestation

CASE STUDY APPLICATION ANSWERS

1. An OB/GYN is an obstetrician/gynecologist who specializes in female reproductive health. These highly trained physicians treat conditions of the reproductive system, including menstruation problems, pregnancy, childbirth, and diseases/disorders unique to females.
2. Placenta previa is a condition in which the placenta, an organ that develops during pregnancy, covers the cervix (opening of the uterus). The placenta usually attaches to the top (superior portion) or side of the uterus. If the placenta attaches to the lower uterine wall, tissue covers the cervix and may result in excessive bleeding during pregnancy (as Paige experienced) or during delivery.
3. Transvaginal ultrasound diagnosed placenta previa.
4. A C-section is a surgical operation in which an incision is made into the pregnant person's abdomen to deliver the fetus. C-sections are performed when a vaginal birth is not recommended, as in Paige's case. If Paige were to have a vaginal birth, the risk of vaginal bleeding and hemorrhage is increased.

End-of-Chapter Exercises

Exercise 15.1 Labeling

Male reproductive system

1. prostate
2. ductus deferens or vas deferens
3. penis
4. glans penis
5. foreskin
6. epididymis
7. seminal gland
8. testis
9. scrotum

Female reproductive system

1. uterine tube
2. ovary
3. uterus
4. urinary bladder
5. clitoris
6. labium minus
7. labium majus
8. cervix
9. rectum
10. anus
11. vagina
12. urethra

Exercise 15.2 Word Parts

1. *amenorrhea*
   prefix: a- (without)
   root: men/o (menses)
   suffix: -rrhea (flowing, discharge)
   definition: absence of menstruation
2. *azoospermia*
   prefix: a- (without)
   prefix: zoo- (animal, living being)
   root: sperm/o (sperm)
   suffix: -ia (condition of)
   definition: absence of sperm in the semen
3. *dysmenorrhea*
   prefix: dys- (bad, difficult)
   root: men/o (menses)
   suffix: -rrhea (flowing, discharge)
   definition: painful menstruation
4. *menorrhagia*
   root: men/o (menses)
   suffix: -rrhagia (rapid flow of blood)
   definition: increased amount and duration of flow
5. *prostatitis*
   root: prostat/o (prostate)
   suffix: -itis (inflammation)
   definition: inflammation of the prostate
6. *hysterotomy*
   root: hyster/o (uterus)
   suffix: -tomy (incision into)
   definition: incision of the uterus
7. *mastectomy*
   root: mast/o (breast)
   suffix: -ectomy (excision)
   definition: removal of a breast
8. *neonatology*
   prefix: neo- (new)
   root: nat/o (birth)
   suffix: -logy (study of)
   definition: medical specialty dealing with newborns

Exercise 15.3 Word Building

1. cystocele
2. hysteralgia
3. mastitis
4. orchiopathy
5. amniocentesis
6. mammography
7. laparoscopy

8. oophorotomy
9. uteropexy
10. gynecologist

Exercise 15.4 Matching

1. d
2. o
3. e
4. i
5. a
6. g
7. c
8. m
9. b
10. k
11. n
12. f
13. h
14. l
15. j

Exercise 15.5 Multiple Choice

1. a
2. b
3. a
4. d
5. b
6. b
7. c
8. a
9. d

Exercise 15.6 Fill in the Blank

1. sperm
2. oocyte
3. testosterone
4. seminal glands or seminal vesicles
5. endometrium
6. embryo
7. ectopic
8. cervix
9. ova
10. ovaries

Exercise 15.7 Abbreviations

1. benign prostatic hyperplasia
2. gravida
3. human immunodeficiency virus
4. estimated date of delivery
5. cesarean section
6. obstetrics
7. estimated date of confinement
8. sexually transmitted disease
9. gynecology
10. pelvic inflammatory disease
11. herpes simplex virus
12. A
13. STI
14. TURP
15. GC
16. LMP
17. D&C
18. P
19. HPV

Exercise 15.8 Spelling

1. d
2. c
3. a
4. b
5. c
6. a
7. b
8. d
9. b
10. c

Exercise 15.9 Medical Report

1. Gravida II means that she has had two pregnancies. Para I means that she has had one birth after 20 weeks.
2. An amniocentesis is a transabdominal puncture of the amniotic sac to remove amniotic fluid for testing.
3. Intrauterine means within the uterus.

Reflection answers will vary.

Appendix B

Glossary of Word Parts with Meanings

Word Part	Meaning
ab-	away from, outside of, beyond
abdomin/o	abdomen
-ac	converts a root or noun to an adjective
acous/o acoust/o acus/o	hearing
acr/o	extremities
ad-	toward, near to
aden/o	gland
adeno-	glandlike
adren/o	adrenal glands
adrenal/o	adrenal glands
adip/o	fat
-al	adjective suffix
albin/o	white
-algia	pain
aliment/o	nutrition
amni/o	amnion
-amphi	both sides
a-, an-	not; without
-an	converts a root or noun to an adjective
-aneous	converts a root or noun to an adjective
angi/o	blood vessel
ankyl/o	stiff, fused, closed
ante-	before
anter/o	front, anterior

Word Part	Meaning
anti-	against, opposed
aort/o	aorta
-ar	converts a root or noun to an adjective
arachn/o	spider
arter/i/o	artery
ather/o	fatty
arthr/o	joint
aspir/o	breathe in
atri/o	atrium
-ary	converts a root or noun to an adjective
audi/o	sound
aur/o	ear
auricul/o	ear
balan/o	glans penis
bi-	two
blephar/o	eyelid
brachi/o	arm
brady-	slow
bronch/o bronchi/o	bronchus
bucc/o	cheek
calcane/o	calcaneus, heel bone
calc/i	calcium
card/i/o	heart
carp/o	wrist

Word Part	Meaning
-cele	protrusion, hernia
-centesis	surgical puncture
cephal/o	head
cerebell/o	cerebellum
cerebr/o	cerebrum; brain
cerv/o cervic/o	neck, cervix
cheil/o	lip
chol/e, chol/o	bile, gall
cholangi/o	bile duct
cholecyst/o	gallbladder
choledoch/o	common bile duct
chondr/o	cartilage
circum/o	around
cirrh/o	yellow
col/o, colon/o	colon
colp/o	vagina
con-	with
conjunctiv/o	conjunctiva (*conjunctivae*, plural)
contra-	against
corne/o	horny
coron/o	crown; encircling, such as in the coronary blood vessels encircling the heart
cortic/o	outer layer or covering
cost/o	rib
crani/o	cranium, skull
crin/o	to separate or secrete
cutane/o	skin
cyan/o	blue
cyst/o	bladder
-cyte, cyt/o	cell
dacry/o	tears, lacrimal sac, or lacrimal duct
dactyl/o	finger, toe
de-	without, not
dent/i, dent/o	teeth
derm/o dermat/o	skin

Word Part	Meaning
-desis	surgical binding
di-, dipl-	two, twice
dipl/o	two, double
dia-	across, through
dis-	remove
diverticul/o	diverticulum
dors/o	back
duoden/o	duodenum
-dynia	pain
dys-	painful, bad, difficult
-eal	converts a root or noun to an adjective
ec-, ecto-	outside
-ectomy	surgical removal
-ectasia -ectasis	expansion or dilation
-edema	excessive fluid
electr/o	electricity
-emesis	vomiting
-emia	blood
en-	inside
enchephal/o	brain
endo-	within, inner
endocrin/o	secreting internally
enter/o	intestine
-eous	converts a root or noun to an adjective
epi-	upon, above, in addition
erythr/o	red
esophag/o	esophagus
ex-, exo-	outside
extra-	beyond
fasci/o	fibrous membrane
femur/o	femur, thighbone
fer/o	to carry
fibr/o	fiber
gangli/o	ganglia (*ganglion*, singular)
ganglion/o	ganglia (*ganglion*, singular)

Word Part	Meaning
gastr/o	stomach
-gen, -genic	origin, cause, formation
-genesis	origin, producing
gen/o	origin, cause, formation
ger/o/onto	old age
gingiv/o	gums
gli/o	glue
glomerul/o	glomerulus
gloss/o	tongue
gluc/o	sugar, glucose, glycogen
glyc/o	sugar, glucose, glycogen
gonad/o	gonads, sex glands
-gram	a recording, usually by an instrument; written record of something
-graph	the instrument for making a recording
-graphy	act of graphic or pictorial recording
gynec/o	woman, female
hem/a/to	blood
hemi-	half
hem/o	blood
hemat/o	blood
hepat/o	liver
humer/o	humerus, upper arm bone
hydr/o	water
hyper-	above, beyond normal
hypo-	low, below, below normal
hypophys/o	pituitary gland
hyster/o	uterus
-iac	converts a root or noun to an adjective
-ian	specialist
-iasis	a condition or state
-iatric	converts a root or noun to an adjective
-iatrics	medical specialty
iatr/o	physician

Word Part	Meaning
-iatry	medical specialty
-ic	suffix that converts a noun to an adjective
-ical	converts a root or noun to an adjective
ichthy/o	dry, scaly
-ics	medical specialty
ile/o	ileum
immun/o	immune system
-ine	suffix used in the formation of names of chemical substances
infra-	inside or below
inguin/o	groin
inter-	between
intra-	inside, within
irid/o	iris
-ism	a condition of; a process; or a state of
-ist	specialist in a field of study
-itis	inflammation
jaund/o	yellow
jejun/o	jejunum
kerat/o	horn, cornea
kine-kinesi/o	movement
-kinesia	movement
kyph/o	hump
lacrim/o	tear, lacrimal apparatus
lact/o	milk
lapar/o	abdomen
laryng/o	larynx
ligament/o	ligament
-lith	stone, calculus, calcification
lob/o	lobe
-logy	study of
lord/o	swayback, curve
lumb/o	lower back
lymph/o	lymph or lymphatic system

Word Part	Meaning
lymphaden/o	lymph nodes
lymphangia/o	lymph vessels
lymphat/o	lymph or lymphatic system
-lysis	disintegration, breaking down
macro-	big
-malacia	softening
mamm/o	breast
-mania	mental abnormality or obsession
mast/o	breast
-megaly	enlargement
melan/o	black
meningi/o	membrane
men/o	menses, menstruation
ment/o	referring to the mind
meso-	middle
meta-	beyond
-meter	device for measuring
metr/o	uterus
-metry	act of measuring
micro-	small
-mnesia	memory
mono-	one
muscul/o	muscle
myc/o	fungus
my/o	muscle
myel/o	spinal cord and medulla oblongata; bone marrow
myring/o	tympanic membrane (eardrum)
nas/o	nose
natal	birth; born
nat/o	birth
neo-	new
nephr/o	kidney
neur/o	nerve, nerve tissue
noct/o	night
ocul/o	eye

Word Part	Meaning
-oid	forming adjectives and nouns denoting a form or resemblance to
olig-	little, few, scant
oligo-	little, few, scant
-oma	tumor
onych/o	nail
oophor/o	ovary, egg-bearing
ophthalm/o	eye
-opia	vision
-opsy	examination
opt/o	light, eye, vision
orch/o	testes
orchi/o	testes
orchid/o	testes
or/o	mouth, opening
-orth/o	correct, straight
-osis	abnormal condition; condition of
oste/o	bone
-otic	converts a root or noun to an adjective
ot/o	ear
-ous	converts a root or noun to an adjective
ovari/o	ovary, egg-bearing
-oxia	oxygen
pan-	all or everywhere
panceat/o	pancreas
para-	alongside, near; disordered function
parathyr/o	parathyroid gland
parathyroid/o	parathyroid gland
-paresis	partial or incomplete paralysis
path/o	disease
-pathy	disease
ped/ia	child
ped/o	foot, child
pelv/o	pelvis
-penia	reduction of size or quantity

Word Part	Meaning
-pepsia	digestion
peri-	around, surrounding
-pexy	surgical fixation
phac/o	lens
phag/o	eating, swallowing
-phagia	eat or swallow
phalang/o	bones of fingers and toes
pharyng/o	pharynx
-phasia	speech
phleb/o	vein
-phobia	fear
-phonia	voice
phren/o	diaphragm
-phylaxis	protection
-physis	growth
pil/o	hair
-plasia	abnormal formation
-plasty	surgical repair
-plegia	paralysis
pleur/o	rib, side, pleura
-pnea	breathing
pneumo-	lungs, air
pneumon/o	lungs, air
-poesis	producing
poly-	many
-porosis	porous condition
post-	after
poster/o	posterior, back
pre-	before
presby/o	old age
proct/o	anus and rectum
prostat/o	prostate gland
proxim/o	near
-ptosis	downward displacement
psych/o	mind
pulmon/o	lung

Word Part	Meaning
pupil/o	pupil
pyel/o	pelvis
pylor/o	pylorus
py/o	pus
quadri-	four
rect/o	rectum
ren/o	kidney
retin/o	retina
retro-	backward, behind
rhin/o	nose
-rrhage	flowing forth
-rrhapy	suture
-rrhea	discharge
-rrhexis	rupture
salping/o	tube, uterine tube
schiz/o	to split
scler/o	hard; relating to the sclera
-sclerosis	hardness
-scope	viewing; an instrument used for viewing
-scopy	act of viewing, to visually examine
seb/o	sebum
semi-	half, partial
sial/o	salivary glands
sigmoid/o	sigmoid colon
sinus/o	sinus cavity
skelet/o	skeleton
-spasm	muscular contraction
sperm/o	sperm
spermat/o	sperm
spin/o	spine
splen/o	spleen
spondyl/o	vertebrae
staped/o	stapes (smallest ear bone)
-stasis	level; unchanging
-stenosis	a narrowing

Word Part	Meaning
sthen/o	strength
stomat/o	mouth
-stomy	artificial or surgical opening
sub-	below
sudor-	sweat
super/o	superior
sym-	with
syn-	with, joined together
tachy-	rapid
tend/o	tendon; to stretch
tendin/o	tendon; to stretch
tetra-	four
thorac/o	thorax, chest
thorac/l	thorax, chest
thoracic/o	thorax, chest
thromb/o	clot
thym/o	thymus
thyr/o	thyroid gland
thyroid/o	thyroid gland
-tic	converts a root or noun to an adjective
-tome	instrument for cutting
-tomy	incision
ton/o	tone
tonsill/o	tonsil
trache/o	trachea

Word Part	Meaning
trans-	across
tri-	three
-tripsy	crushing
-tropin	suffix meaning nourishment or stimulation
tympan/o	eardrum
-ular	converts a root or noun to an adjective
uni-	one
ur/o, urin/o	urine
ureter/o	ureter
urethr/o	urethra
uter/o	uterus
uve/o	denoting the pigmented middle eye layer
vagin/o	vagina
valv/o	valve
varic/o	dilated
vas/o	vessel, vas deferens
ven/o	vein
ventricul/o	ventricle
vertebr/o	vertebrae
vulv/o	vulva
xanth/o	yellow
xer/o	dry
zygo-	joining, pairing, yoked together

Appendix C

Glossary of Abbreviations

Abbreviation	Meaning
A	abortus
ABG	arterial blood gas
ACE	angiotensin-converting enzyme
ACL	anterior cruciate ligament
ACTH	adrenocorticotropic hormone
AD	Alzheimer's disease
AD	right ear
ADH	antidiuretic hormone
ADR	adverse drug reaction
A-fib	atrial fibrillation
AIDS	acquired immunodeficiency syndrome
ALS	amyotrophic lateral sclerosis
ARB	angiotensin II receptor blocker
ARF	acute renal failure
AS	left ear
AU	both ears
AV	atrioventricular
BE	barium enema
BM	bowel movement
BP	blood pressure
BPH	benign prostatic hyperplasia
BSA	body surface area
BUN	blood urea nitrogen
C (C1–C7)	cervical; cervical vertebrae 1 through 7
CABG	coronary artery bypass graft
CAD	coronary artery disease

Abbreviation	Meaning
CAPD	continuous ambulatory peritoneal dialysis
CCB	calcium channel blocker
CCU	cardiac care unit
CF	cystic fibrosis
CHF	congestive heart failure
CNS	central nervous system
c/o	complains of
CO_2	carbon dioxide
COPD	chronic obstructive pulmonary disease
CP	cerebral palsy
CRF	chronic renal failure
CRP	C-reactive protein
CS	cesarean section
C-section	cesarean section
CSF	cerebrospinal fluid
CT	calcitonin
CT	computed tomography
CVA	cerebrovascular accident
CXA	chest X-ray
D&C	dilation and curettage
DDP-4	dipeptidyl peptidase-4
DIC	disseminated intravascular coagulation
DM	diabetes mellitus
DO	doctor of osteopathic medicine
DVT	deep vein thrombosis
EBV	Epstein–Barr virus

Abbreviation	Meaning
ECG	electrocardiogram, electrocardiograph, electrocardiography, or cardiogram
ECT	electroconvulsive therapy
EDC	estimated date of confinement (due date)
EDD	estimated date of delivery (due date)
EEG	electroencephalography
EGD	esophagogastroduodenoscopy
EKG	electrocardiogram, electrocardiograph, electrocardiography
EMG	electromyography
EOM	extra-ocular movement
ERV	expiratory reserve volume
ESRD	end-stage renal disease
F	Fahrenheit
FBS	fasting blood sugar
FSH	follicle-stimulating hormone
Fx	fracture
G	gravida
GC	gonorrhea
GERD	gastroesophageal reflux disease
GFR	glomerular filtration rate
GH	growth hormone
GI	gastrointestinal
GP	general practitioner
GTT	glucose tolerance test
GYN	gynecology
Hb	hemoglobin (protein in the blood that carries oxygen)
HbA$_{1c}$	hemoglobin A$_{1c}$ (glycosylated hemoglobin)
HCl	hydrochloric acid
HDL	high-density lipoprotein
HIV	human immunodeficiency virus
HPV	human papillomavirus
HR	heart rate
HRT	hormone replacement therapy
HSV	herpes simplex virus

Abbreviation	Meaning
HTN	hypertension
IBD	irritable bowel disease
IBS	irritable bowel syndrome
ICP	intracranial pressure
ICU	intensive care unit
IM	intramuscular
IOP	intra-ocular pressure
IRV	inspiratory reserve volume
IVP	intravenous pyelogram
I&D	incision and drainage
KUB	kidneys, ureter, and bladder
L (L1–L5)	lumbar; lumbar vertebrae 1 through 5
LASIK	laser-assisted in situ keratomileusis
LES	lower esophageal sphincter
LDL	low-density lipoprotein
LGI	lower gastrointestinal
LH	luteinizing hormone
LLQ	left lower quadrant (of abdomen)
LMP	last menstrual period
LP	lumbar puncture
LUQ	left upper quadrant (of abdomen)
MD	muscular dystrophy
MG	myasthenia gravis
MI	myocardial infarction
MRI	magnetic resonance imaging
MS	multiple sclerosis
MSH	melanocyte-stimulating hormone
NG	nasogastric
NPO	nothing by mouth
NSAID	nonsteroidal anti-inflammatory drug
O$_2$	oxygen
OB	obstetrics
OCD	obsessive–compulsive disorder
OD	right eye
O.D.	doctor of optometry
OM	otitis media

Abbreviation	Meaning
OS	left eye
OU	both eyes
OXT	oxytocin
P	para
P	pulse
PA	physician assistant
Pap smear	Papanicolaou smear
PE	pulmonary embolism
PID	pelvic inflammatory disease
PD	Parkinson's disease
PFT	pulmonary function test
PNS	peripheral nervous system
PO	per os or by mouth
PPI	proton pump inhibitor
PRL	prolactin
PT	physical therapy
PTCA	percutaneous transluminal coronary angioplasty
PTH	parathyroid hormone
PTSD	posttraumatic stress disorder
R	respiration
RA	rheumatoid arthritis
RBC	red blood cell
Rh+, Rh-	symbol for Rh blood group; Rh positive, Rh negative
RICE	rest, ice, compression, elevation
RLQ	right lower quadrant (of abdomen)
ROM	range of motion
RUQ	right upper quadrant (of abdomen)
RV	residual volume (as measured with test equipment)
S	sacral
SA	sinoatrial

Abbreviation	Meaning
SLE	systemic lupus erythematosus
SNRI	serotonin and norepinephrine reuptake inhibitor
SOB	shortness of breath
SSRI	selective serotonin reuptake inhibitor
STD	sexually transmitted disease
STI	sexually transmitted infection
T	temperature
T (T1–T12)	thoracic; thoracic vertebrae 1 through 12
T_3	triiodothyronine
T_4	thyroxine tetraiodothyronine
T and A	tonsillectomy and adenoidectomy
TB	tuberculosis
THR	total hip replacement
TIA	transient ischemic attack
TKA	total knee arthroplasty
TKR	total knee replacement
TLC	total lung capacity
TPN	total parenteral nutrition
TURP	transurethral resection of the prostate
UA	urinalysis
UACR	urine albumin-to-creatinine ratio
UC	ulcerative colitis
UGI	upper gastrointestinal
UGIS	upper gastrointestinal series
URI	upper respiratory infection
US	urinalysis
UTI	urinary tract infection
UV	ultraviolet
VC	vital capacity
WBC	white blood cell

Appendix D

Error-Prone Abbreviations, Symbols, and Dose Designations

This list is assembled from the Institute for Safe Medication Practices (ISMP), a nonprofit organization whose mission is to educate consumers and the healthcare community about safe medication practices.

The abbreviations, symbols, and dose designations found in this table have been reported to ISMP through the ISMP National Medication Errors Reporting Program (ISMP MERP) as being frequently misinterpreted and involved in harmful medication errors. They should NEVER be used when communicating medical information. This includes internal communications, telephone/verbal prescriptions, computer-generated labels, labels for drug storage bins, medication administration records, as well as pharmacy and prescriber computer order entry screens.

Abbreviations	Intended Meaning	Misinterpretation	Correction
μg	Microgram	Mistaken as "mg"	Use "mcg"
AD, AS, AU	right ear, left ear, each ear	Mistaken as OD, OS, OU (right eye, left eye, each eye)	Use "right ear," "left ear," or "each ear"
OD, OS, OU	right eye, left eye, each eye	Mistaken as AD, AS, AU (right ear, left ear, each ear)	Use "right eye," "left eye," or "each eye"
BT	bedtime	Mistaken as "BID" (twice daily)	Use "bedtime"
cc	cubic centimeters	Mistaken as "u" (units)	Use "mL"
D/C	discharge or discontinue	Premature discontinuation of medications if D/C (intended to mean "discharge") has been misinterpreted as "discontinued" when followed by a list of discharge medications	Use "discharge" and "discontinue"
IJ	injection	Mistaken as "IV" or "intrajugular"	Use "injection"
IN	intranasal	Mistaken as "IM" or "IV"	Use "intranasal" or "NAS"
HS hs	half-strength at bedtime, hours of sleep	Mistaken as bedtime Mistaken as half-strength	Use "half-strength" or "bedtime"
IU*	international unit	Mistaken as IV (intravenous) or 10 (ten)	Use "units"
o.d. or OD	once daily	Mistaken as "right eye" (OD-oculus dexter), leading to oral liquid medications administered in the eye	Use "daily"
OJ	orange juice	Mistaken as OD or OS (right or left eye); drugs meant to be diluted in orange juice may be given in the eye	Use "orange juice"

Abbreviations	Intended Meaning	Misinterpretation	Correction
Per os	by mouth, orally	The "os" can be mistaken as "left eye" (OS-oculus sinister)	Use "PO," "by mouth," or "orally"
q.d. or QD*	every day	Mistaken as q.i.d., especially if the period after the "q" or the tail of the "q" is misunderstood as an "i"	Use "daily"
qhs	nightly at bedtime	Mistaken as "qhr" or every hour	Use "nightly"
qn	nightly or at bedtime	Mistaken as "qh" (every hour)	Use "nightly" or "at bedtime"
q.o.d. or QOD*	every other day	Mistaken as "q.d." (daily) or "q.i.d. " (four times daily) if the "o" is poorly written	Use "every other day"
q1d	daily	Mistaken as q.i.d. (four times daily)	Use "daily"
q6PM, etc.	every evening at 6 PM	Mistaken as every 6 hours	Use "daily at 6:00 AM" or "6:00 PM daily"
SC, SQ, sub q	subcutaneous	SC mistaken as SL (sublingual); SQ mistaken as "5 every;" the "q" in "sub q" has been mistaken as "every" (e.g., a heparin dose ordered "sub q 2 hours before surgery" misunderstood as every 2 hours before surgery)	Use "subcut" or "subcutaneously"
ss	sliding scale (insulin) or ½ (apothecary)	Mistaken as "55"	Spell out "sliding scale;" use "one-half" or "½"
SSRI SSI	sliding scale regular insulin sliding scale insulin	Mistaken as selective serotonin reuptake inhibitor Mistaken as Strong Solution of Iodine (Lugol's)	Spell out "sliding scale (insulin)"
i/d	one daily	Mistaken as "tid"	Use "1 daily"
TIW or tiw	3 times a week	Mistaken as "3 times a day" or "twice in a week"	Use "3 times weekly"
U or u*	unit	Mistaken as the number 0 or 4, causing a 10-fold overdose or greater (e.g., 4U seen as "40" or 4u seen as "44"); mistaken as "cc" so dose given in volume instead of units (e.g., 4u seen as 4cc)	Use "unit"
UD	as directed ("ut dictum")	Mistaken as unit dose (e.g., diltiazem 125 mg IV infusion "UD" misinterpreted as meaning to give the entire infusion as a unit [bolus] dose)	Use "as directed"
Dose Designations and Other Information	**Intended Meaning**	**Misinterpretation**	**Correction**
Trailing zero after decimal point (e.g., 1.0 mg)*	1 mg	Mistaken as 10 mg if the decimal point is not seen	Do not use trailing zeros for doses expressed in whole numbers
"Naked" decimal point (e.g., .5 mg)*	0.5 mg	Mistaken as 5 mg if the decimal point is not seen	Use zero before a decimal point when the dose is less than a whole unit
Abbreviations such as mg. or mL. with a period following the abbreviation	mg mL	The period is unnecessary and could be mistaken as the number 1 if written poorly	Use mg, mL, etc. without a terminal period

Dose, Designations, and Other Information	Intended Meaning	Misinterpretation	Correction
Drug name and dose run together (especially problematic for drug names that end in "l" such as Inderal 40 mg; Tegretol300 mg)	Inderal 40 mg Tegretol 300 mg	Mistaken as Inderal 140 mg Mistaken as Tegretol 1300 mg	Place adequate space between the drug name, dose, and unit of measure
Numerical dose and unit of measure run together (e.g., 10mg, 100mL)	10 mg 100 mL	The "m" is sometimes mistaken as a zero or as two zeros, risking a 10- to 100-fold overdose	Place adequate space between the dose and unit of measure
Large doses without properly placed commas (e.g., 100000 units; 1000000 units)	100,000 units 1,000,000 units	100000 has been mistaken as 10,000 or 1,000,000; 1000000 has been mistaken as 100,000	Use commas for dosing units at or above 1,000, or use words such as 100 "thousand" or 1 "million" to improve readability"

Drug Name Abbreviations	Intended Meaning	Misinterpretation	Correction
APAP	acetaminophen	Not recognized as acetaminophen	Use complete drug name
ARA A	vidarabine	Mistaken as cytarabine (ARA C)	Use complete drug name
AZT	zidovudine (Retrovir)	Mistaken as azathioprine or aztreonam	Use complete drug name
CPZ	Compazine (prochlorperazine)	Mistaken as chlorpromazine	Use complete drug name
DPT	Demerol–Phenergan–Thorazine	Mistaken as diphtheria–pertussis–tetanus (vaccine)	Use complete drug name
DTO	diluted tincture of opium, or deodorized tincture of opium (Paregoric)	Mistaken as tincture of opium	Use complete drug name
HCl	hydrochloric acid or hydrochloride	Mistaken as potassium chloride (The "H" is misinterpreted as "K.")	Use complete drug name unless expressed as a salt of a drug
HCT	hydrocortisone	Mistaken as hydrochlorothiazide	Use complete drug name
HCTZ	hydrochlorothiazide	Mistaken as hydrocortisone (seen as HCT250 mg)	Use complete drug name
MgSO4*	magnesium sulfate	Mistaken as morphine sulfate	Use complete drug name
MS, MSO4*	morphine sulfate	Mistaken as magnesium sulfate	Use complete drug name
MTX	methotrexate	Mistaken as mitoxantrone	Use complete drug name
NoAC	novel/new oral anticoagulant	No anticoagulant	Use complete drug name
PCA	procainamide	Mistaken as patient-controlled analgesia	Use complete drug name
PTU	propylthiouracil	Mistaken as mercaptopurine	Use complete drug name
T3	Tylenol with codeine No. 3	Mistaken as liothyronine	Use complete drug name
TAC	triamcinolone	Mistaken as tetracaine, adrenaline, cocaine	Use complete drug name

Drug Name Abbreviations	Intended Meaning	Misinterpretation	Correction
TNK	TNKase	Mistaken as "TPA"	Use complete drug name
TPA or tPA	tissue plasminogen activator, Activase (alteplase)	Mistaken as TNKase (tenecteplase), or less often as another tissue plasminogen activator, Retavase (retaplase)	Use complete drug names
ZnSO4	zinc sulfate	Mistaken as morphine sulfate	Use complete drug name

Stemmed Drug Names	Intended Meaning	Misinterpretation	Correction
"Nitro" drip	nitroglycerin infusion	Mistaken as sodium nitroprusside infusion	Use complete drug name
"Norflox"	norfloxacin	Mistaken as Norflex	Use complete drug name
"IV Vanc"	intravenous vancomycin	Mistaken as Invanz	Use complete drug name

Symbols	Intended Meaning	Misinterpretation	Correction
ʒ	dram	Symbol for dram mistaken as "3"	Use the metric system
♏	Minim	Symbol for minim mistaken as "mL"	Use the metric system
×3d	for three days	Mistaken as "3 doses"	Use "for three days"
> and <	more than and less than	Mistaken as opposite of intended; mistakenly use incorrect symbol; "< 10" mistaken as "40"	Use "more than" or "less than"
/ (slash mark)	separates two doses or indicates "per"	Mistaken as the number 1 (e.g., "25 units/10 units" misread as "25 units and 110" units)	Use "per" rather than a slash mark to separate doses
@	at	Mistaken as "2"	Use "at"
&	and	Mistaken as "2"	Use "and"
+	plus or and	Mistaken as "4"	Use "and"
°	hour	Mistaken as a zero (e.g., q2° seen as q 20)	Use "hr," "h," or "hour"
φ or ∅	zero, null sign	Mistaken as numerals 4, 6, 8, and 9	Use 0 or zero, or describe intent using whole words

Appendix E

Top 100 Prescribed Medications

This is a listing of the top 100 prescribed medications in the United States.

Rank	Generic Name	Type	Class/Use
1	lisinopril	angiotensin-converting enzyme (ACE) inhibitor	antihypertensive
2	levothyroxine	thyroid hormone	hypothyroidism
3	atorvastatin	HMG-CoA reductase inhibitor	antihyperlipidemic
4	metformin	biguanide	antidiabetic
5	simvastatin	HMG-CoA reductase inhibitor	antihyperlipidemic
6	omeprazole	proton pump inhibitor (PPI)	anti-gastroesophageal reflux disease (GERD)
7	amlodipine besylate	calcium channel blocker (CCB)	antihypertensive
8	metoprolol	beta blocker	antihypertensive
9	acetaminophen hydrocodone	opioid	analgesic
10	albuterol	beta-2 agonist	bronchodilator
11	hydrochlorothiazide	diuretic	antihypertensive
12	losartan	angiotensin II receptor blocker (ARB)	antihypertensive
13	gabapentin	anticonvulsant	anticonvulsant, seizures, nerve pain
14	sertraline	selective serotonin reuptake inhibitor (SSRI)	antidepressant
15	furosemide	loop diuretic	antihypertensive
16	acetaminophen	analgesic	analgesic
17	atenolol	beta blocker	antihypertensive
18	pravastatin	HMG-CoA reductase inhibitor	antihyperlipidemic
19	amoxicillin	antibiotic	antibiotic
20	fluoxetine	selective serotonin reuptake inhibitor (SSRI)	antidepressant
21	citalopram	selective serotonin reuptake inhibitor (SSRI)	antidepressant

Rank	Generic Name	Type	Class/Use
22	trazodone	selective serotonin reuptake inhibitor (SSRI)	antidepressant
23	alprazolam	benzodiazepine	antianxiety
24	fluticasone	corticosteroid	nasal spray
25	bupropion	dopamine/norepinephrine reuptake inhibitor	antidepressant
26	carvedilol	beta blocker	antihypertensive
27	potassium chloride	electrolyte supplement	electrolyte supplement
28	tramadol	opioid	analgesic
29	pantoprazole	proton pump inhibitor (PPI)	anti-gastroesophageal reflux disease (GERD)
30	montelukast	leukotriene receptor antagonist	anti-asthmatic
31	escitalopram	selective serotonin reuptake inhibitor (SSRI)	antidepressant
32	prednisone	corticosteroid	anti-inflammatory
33	rosuvastatin	HMG-CoA reductase inhibitor	antihyperlipidemic
34	ibuprofen	non-steroidal anti-inflammatory drug (NSAID)	analgesic
35	meloxicam	nonsteroidal anti-inflammatory drug (NSAID)	analgesic
36	insulin glargine	antidiabetic	antidiabetic
37	hydrochlorothiazide and lisinopril	angiotensin-converting enzyme (ACE) inhibitor and diuretic	antihypertensive
38	clonazepam	benzodiazepine	anticonvulsant
39	aspirin	salicylate	antiplatelet, analgesic
40	clopidogrel	antiplatelet	antiplatelet
41	glipizide	sulfonylurea	antidiabetic
42	warfarin	anticoagulant	anticoagulant
43	cyclobenzaprine	muscle relaxant	muscle spasms, analgesic
44	insulin human	antidiabetic	antidiabetic
45	tamsulosin	alpha-1-antagonist	urinary retention
46	zolpidem	hypnotic	hypnotic
47	ethinyl estradiol and norgestimate	contraceptive	contraceptive
48	duloxetine	serotonin and norepinephrine reuptake inhibitor (SNRI)	antidepressant
49	ranitidine	histamine H2 antagonist	anti-ulcer
50	venlafaxine	serotonin and norepinephrine reuptake inhibitor (SNRI)	antidepressant

Rank	Generic Name	Type	Class/Use
51	fluticasone and salmeterol	beta-2 agonist, corticosteroid	asthma
52	oxycodone	opioid	analgesic
53	azithromycin	serotonin and norepinephrine reuptake inhibitor (SNRI)	antidepressant
54	amphetamine	central nervous system (CNS) stimulant	stimulant
55	lorazepam	benzodiazepine	anticonvulsant, anti-anxiety
56	allopurinol	xanthine oxidase inhibitor	antigout
57	paroxetine	serotonin and norepinephrine reuptake inhibitor (SNRI)	antidepressant
58	methylphenidate	central nervous system (CNS) stimulant	stimulant
59	estradiol	estrogen derivative	hormonal issues
60	hydrochlorothiazide and losartan K	angiotensin II receptor blocker (ARB) and diuretic	antihypertensive
61	ethinyl estradiol and norethindrone	contraceptive	contraceptive
62	fenofibrate	antihyperlipidemic	antihyperlipidemic
63	propranolol	beta blocker	antianginal
64	glimepiride	sulfonylurea	antidiabetic
65	ergocalciferol	vitamin D analog	prevent and treat vitamin D deficiency
66	esomeprazole	proton pump inhibitor (PPI)	anti-gastroesophageal reflux disease (GERD)
67	spironolactone	diuretic	antihypertensive
68	loratadine	histamine H1 antagonist	antihistamine
69	naproxen	non-steroidal anti-inflammatory drug (NSAID)	analgesic
70	lamotrigine	anticonvulsant	anticonvulsant
71	hydrochlorothiazide/ triamterene	diuretic/thiazide	antihypertensive
72	cetirizine	histamine H1 antagonist	antihistamine
73	sulfamethoxazole; trimethoprim	antibiotic	antibiotic
74	lovastatin	HMG-CoA reductase inhibitor	antihyperlipidemic
75	diltiazem	calcium channel blocker (CCB)	anti-anginal
76	clonidine	alpha-2 agonist	antihypertensive
77	topiramate	anticonvulsant	anticonvulsant
78	doxycycline	anti-infective	antibiotic
79	pregabalin	anticonvulsant	anticonvulsant

Rank	Generic Name	Type	Class/Use
80	folic acid	essential vitamin	essential vitamin
81	alendronate sodium	bisphosphonate	bone health
82	hydrocodone bitartrate	opioid	analgesic
83	amitriptyline	tricyclic antidepressant (TCA)	antidepressant
84	diclofenac	non-steroidal anti-inflammatory drug (NSAID)	analgesic
85	insulin aspart	antidiabetic	antidiabetic
86	tiotropium	anticholinergic	asthma, chronic obstructive pulmonary disease (COPD)
87	quetiapine fumarate	antipsychotic	antipsychotic
88	enalapril	angiotensin-converting enzyme (ACE) inhibitor	antihypertensive
89	polymyxin B sulfate	antibiotic	antibiotic
90	sitagliptin phosphate	dipeptidyl peptidase-4 (DDP-4) inhibitor	antidiabetic
91	diazepam	benzodiazepine	anticonvulsant, antianxiety
92	latanoprost	antiglaucoma	ophthalmic
93	ciprofloxacin	antibiotic	antibiotic
94	budesonide and formoterol	beta-2 agonist, corticosteroid	asthma, corticosteroid
95	hydroxyzine	histamine H1 antagonist	antihistamine
96	ethinyl estradiol and levonorgestrel	contraceptive	contraceptive
97	docusate	stool softener	laxative
98	valsartan	angiotensin II receptor blocker (ARB)	antihypertensive
99	finasteride	5 alpha-reductase inhibitor	urinary retention
100	ondansetron	5HT3 antagonist	antiemetic

Fuentes AV, Pineda MD, Venkata KCN. Comprehension of top 200 prescribed drugs in the US as a resource for pharmacy teaching, training and practice. *Pharmacy* (Basel). 2018 May 14;6(2):43. doi: 10.3390/pharmacy6020043. PMID: 29757930; PMCID: PMC6025009.

Index

A

Abbreviations
  abdominopelvic quadrants, 35*t*
  body organization, 35*t*
  cardiovascular system, 182*t*
  digestive system, 246*t*
  endocrine system, 158*t*
  hearing, 135, 135*t*
  immunity, 203*t*
  integumentary system, 46*t*
  lymphatic system, 203*t*
  muscular system, 93*t*
  nervous system, 111*t*
  reproductive system, 289*t*
  respiratory system, 223*t*
  sight, 135, 135*t*
  urinary system, 265*t*
Abdominal aorta, 262*f*
Abdominal cavity, 32, 32*f*
Abdominopelvic cavity, 32–34, 32*f*
  four quadrants of, 33*f*, 34, 34*t*
  nine regions of, 33, 33*f*, 34*t*
ABGs (arterial blood gases), 222
Abnormal breath sounds, 221
Abortus (A), defined, 286
Absence seizure, 110
Absorption, 239
Accessory organs, of digestive system, 243, 244*f*, 245
Accommodation, 130, 130*f*
Acetabulum, 64, 66*f*
ACL (anterior cruciate ligament), 71
Acne, 44
Acquired immunity, 203
Acquired immunodeficiency syndrome (AIDS), 203
Acromegaly, 156
Active immunity, 202
AD (Alzheimer's disease), 109, 110
Adaptive immunity, 202
Addison's disease, 157, 157*f*, 158
Adenohypophysis, 152
Adenoids, 219, 219*f*
Adenoma, 156
ADH (antidiuretic hormone), 155
Adipose tissue, 40, 41*f*

Adjectives, suffixes that denote, 15–16, 16*t*, 18*t*–19*t*
Adrenal cortex, 155, 155*f*
Adrenal glands, 152, 153*f*, 153*t*–154*t*, 155, 155*f*, 157–158, 157*f*
Adrenal medulla, 155, 155*f*
Adrenaline, 155
AIDS (acquired immunodeficiency syndrome), 203
Aldosterone, 155
Alimentary canal. *See* Gastrointestinal tract
Allergists, 203
Allergy, 203
Alopecia, 44
ALS (amyotrophic lateral sclerosis), 90, 92, 109, 110
Alveoli, 215, 216*f*, 217*f*, 219
Alzheimer's disease (AD), 109, 110
Amenorrhea, 288
Amniocentesis, 288, 288*f*
Amnion, 284, 285*f*
Amniotic fluid, 284, 285*f*
Amniotic sac, 284
Amphiarthrosis, 67
Amyotrophic lateral sclerosis (ALS), 90, 92, 109, 110
Anacusis, 133
Anaphylaxis, 203
Anatomical position, 30, 30*f*, 31*t*, 35*t*
Anatomical terms of location, 30, 32, 33, 34*f*, 35*t*
Anatomy, 27
Androgens, 155, 282
Anemia, 180
Ankle bones, 64, 65, 67*f*
Anorchism, 288
Anorexia, 221, 245
Antagonist, 88
Anteflexion, of uterus, 287, 287*f*
Anterior chamber, 129*f*, 130
Anterior cruciate ligament (ACL), 71
Anterior lobe, of pituitary gland, 152, 153*t*–154*t*
Anterior position, 30, 31*f*
Anteversion, of uterus, 287, 287*f*
Antiarrhythmics, 180
Antibiotics, 46
Anti-body, 202

Antidiuretic hormone (ADH), 155
Antifungals, 46
Antigen, 202
Antihistamines, 222
Anti-inflammatory, 46
Antipruritics, 46
Antiseptics, 46
Antiviral agents, 203
Anus, 240*f*, 243, 243*f*, 244*f*, 283*f*, 285*f*
Anxiety disorders, 110
Aorta, 172*f*, 174, 175*f*, 176*f*
Aortic valve, 175, 175*f*
Apex, 173, 220, 220*f*
Apnea, 221
Appendicitis, 244
Appendicular skeleton, 61, 61*f*, 63–67, 66*f*, 67*f*
Appendix, 10, 201, 242, 243, 243*f*, 244
Aqueous humor, 130
Arachnoid mater, 107, 108*f*
Areola, 283, 284*f*
Arrector pili muscles, 41, 41*f*
Arrhythmias, 179–180
Arterial blood gases (ABGs), 222
Arterial stent, 180, 181*f*
Arteries, 41*f*, 171, 177, 178*f*
  blocked, 182*f*
Arterioles, 177, 178*f*
Arteriosclerosis, 179, 179*f*, 180
Arthritis, 70, 203
Arthrocentesis, 70
Articulations. *See* Joints
Ascending colon, 243, 243*f*, 244*f*
Asthma, 222
Astigmatism, 131
Astrocytoma, 109
Atelectasis, 222
Atherosclerosis, 179, 179*f*, 180
Atrial fibrillation, 180
Atrial systole, of cardiac cycle, 177*f*
Atrioventricular bundle, 176, 176*f*
Atrioventricular (AV) node, 175*f*, 176, 176*f*
Atrioventricular (AV) valves, 174
Atrium, 172*f*, 174, 175*f*, 176*f*
Audiologist, 135
Audiology, 135
Auditory ossicles, 133, 134, 134*f*
Auditory tube, 133, 134*f*

Auricle, 134f
Autoimmune diseases, 203
Autonomic nervous system, 103, 104f, 107
AV node (atrioventricular node), 175f,
    176, 176f
AV valves (atrioventricular valves), 174
Avascular tissue, 41
Axial skeleton, 61, 61f, 62–63, 63f,
    64f, 65f
Axon, 106
Azoospermia, 288

B

B lymphocytes, 199
Back bones, 63
Back, divisions of, 34, 34f
Balanitis, 287
Ball-and-socket joint, 67
Barium enema (BE), 244
Basal cell carcinoma, 43, 44f
Base, 220, 220f
Basophils, 178
BE (barium enema), 244
Bedsores, 44
Behavioral disorders, nervous system, 110
Benign prostatic hyperplasia (BPH), 288
Benign skin cancers, 43
Benign tumors, of uterus, 287
Bicuspid valve. See Mitral valve
Bilateral oophorectomy, 288
Bilateral salpingo-oophorectomy, 288
Bile, 243
Bile duct, 240f, 243
Biopsy, 45
    cone, 288
    of skin, 45
Biopsy needle, 288f
Bipolar disorder, 110
Bladder. See Gallbladder; See Urinary
    bladder
Blepharoptosis, 131
Blind spot, 130
Blocked artery, 182f
Blood, 171, 178, 178t
    capillaries, 171, 177, 178f, 215, 216f,
        217f
    disorders, cardiovascular system, 180
    flow, of heart, 174–175, 175f
    groups, 178, 178t
Blood clots, 179
Blood pressure (BP), 177–178, 261
Blood pressure (BP) cuff, 178
Blood urea nitrogen (BUN), 265
Blood vessels, 171, 177–178, 178f
Body, 242, 242f
Body organization, 27–38
    abbreviations, 35t
    anatomic position, 30, 30f, 31t, 35t
    case study of, 27, 36
    cavities and divisions of, 32–35, 32f, 36t
    directional terms, 30, 31f, 31t, 35t

exercises for, 37–38
    levels of, 28, 28t, 29f
    navigating, 29–32
    planes, 32, 32f
    study table, 35t–36t
    word elements related to, 28, 28t
Body surface area (BSA), 42
Bolus, 242
Bones. See Skeletal system
Bony labyrinth, 133
Bowman's capsule, 263
BP (blood pressure), 177–178, 261
BPH (benign prostatic hyperplasia), 288
Bradycardia, 179
Bradypnea, 221
Brain, 103, 104f, 105, 108f
    sagittal section of, 107f
Brain trauma, 108–109, 109f
Brainstem, 107
Breasts. See Mammary glands
Breathing, 220f
    abnormalities in, 221
    dome-shaped muscle, 216
Bronchi, 215, 216f, 217f, 219
Bronchial tree, 219, 219f
Bronchioles, 215, 216f, 217f, 219,
    219f, 220f
Bronchodilator, 223
Bronchoscopy, 222, 222f
Bruxism, 244
BSA (body surface area), 42
Bulbo-urethral glands, 281, 281f, 282f
Bulimia, 245
Bulla, 42f, 43
BUN (blood urea nitrogen), 265
Bundle branches, 176, 176f
Bundle of His, 176, 176f
Burns, 42, 42t
Bursae, 67

C

CABG (coronary artery bypass graft),
    180, 182f
CAD (coronary artery disease), 179, 179f
Calcaneus, 65, 67f
Calcitonin, 153t–154t, 155
Calyx, 263, 263f
Cancer. See also Tumors
    of reproductive system, 288
    of skin, 43, 44f
Capillaries
    blood, 171, 177, 178f, 215, 216f, 217f
    lymph, 201, 202f
Capitate, 66f
Cardia, 242, 242f
Cardiac ablation, 180
Cardiac catheterization, 179
Cardiac cycle, 176, 177f
Cardiac muscle, 90, 90f
Cardiac notch, 220, 220f
Cardiac sphincter, 242

Cardiologists, 180
Cardiothoracic surgeons, 180
Cardiovascular surgeons, 180
Cardiovascular system, 171–197
    abbreviations, 182t
    case study, 171, 191–192
    diagnostic tests, 180
    disorders related to, 179–180
        of arrhythmias, 179–180
        blood clots, 179
        blood disorders, 180
        congestive heart failure, 179
        coronary artery disease, 179, 179f
        hypertension, 180
        myocardial infarction, 179
        thrombosis, 179
    exercises, 192–197
    lymphatic system in relation to, 201
    overview of, 171, 172f
    practice and practitioners, 180
    structure and function of, 173–178
        blood, 178, 178t
        blood vessels, 177–178, 178f
        heart, 173–175, 174f, 175f
        heartbeat, 175–176, 176f, 177f
    study table, 182t–191t
    surgical procedures, 180
    treatments, 180
    word elements related to, 172,
        172t–173t
Cardioversion, 180
Carpal bones, 64
Carpal tunnel syndrome, 90, 91f
Cartilage, 67
Cataract, 131, 132f
Catheter, 181f
Caudal position, 30, 31f
Cavities. See also Dental caries
    abdominal, 32, 32f
    abdominopelvic, 32–34, 32f
    and divisions of body, 32–35, 32f, 36t
Cecum, 242, 243f
Cell body, 106
Cells, 28
    elements of, 28, 29f
    membrane, 28, 29f
    structure of, 29f
Central nervous system (CNS), 103, 104f
Cephalic position, 30, 31f
Cerebellum, 106f, 107, 107f
Cerebral aneurysm, 109
Cerebral cortex, 107
Cerebrospinal fluid (CSF), 107
Cerebrovascular accident (CVA), 109, 109f
Cerebrum, 106
Cerumen, 133
Cervical vertebrae, 65f
Cervicitis, 286
Cervix, 34, 34f, 35t, 283, 283f, 285f
CF (cystic fibrosis), 222
Cheyne-Stokes respiration, 221
CHF (congestive heart failure), 179
Chlamydia, 286

Cholangiolitis, 245
Cholecystitis. *See* Gallbladder
Choledocholithiasis, 245
Cholelithiasis, 245
Chondrosarcoma, 70
Choroid, 129*f*, 130, 132*f*
Chronic bronchitis, 222
Chronic disorders, muscular system, 90
Chronic obstructive pulmonary disease
 (COPD), 222
Chyme, 242
Ciliary body, 130
Circulation, of heart, 171
Circumcision, 289
Cirrhosis, 245
Clavicle, 64
Clitoris, 283, 283*f*
Closed fracture, 67, 69, 69*f*
Clotting disorders, 180
CNS (central nervous system), 103, 104*f*
Coccygeal vertebrae, 65*f*
Coccyx, 34, 34*f*, 35*t*, 63, 65*f*
Cochlea, 133, 134*f*
Cold, common, 221
Collarbone, 64
Collecting duct, 263
Colon, 242–243
 ascending, 243, 243*f*
 descending, 243, 243*f*
Colonoscope, 245
Colonoscopy, 245
Colostomy, 245
Colposcope, 288
Colposcopy, 288
Combining form, 2, 3
Comminuted fracture, 69, 69*f*
Common cold, 221
Compact bone, 62, 62*f*
Compound fracture, 67, 69, 69*f*
Compression fracture, 70
Computed tomography (CT), 110
Concussion, 108
Conducting system, of heart, 175, 176*f*
Conductive hearing loss, 133
Cone biopsy, 288
Cones, 130
Congestive heart failure (CHF), 179
Conjunctiva, 128, 129, 129*f*
Conjunctivitis, 131
Connective tissue, 40
Contact dermatitis, 43
COPD (chronic obstructive pulmonary
 disease), 222
Corium. *See* Dermis
Cornea, 129, 129*f*, 130
Coronal plane, 32, 32*f*
Coronal suture, 63, 63*f*
Coronary artery, 181*f*
Coronary artery bypass graft (CABG),
 180, 182*f*
Coronary artery disease (CAD), 179, 179*f*
Coronary sinus, 174
Cortex, 153*t*–154*t*

Corticosteroids, 158, 203
Cortisol, 153*t*–154*t*, 155, 157
Costal cartilage, 64*f*
Cowper's glands. *See* Bulbo-urethral
 glands
Coxal bone, 64
Crackles. *See* Rales
Cranial bones, 62, 63, 63*f*
Cranial cavity, 32, 32*f*
Cranial nerves, 104*f*
Cranial position, 30, 31*f*
Cranial sutures, 63, 63*f*
Cranium, 62
Crohn's disease, 244
Croup, 221
Cryogenic surgery, 45
Cryosurgery, 45
Cryotherapy, 45
Cryptorchidism, 288
CSF (cerebrospinal fluid), 107
CT (computed tomography), 110
CTDs (cumulative trauma disorders),
 90–91, 91*f*, 92*f*
Cuboid, 65, 67*f*
Cumulative trauma disorders (CTDs),
 90–91, 91*f*, 92*f*
Cuneiform, 65, 67*f*
Cushing's syndrome, 157
Cutaneous, 39
Cuticle, 42, 42*f*
CVA (cerebrovascular accident), 109, 109*f*
Cystalgia, 264
Cystectomy, 264
Cystic fibrosis (CF), 222
Cystitis, 264
Cystocele, 287
Cystopexy, 264
Cytoplasm, 28, 29*f*

D

DA (dopamine), 110
Dacryocystitis, 131
D&C (dilation and curettage), 288
Deaf, 133
Debridement, 45
Decongestants, 223
Decubitus, 44
Demyelination, 110
Dendrites, 106
Dental caries, 244
Depressed lesions, skin, 42*f*, 43
Depression, 110
Dermatologist, 46
Dermatology, 46
Dermatoplasty, 46
Dermis, 40, 41, 41*f*
Descending colon, 243, 243*f*, 244*f*
Diabetes insipidus, 156
Diabetes mellitus (DM), 158
Diagnosis, 3, 4
Diagnostic terms, suffixes and, 14, 15*t*

Diagnostic tests
 cardiovascular system, 180
 digestive system, 245–246
 endocrine system, 158
 eye, 132
 hearing, 134
 integumentary system, 45–46
 lymphatic system, 203
 muscular system, 91–92
 nervous system, 110
 reproductive system, 288–289
 respiratory system, 222–223
 sight, 132
 skeletal system, 70
 urinary system, 264–265
Diaphragm, 216, 216*f*, 220, 220*f*, 245*f*
Diaphysis, 62, 62*f*
Diarthrosis. *See* Synovial joints
Diastole, 176
Diastolic pressure, 178
DIC (disseminated intravascular
 coagulation), 180
Diencephalon, 107
Digestion, 239, 243
Digestive system, 239–260
 abbreviations, 246*t*
 accessory organs of, 243, 244*f*, 245
 case study, 239
 diagnostic tests, 245–246
 disorders of, 244–245
  accessory organ disorders, 245
  lower GI tract disorders, 244–245
  upper GI tract disorders, 244
 exercises, 255–260
 overview of, 239–240
 practice and practitioners, 246
 structure and function of, 240*f*,
  241–244
  accessory organs, 243, 244*f*
  gallbladder, 243
  large intestine, 242–243, 243*f*, 244*f*
  liver, 243
  lower GI tract, 239–240, 244–245
  mouth, 242
  pancreas, 243
  pharynx and esophagus, 242
  salivary glands, 243
  small intestine, 242, 243*f*, 244*f*
  stomach, 242
  upper GI tract, 239–240, 244
 study table, 246*t*–249*t*
 surgical procedures, 245–246
 treatments, 245–246
 word elements related to, 240,
  240*t*–241*t*
Digestive tract, 239
Dilation and curettage (D&C), 288
Direction, prefixes of, 11, 11*t*
Directional terms, 30, 31*f*, 31*t*, 35*t*
Disorders
 cardiovascular system, 179–180
  of arrhythmias, 179–180
  blood clots, 179

Disorders (*continued*)
- blood disorders, 180
  - congestive heart failure, 179
  - coronary artery disease, 179, 179f
  - hypertension, 180
  - myocardial infarction, 179
  - thrombosis, 179
- digestive system, 244–245
- endocrine system, 156–158
  - adrenal gland, 157–158, 157f
  - pancreas, 158
  - pituitary gland, 156, 156f
  - thyroid gland, 156–157, 157f
- hearing, 133–134
- immunity, 202–203, 203f
- integumentary system, 42–45
  - burns, 42, 42t
  - inflammatory disorders, 43, 43f
  - other disorders, 44, 45f
  - skin cancer, 43, 44f
  - skin infections, 44, 44f, 45f
  - skin lesions, 42–43, 42f
- lymphatic system, 202–203, 203f
- muscular system, 90–91
- nervous system, 108–110
  - behavioral disorders, 110
  - brain trauma, 108–109, 109f
  - seizure disorders, 110
  - systemic degenerative diseases, 109–110
  - trauma, 108–109, 109f
  - tumors, 109
  - vascular insults, 109, 109f
- reproductive system, 286–288
  - affect males, 288
  - female structural abnormalities, 287, 287f
  - inflammation, 286–287
  - menstrual cycle disorders, 288
  - sexually transmitted diseases, 286
  - tumors, 287–288
- respiratory system, 221–222
  - abnormal breath sounds, 221
  - expansion disorders, 222
  - infectious disorders, 221
  - obstructive lung diseases, 221–222
- sight, 131–132
  - eyelid disorder, 131
  - infection, 131
  - other disorders, 131–132
  - refractive errors, 131, 131f
- skeletal system, 67–70, 70f
- urinary system, 264
Disseminated intravascular coagulation (DIC), 180
Distal epiphysis, 62f
Distal phalanges, 66f
Distal phalanx, 66f
Distal position, 30, 31f
Diverticula, 245
Diverticulitis, 245
Diverticulosis, 245

DM (diabetes mellitus), 158
Dopamine (DA), 110
Dorsal cavity, 30, 31f
Drugs. *See* Pharmacology
Dry eyes. *See* Xerophthalmia
Duchenne dystrophy, 90
Ductus deferens, 281f, 282, 282f
Due date, 286
Duodenoscopy, 245
Duodenostomy, 245
Duodenum, 242, 242f, 243, 243f, 244f, 245, 246
Dura mater, 107, 108f
Dyscrasia, 180
Dysmenorrhea, 288
Dyspepsia, 245
Dysphagia, 90, 244
Dysphonia, 221
Dyspnea, 221
Dysuria, 264

E

Ear. *See* Hearing
Earwax. *See* Cerumen
EBV (Epstein–Barr virus), 203
ECG. *See* Electrocardiogram
Echocardiography, 179
Ectopic pregnancy, 286
Ectropion, 131
Eczema, 43, 43f
Edaravone (Radicava), 92
EDC (estimated date of confinement), 286
EDD (estimated date of delivery), 286
EEG (electroencephalography), 110
EGD (esophagogastroduodenoscopy), 245
Ejaculatory duct, 281f, 282, 282f
Electrocardiogram (ECG, EKG), 176, 179
Electrocardiograph, 176
Electroencephalography (EEG), 110
Elevated lesions, skin, 42f, 43
Elimination, defined, 239
Embolus, 179
Embryo, 284
Emphysema, 222
Emulsification, 243
Endarterectomy, 180
Endocardium, 173, 174f, 175f
Endocrine system
- abbreviations, 158t
- case study, 151, 165
- diagnostic tests, 158
- disorders related to, 156–158
  - adrenal gland, 157–158, 157f
  - pancreas, 158
  - pituitary gland, 156, 156f
  - thyroid gland, 156–157, 157f
- exercises, 166–170
- overview of, 151
- pharmacology for, 158
- practice and practitioners, 158

- structure and function of, 152–156, 153f, 153t–154t
  - adrenal glands, 155, 155f
  - gonads, 156
  - pancreas, 156
  - parathyroid glands, 155, 155f
  - pituitary gland, 152–155
  - thyroid gland, 155, 155f
- study table, 159t–165t
- surgical procedures, 158
- treatments, 158
- word elements related to, 151–152, 152t
Endocrinologist, 158
Endocrinology, 158
Endometriosis, 288
Endometrium, 283, 288
Endosteum, 62, 62f
End-stage renal disease (ESRD), 264
Enteroscope, 245
Enteroscopy, 245
Entropion, 131
Eosinophils, 178
Epicardium, 173, 175f
Epicondylitis, 91, 92f
Epidermis, 40–41, 41f
Epididymis, 281f, 282, 282f
Epididymitis, 287
Epidural hematoma, 108f, 109f
Epigastric regions, 33, 33f, 34t
Epiglottis, 218f, 219, 219f, 221
Epilepsy, 110
Epinephrine. *See* Adrenaline
Epiphyseal plate, 62, 62f
Epiphysis, 62
- distal, 62f
- proximal, 62f
Epithelial tissue, 40, 41
Epstein–Barr virus (EBV), 203
Erection, 282
Eructation, 245
ERV (expiratory reserve volume), 222t
Erythema, 44
Erythematous, 43
Erythrocytes. *See* Red blood cells
Esophageal hiatus, 245f
Esophageal sphincter, lower. *See* Cardiac sphincter
Esophagitis, 244
Esophagogastroduodenoscopy (EGD), 245
Esophagus, 218f, 239, 240f, 242, 242f, 244, 244f, 245f
ESRD (end-stage renal disease), 264
Estimated date of confinement (EDC), 286
Estimated date of delivery (EDD), 286
Estrogen, 156
Ethmoidal sinus, 218f
Etymology, 2, 4
Eupnea, 221
Exhaled air, respiratory system, 215, 217f
Exocrine glands, 151

Exophthalmos, 157, 157*f*
Expansion disorders, of respiratory system, 222
Expiratory reserve volume (ERV), 222*t*
External acoustic meatus, 134*f*
External ear, 133, 134*f*
External genitalia, 281
   female reproductive system, 283
   male reproductive system, 281
External respiration, 215
External urethral sphincter, 264
Extraocular muscles, 128
Eye. *See* Sight
Eyeball
   protective structures of, 129, 129*f*
   structures of, 129, 129*f*
Eyebrow, 128, 129, 129*f*
Eyelashes, 128, 129, 129*f*
Eyelid disorder, 131
Eyelids, 128, 129

F

Facial bones, 62, 63*f*
Fallopian tubes, 283
False ribs, 63, 64*f*
Fascia, 88
Fascicle, 88
Fat tissue, 40
Female reproductive system
   infections of, 286
   pregnancy, 284–286, 285*f*
   structural abnormalities, 287, 287*f*
   structure and function of, 283–284, 283*f*, 284*f*
Femur, 64, 66*f*
Fertilization, 279, 283, 284, 286, 288
Fetus, 284, 285*f*
Fibrillation, 179
Fibroids, 287
Fibroleiomyomas, 287
Fibromyalgia, 90
Fibrous capsule, 263, 263*f*
Fibrous layer, eye, 129
Fibula, 64, 66*f*, 67*f*
Fingers, nail, 42, 42*f*
Fissure, 42*f*, 43
Flat lesions, skin, 42*f*, 43
Floating bone, 64
Floating ribs, 63, 64*f*
Flu. *See* Influenza
Foot bones, 65, 67*f*
Foreskin, 281, 281*f*
Fourth ventricle, 107*f*
Fovea centralis, 130, 130*f*
Fracture, 67, 69, 69*f*
Free edge, 42, 42*f*
Frontal bone, 62, 63*f*
Frontal lobe, 106, 107*f*
Frontal plane, 32, 32*f*
Frontal sinus, 218*f*

Function. *See* Structure and function
Fundus, 242, 242*f*, 283
Funny bone, 64

G

Gallbladder, 239, 240*f*, 243, 244*f*, 245
Gallstones. *See* Cholelithiasis
Gametes, 279
Ganglia, 106
Ganglion, 106
Gastritis, 244
Gastroenterologists, 246
Gastroenterology, 246
Gastroesophageal reflux disease (GERD), 244
Gastrointestinal (GI) tract, 239
   lower, 239–240, 244–245
   pathway of food through, 243, 244*f*
   upper, 239–240, 244
Gastroscope, 245
Gastroscopy, 245
Gastrostomy, 246
GC (gonorrhea), 286
Generalized tonic–clonic seizure, 110
Genitalia, external, 281
   female reproductive system, 283
   male reproductive system, 281
GERD (gastroesophageal reflux disease), 244
Gestation, 284
Gestational diabetes, 158
GFR (glomerular filtration rate), 265
GH (growth hormone), 156
GI tract. *See* Gastrointestinal tract
Gigantism, 156
Gingivitis, 244
Glands
   of endocrine system, 151, 152, 153*f*, 153*t*–154*t*
   within skin, 39, 41
Glans penis, 281, 281*f*
Glaucoma, 131
Glomerular capsule, 263
Glomerular filtration rate (GFR), 265
Glomerulonephritis, 264
Glomerulus, 263
Glottis, 219, 219*f*
Glucagon, 153*t*–154*t*, 156
Glycosuria, 158
Goiter, 157, 157*f*
Golfer's elbow. *See* Epicondylitis
Gonads, 156, 279
Gonorrhea (GC), 286
Grandmal seizure, 110
Graves' disease, 157, 157*f*, 158
Gravida (G), defined, 285
Greenstick fracture, 69, 69*f*
Growth hormone (GH), 156
Growth plate, 62
Gynecologists, 289
Gynecology (GYN), 289

H

Hair, 41*f*
Hair follicles, 41, 41*f*
Hamate, 66*f*
Hamstring injury, 91
Hand bones, 66*f*
Hearing, 127–144
   abbreviation, 135, 135*t*
   case study, 127, 144
   diagnostic tests, 134
   disorders of ear, 133–134
   exercises, 145–150
   overview of, 127–128
   practice and practitioners of, 135
   structure and function of, 133, 134*f*
   study table, 135*t*–144*t*
   surgical procedures, 134
   treatments, 134
   word elements related to, 132–133, 133*t*
Heart, 173–175, 174*f*, 175*f*
   blood flow of, 174–175, 175*f*
   conducting system of, 175, 176*f*
   pacemaker of, 176
   wall layers, 174*f*
Heart attack. *See* Myocardial infarction
Heart muscle. *See* Cardiac muscle
Heart rate (HR), 176
Heartbeat, 175–176, 176*f*, 177*f*
Heel bone, 65
Hematologists, 180, 203
Hematoma, 109*f*
Hemiparesis, 91
Hemiplegia, 91
Hemoglobin (Hb), 178
Hemolysis, 201
Hemophilia, 180
Hemoptysis, 221
Hemorrhage, 109*f*
Hemorrhoids, 245
Hepatitis, 245
Hernia
   hiatal, 244, 245*f*
   inguinal, 245
Herniated disc, 70
Herpes simplex virus (HSV), 286
Herpes zoster. *See* Shingles
Hiatal hernia, 244, 245*f*
Hilum, 263, 263*f*
Hip bone, 64, 66*f*
HIV (human immunodeficiency virus), 286
Hodgkin's lymphoma, 203
Homeostasis, 103, 151
Hordeolum, 131
Horizontal plane, 32, 32*f*
Hormone replacement therapy (HRT), 158
Hormones, 151, 153*t*–154*t*
HPV (human papilloma virus), 286

HR (heart rate), 176
HRT (hormone replacement therapy), 158
HSV (herpes simplex virus), 286
Human immunodeficiency virus (HIV), 286
Human papilloma virus (HPV), 286
Humerus, 64, 66f
Humpback, 70
Hydrocele, 288
Hyoid bone, 155f
Hyperemesis, 245
Hyperglycemia, 158
Hyperlipidemia, 179
Hyperopia, 131, 131f
Hypertension, 180
    secondary, 180
Hyperthyroidism, 156
Hypochondriac regions, 33, 33f, 34t
Hypodermis, 40, 41f
Hypogastric regions, 33, 33f, 34t
Hypophysis. See Pituitary gland
Hypothalamus, 107, 107f, 152
Hypothyroidism, 156
Hysterectomy, 288
Hysterosalpingography, 288

I

IBD (inflammatory bowel disease), 245
IBS (irritable bowel syndrome), 245
Ichthyosis, 44
Icterus. See Jaundice
I&D (incision and drainage), 46
Ileocecal sphincter, 242
Ileostomy, 246
Ileum, 242, 243f, 244f
Ilium, 64, 66f
Immunity, 199–214. See also Lymphatic
        system
    abbreviations, 203t
    acquired, 203
    active, 202
    adaptive, 202
    case study, 199, 209
    disorders related to, 202–203, 203f
    exercises, 209–214
    innate, 202
    natural, 202
    overview of, 199–200
    study table, 204t–209t
    types of, 202f
    word elements related to, 200–201,
        201t
Immunization, 203
Immunologist, 203
Immunology, 203
Immunosuppressants, 203
Impacted cerumen, 133
Impetigo, 44, 44f
Incision and drainage (I&D), 46
Incontinence, 264
Incus, 133, 134f

Infection
    eye, 131
    reproductive system, 286
    respiratory system, 221
    of skin, 44, 44f, 45f
    urinary tract, 264
Infectious mononucleosis, 203
Infectious rhinitis. See Common cold
Inferior lobe, of lungs, 220, 220f
Inferior parathyroid glands, 155f
Inferior position, 30, 31f
Inferior vena cava, 172f, 174, 175f, 262f
Inflammation, 286–287
Inflammatory bowel disease (IBD), 245
Inflammatory disorders, of
        integumentary system, 43, 43f
Influenza, 221
Inguinal hernia, 245
Inguinal regions, 33, 33f, 34t
Inhaled air, respiratory system, 215, 217f
Innate immunity, 202
Inner layer, eye, 129
Inspiratory reserve volume (IRV), 222t
Insulin, 156
Integumentary system, 39–57
    abbreviations, 46t
    case study, 39, 51
    diagnostic tests for, 45–46
    disorders related to, 42–45
        burns, 42, 42t
        inflammatory disorders, 43, 43f
        other disorders, 44, 45f
        skin cancer, 43, 44f
        skin infections, 44, 44f, 45f
        skin lesions, 42–43, 42f
    exercises for, 52–57
    nonsurgical treatments, 47
    overview of, 39
    pharmacology for, 45
    practice and practitioners, 46
    structure and function of, 40–42, 41f,
        42f
    study table, 46t–51t
    surgical procedures of, 45–46
    topical medications, 46
    treatments of, 45–46
    word elements related to, 40, 40t
Interatrial septum, 174
Intermediate cuneiform, 65, 67f
Intermediate lobe, of pituitary gland,
        153t–154t
Intermodal pathways, 175
Internal ear, 133, 134f
Internal respiration, 215
Internal right eye, structures, 130, 130f
Internal thoracic artery, 182f
Internal urethral sphincter, 263
Internist, 246
Internodal pathways, 176f
Interstitial fluid, 201
Interventricular septum, 174, 175f
Intestinal obstruction, 245
Intraocular pressure (IOP), 132

Intravenous pyelogram (IVP), 265
Intussusception, 245
IOP (intraocular pressure), 132
Iris, 129f, 130
Irritable bowel syndrome (IBS), 245
IRV (inspiratory reserve volume), 222t
Ischemia, 179
Ischium, 64, 66f
Islets of Langerhans, 153t–154t, 156
IVP (intravenous pyelogram), 265

J

Jaundice, 245
Jejunum, 242, 243f, 244f
Joint disorders, 70
Joints, 62, 67, 68f, 68t–69t

K

Keratin, 41
Keratitis, 131
Kidneys, 152, 155, 155f, 261, 262f, 263
Kinesiologists, 71, 92
Kneecap, 64
Kussmaul respiration, 221
Kyphosis, 70, 70f

L

Labium majus, 283, 283f
Labium minus, 283, 283f
Labyrinth, 134
Labyrinthitis, 134
Labyrinthotomy, 134
Lacrimal apparatus, 128, 129f
Lacrimal ducts, 129, 129f
Lacrimal gland, 129, 129f
Lacrimal sac, 129, 129f
Lactation, 284
Lactiferous ducts, 283, 284f
LAD (left anterior descending) artery,
        182f
Lambdoid suture, 63, 63f
Language sense, 2
Laparoscopy, 288
Large intestine, 239, 240f, 242–243,
        243f, 244f
Laryngitis, 221
Laryngopharynx, 218f, 219
Laryngotracheobronchitis, 221
Larynx, 155f, 215, 216f, 217f, 218f, 219,
        220f
Laser-assisted in situ keratomileusis
        (LASIK), 132
Last menstrual period (LMP), 286
Lateral angle of eye, 129
Lateral canthus, 129
Lateral cuneiform, 65, 67f

Lateral epicondylitis, 92f
Lateral malleolus, 65, 67f
Lateral position, 30, 31f
Left anterior descending (LAD) artery, 182f
Left atrioventricular valve, 174
Left atrium, 172f, 174, 175f, 176f
Left bronchus, 219, 219f
Left pulmonary arteries, 175f
Left pulmonary veins, 175f
Left subclavian artery, 182f
Left ventricle, 172f, 174, 175f, 176f
Left ventricular hypertrophy, 180
Lens, 129f, 130, 130f
Leptomeninx, 107
LES (lower esophageal sphincter), 242, 242f
Lesions, 42, 109
    skin, 42–43, 42f
        depressed, 42f, 43
        elevated, 42f, 43
        flat, 42f, 43
Leukemia, 180
Leukocytes. *See* White blood cells
LGI (lower gastrointestinal) tract, 239–240, 244–245
Ligaments, 62, 88
Lingual tonsils, 219, 219f
Liver, 239, 240f, 243, 244f, 245
LMP (last menstrual period), 286
Lobes, of lungs, 220, 220f
Lobules of mammary gland, 284, 284f
Lordosis, 70, 70f
Lou Gehrig's disease. *See* Amyotrophic lateral sclerosis
Lower esophageal sphincter (LES), 242, 242f
Lower extremity, 64
Lower eyelid, 129f
Lower gastrointestinal (LGI) tract, 239–240, 244–245
Lower limb bones, 66f
Lower lobe, of lungs, 220
Lower respiratory tract, 215, 216f
LP (lumbar puncture), 111, 111f
Lumbar, 33, 33f, 34f, 34t, 35, 35t
Lumbar puncture (LP), 111, 111f
Lumbar vertebrae, 65f
Lumen, 177
Lunate, 66f
Lungs, 172f, 174f, 215, 216f, 219–220, 220f, 222, 222f
Lunula, 42, 42f
Lymph, 199
    flow, 202f
Lymph capillaries, 201, 202f
Lymph nodes, 201, 284f
Lymphadenectomy, 203
Lymphadenitis, 202
Lymphadenopathy, 203
Lymphangiectomy, 203
Lymphatic duct, 199
Lymphatic system, 199–214
    abbreviations, 203t

case study, 199, 209
diagnostic tests, 203
disorders related to, 202–203, 203f
exercises, 209–214
lymphatic organs, 201
overview of, 199–200, 200f
practice and practitioners, 203
structure and function of, 201–202, 202f
study table, 204t–209t
surgical procedures, 203
treatments, 203
word elements related to, 200–201, 201t
Lymphatic tissue, 218
Lymphatic trunks, 201
Lymphedema, 202, 203f
Lymphocytes, 178, 199, 201

M

Macrophages, 201
Macula, 130, 130f
Macule, 42f, 43
Magnetic resonance imaging (MRI), 111
Male gametes, 279
Male reproductive system
    disorders, 288
    structure and function of, 281–282, 281f, 282f
Malignant melanoma, 43, 44f
Malignant skin cancers, 43
Malleolus, 67f
Malleus, 133, 134f
Mammary glands, 284
    frontal view of, 284f
    lobules of, 284f
Mammography, 288
Mandible, 62, 63f
Manubrium, 63, 64f
Marrow tissue, 62
Mastectomy, 288
Mastication, 242
Mastitis, 286
Mastoidectomy, 134
Mastoiditis, 134
Maxilla, 62, 63f
Maxillary sinus, 218f
MD (muscular dystrophy), 90
Medial angle of eye, 129, 129f
Medial canthus, 129
Medial cuneiform, 65, 67f
Medial epicondylitis, 92f
Medial malleolus, 65, 67f
Medial position, 30, 31f
Medical conditions, suffixes that signify, 13, 13t–14t, 18t–19t
Medical terms, 1–6. *See also* Word elements
    analyzing, 3–5, 4t, 5t
    case study of, 1, 6
    combining form, 2, 3

common elements, 3
exercises for, 6–7
language sense, 2
pronunciation of, 2, 3
value of standardized, 2f
Medulla, 153t–154t
Medulla oblongata, 106f, 107, 107f
Medullary cavity, 62, 62f
Meiosis, 281, 282
Melanin, 41
Melanocytes, 41
Melanoma, 43
Menarche, 284
Ménière's syndrome, 134
Meninges, 107
Meningioma, 109
Menopause, 284
Menorrhagia, 288
Menstrual cycle, 284
    disorders, 288
Menstrual period, 288
Menstrual phase, 284
Menstruation, 283, 288
Mesencephalon, 107
Metacarpals, 64, 66f
Metatarsals, 65, 66f, 67f
MG (myasthenia gravis), 90
MI (myocardial infarction), 179
Microphages, 201
Micturition reflex, 263
Midbrain. *See* Mesencephalon
Middle ear, 133, 134f
Middle lobe, of lungs, 220, 220f
Middle phalanges, 66f
Mitochondria, 28, 29f
Mitral valve, 175, 175f
Monocytes, 178, 201
Mood disorders, 110
Mouth. *See* Oral cavity
MRI (magnetic resonance imaging), 111
MS (multiple sclerosis), 109, 110
Mucus, 218
Multiple sclerosis (MS), 109, 110
Muscle cells, 88
Muscle fibers, 88
Muscle movement, 91
Muscle tissue, 88, 89f, 90f
Muscles
    arrector pili, 41, 41f
    cardiac, 90, 90f
    extraocular, 128
    skeletal, 88, 89f, 90f
    smooth, 88–90, 90f
Muscular dystrophy (MD), 90
Muscular system, 87–102
    abbreviations, 93t
    case study, 87, 97
    chronic disorders, 90
    cumulative trauma disorders and sports injuries, 90–91, 91f, 92f
    diagnostic tests, 91–92
    disorders related to, 90–91
    exercises, 97–102

Muscular system (*continued*)
overview of, 87
paralysis, 91
paresis, 91
practice and practitioners, 92–93
structure and function of, 88–90
cardiac muscle, 90
muscle movement, 91
skeletal muscle, 88, 89f, 90f
smooth muscle, 88–90, 90f
types of muscle tissue, 88, 89f, 90f
study table, 93t–97t
surgical procedures, 91–92
treatments, 91–92
word elements related to, 88, 88t
Myasthenia gravis (MG), 90
Mycobacterium tuberculosis, 221
Myelin, 106
Myocardial infarction (MI), 179
Myocardial muscle. *See* Cardiac muscle
Myocardium, 173, 174f, 175f
Myology, 92
Myometrium, 283
Myopia, 131, 131f
Myringectomy, 134
Myringitis, 134
Myringotomy, 134

N

Nail, 42, 42f
disorders, 44
surface view of, 42f
treatments, 46
Nasal, 216
Nasal bone, 62, 63f
Nasal cavity, 215, 216–218, 216f, 217f, 218, 218f
Nasal septum, 218, 218f
Nasolacrimal duct, 129, 129f
Nasopharynx, 218f, 219
Natural immunity, 202
Navicular, 67f
NCS (nerve conduction study), 111
NCV (nerve conduction velocity), 111
Negation, prefixes of, 13, 13t
Neisseria gonorrhoeae, 286
Neonatologists, 289
Neonatology, 289
Neoplasms. *See* Tumors
Nephritis, 264
Nephrologist, 265
Nephrology, 265
Nephron, 263
Nerve cells, 106
Nerve conduction study (NCS), 111
Nerve conduction velocity (NCV), 111
Nerve tissue, 28
Nerves, 41f, 106
Nervous system, 103–125
abbreviations, 111t
case study, 103, 120

diagnostic tests, 110
disorders of, 108–110
behavioral disorders, 110
brain trauma, 108–109, 109f
seizure disorders, 110
systemic degenerative diseases, 109–110
trauma, 108–109, 109f
tumors, 109
vascular insults, 109, 109f
exercise, 120–125
overview of, 103, 104f
practice and practitioners, 111
structure and function of, 105–108
central nervous system, 104f, 106–107, 106f, 107f
peripheral nervous system, 104f, 107–108, 108f
study table, 112t–119t
surgical procedures, 110
treatments, 110
word elements related to, 105, 105t
Neuroglia, 106
Neurohypophysis, 152
Neurologists, 111
Neurology, 4
Neurons, 106
Neurosurgeons, 111
Neurotransmitter, 106
Neutrophils, 178, 201
Nipple, 283, 284f
Nodule, 42f, 43
Nonstriated muscle. *See* Smooth muscle
Nontraditional word, 3
Noradrenaline, 155
Norepinephrine. *See* Noradrenaline
Nose, 215, 216–218, 216f, 217f, 218f
Nostrils, 216, 218f
Nucleus, 28, 29f, 106
CNS, 106
Number, prefixes of, 12, 12t

O

Obsessive–compulsive disorder (OCD), 110
Obstetricians, 289
Obstetrics (OB), 289
Obstruction, intestinal, 245
Obstructive lung diseases, 221–222
Occipital bone, 62, 63f
Occipital lobe, 106, 107f
Occupational therapists, 71, 92
OCD (obsessive–compulsive disorder), 110
Oligomenorrhea, 288
Oligospermia, 288
Oncologists, 203
Onychectomy, 46
Onychotomy, 46
Oocytes, 279
Oophorectomy, 288
Oophoritis, 286
Open fracture, 67, 69, 69f

Ophthalmologist, 132
Ophthalmology, 132
Ophthalmoscope, 132
Optic disc, 130, 130f
Optic nerve, 129f, 130
Opticians, 132
Optometrist, 132
Optometry, 132
Oral cavity, 218f, 240f, 242, 243, 244, 244f, 246
Orbit, 128
Orchialiga, 288
Orchiectomy, 289
Orchiopathy, 288
Orchioplasty, 289
Orchitis, 287
Organs, 28
Oropharynx, 218f, 219
Orthopedic surgeons, 71, 92
Orthopedics, 70
Orthopnea, 221
Os coxae. *See* Hip bone
Osseous tissue, 62
Ossicles, auditory, 133, 134, 134f
Ossification, 62
Osteoarthritis, 70
Osteoblasts, 62
Osteoclasts, 62
Osteocytes, 62
Osteomalacia, 70
Osteomyelitis, 70
Osteoporosis, 70
Osteosarcoma, 70
Ostomy, 245
Otalgia, 133
Otitis, 133
Otodynia, 133
Otolaryngologists, 223
Otologist, 135
Otology, 135
Otoplasty, 134
Otorhinolaryngologists, 135, 223
Otosclerosis, 134
Otoscope, 135
Ovaries, 152, 153f, 153t–154t, 156, 279, 283, 283f
Ovulation, 284
Ovum, 283
Oxytocin (OXT), 155

P

Pacemaker of heart, 176
Palatine tonsils, 219, 219f
Palpebrae, 129
Pancreas, 152, 153f, 153t–154t, 156, 158, 239, 240f, 243, 244f
Pancreatic islets, 153t–154t, 156
Papanicolaou test (Pap smear), 288
Papule, 42f, 43
Para (P), defined, 286
Paralysis, 91

Paranasal sinuses, 215, 216–218, 216*f*, 218, 218*f*
Paranoia, 110
Paraplegia, 91
Pararenal fat body, 263
Parasympathetic nervous system, 103, 104*f*, 108
Parathormone, 155
Parathyroid glands, 152, 153*f*, 153*t*–154*t*, 155, 155*f*
Parathyroid hormone (PTH), 155
Paresis, 91
Parietal bones, 62, 63*f*
Parietal lobe, 106, 107*f*
Parietal pleura, 220, 220*f*
Parkinson's disease (PD), 109, 110
Paronychia, 44, 45*f*
Parotiditis, 244
Parotitis. *See* Parotiditis
Patella, 64, 66*f*
Patency, of lungs, 221
Patent, 221
Pathogens, 200
PD (Parkinson's disease), 109, 110
Pectoral girdle, 64
Pediatricians, 5, 15, 16, 289
Pediatrics, 289
Pelvic cavity, 32, 32*f*
Pelvic girdle, 64
  bones of, 66*f*
Pelvic inflammatory disease (PID), 286
Penis, 281, 281*f*
Percutaneous transluminal coronary angioplasty (PTCA), 180, 181*f*
Pericardium, 173, 174*f*
Perimetrium, 283
Perinephric fat, 263, 263*f*
Periosteum, 62, 62*f*
Peripheral nervous system (PNS), 103, 104*f*
Peristalsis, 242
Peritonitis, 245
Pertussis, 221
Petit mal seizure, 110
Peyer's patches, 201
PFT (pulmonary function tests), 222
Phagocytes, 201
Phagocytosis, 201
Phalanges, 64, 65, 66*f*, 67*f*
Phalanx, 66*f*
Pharmacology
  for endocrine system, 158
  for integumentary system, 45
  for respiratory system, 222, 223
Pharyngeal tonsils, 219, 219*f*
Pharynx, 216*f*, 217*f*, 218–219, 218*f*, 219*f*, 240*f*, 242, 244*f*
Phimosis, 288
Phobias, 110
Photoreceptors, 130
Physical therapists, 71, 92
Physiology, 27
Pia mater, 107, 108*f*
PID (pelvic inflammatory disease), 286

Pineal gland, 152, 153*f*, 153*t*–154*t*
Pinkeye. *See* Conjunctivitis
Pituitary gland, 107*f*, 152–155, 153*f*, 153*t*–154*t*, 156, 156*f*
Placenta, 284, 285*f*
Planes of body, 32, 32*f*
Plantar fasciitis, 91
Plaque, 42*f*, 43, 181*f*
Plasma, 178
Platelets, 178
Pleura, 219
  parietal, 220, 220*f*
  visceral, 220, 220*f*
Pleural tap, 222
Pneumonia, 221
Pneumothorax, 222
PNS (peripheral nervous system), 103, 104*f*
Polydipsia, 156, 158
Polyphagia, 158
Polyuria, 156, 158
Pons, 106*f*, 107, 107*f*
Pore, 41, 41*f*
Position, prefixes of, 11–12, 11*t*–12*t*
Positional terms, 30, 30*f*, 31*t*, 35*t*
Posterior chamber, 129*f*, 130
Posterior lobe, of pituitary gland, 152, 153*t*–154*t*
Posterior position, 30, 31*f*
Posttraumatic stress disorder (PTSD), 110
Practice and practitioners
  cardiovascular system, 180
  digestive system, 246
  endocrine system, 158
  eye, 132
  hearing, 135
  integumentary system, 46
  lymphatic system, 203
  muscular system, 92–93
  nervous system, 111
  reproductive system, 289
  respiratory system, 223
  sight, 132
  skeletal system, 70–71
  suffixes associated with, 15, 18*t*–19*t*
  urinary system, 265
Prediabetes, 158
Prefixes, 2, 3, 4*t*, 5*t*
  case study of, 9, 19
  categories of, 10–13, 11*t*–13*t*
  of direction, 11, 11*t*
  exercises for, 20–21
  list of, 285–286
  of negation, 13, 13*t*
  of number, 12, 12*t*
  of position, 11–12, 11*t*–12*t*
  of speed, 10, 11*t*
  study table, 16*t*–17*t*
  of time, 10, 11*t*
Pregnancy
  case study, 279, 299
  ectopic, 286
  reproductive system, 284–286, 285*f*
  uterus with fetus, 285*f*

Prepuce, 281
Presbycusis, 133
Presbyopia, 131
Prime mover, 88
Proctologists, 246
Proctology, 246
Progesterone, 156
Prolapsed uterus, 287
Proliferative phase, of menstrual cycle, 284
Prone position, 30
Pronunciation, of medical terms, 2, 3
Prostate, 281, 281*f*
Prostatitis, 287
Proximal epiphysis, 62*f*
Proximal phalanges, 66*f*
Proximal phalanx, 66*f*
Proximal position, 30, 31*f*
Prurigo, 43
Pruritus, 43
Psoriasis, 43, 43*f*
Psychiatrists, 111
Psychologist, 111
Psychotic disorders, 110
PTCA (percutaneous transluminal coronary angioplasty), 180, 181*f*
PTH (parathyroid hormone), 155
PTSD (posttraumatic stress disorder), 110
Pubic symphysis, 66*f*, 285*f*
Pubis, 66*f*
Pubis bone, 64
Pulmonary, 216
Pulmonary arteries, 172*f*, 175, 175*f*
Pulmonary capacities, 222*t*
Pulmonary circuit, 171, 172*f*
Pulmonary function tests (PFT), 222
Pulmonary trunk, 175*f*
Pulmonary valve, 175, 175*f*
Pulmonary veins, 172*f*, 175*f*
Pulmonary volumes, 222*t*
Pulmonologist, 223
Pulmonology, 223
Pulse oximetry, 222
Pupil, 129*f*, 130
Purkinje fibers, 176, 176*f*
Pustule, 42*f*, 43
Pyelonephritis, 264
Pyloric sphincter, 240, 242, 242*f*
Pylorus, 242, 242*f*

Q

Quadrants, of abdominopelvic cavity, 33*f*, 34, 34*t*
Quadriplegia, 91

R

RA (rheumatoid arthritis), 70, 70*f*, 203
Radicava (edaravone), 92
Radius, 64, 66*f*

Rales, 221
Range of motion (ROM), 67
Rectocele, 287
Rectum, 242, 243f, 244f, 245, 281f, 283f, 285f
Red blood cells, 178
Reduction, 70
Refraction, 130
Refractive errors, 131, 131f
Relaxation phase, of cardiac cycle, 177f
Remodeling process, 62
Renal capsule, 262
Renal corpuscle, 263
Renal cortex, 263, 263f
Renal failure, 264
Renal fascia, 263, 263f
Renal medulla, 263, 263f
Renal pelvis, 263, 263f
Renal tubule, 263
Reproductive system, 279–306
    abbreviation, 289t
    case study, 279, 299
    diagnostic tests, 288–289
    disorders related to, 286–288
        affect males, 288
        female structural abnormalities, 287, 287f
        inflammation, 286–287
        menstrual cycle disorders, 288
        sexually transmitted diseases, 286
        tumors, 287–288
    exercises, 300–306
    overview of, 279
    practice and practitioners, 289
    pregnancy, 284–286, 285f
    structure and function of, 280–286
        female reproductive system, 283–284, 283f, 284f
        male reproductive system, 281–282, 281f, 282f
    study table, 289t–299t
    surgical procedures, 288–289
    treatments, 288–289
    word elements related to, 279–280, 280t
Residual volume (RV), 222t
Respiration, 215
Respiratory system, 215–237
    abbreviations, 223t
    case study, 215, 231
    diagnostic tests, 222–223
    disorders related to, 221–222
        abnormal breath sounds, 221
        expansion disorders, 222
        infectious disorders, 221
        obstructive lung diseases, 221–222
    exercises, 232–237
    inhaled/exhaled air pathway, 215, 217f
    overview of, 215, 216f, 217f
    pharmacology for, 222, 223
    practice and practitioners, 223
    structure and function of, 216–221, 216f
        bronchi, bronchioles, and alveoli, 216f, 217f, 219, 219f

diaphragm, 220, 220f
larynx, 219, 219f
lungs, 219–220, 220f
nasal cavity, 216–218, 218f
nose, 216–218
paranasal sinuses, 216–218, 218f
pharynx, 218–219, 219f
tonsils, 218–219, 219f
trachea, 219, 219f
    study table, 224t–231t
    surgical procedures, 222–223
    treatments, 222–223
    word elements related to, 216, 217t
Respiratory therapists, 223
Retention, 264
Retina, 129f, 130
Retinal detachment, 132f
Retinal tear, 132f
Retroflexion, of uterus, 287, 287f
Retroversion, of uterus, 287, 287f
Rh factor, 178
Rh negative (Rh⁻), 178
Rh positive (Rh⁺), 178
Rheumatoid arthritis (RA), 70, 70f, 203
Rheumatologist, 71, 97
Rhinitis. See Cold, common
Rhinoviruses, 221
Rhonchi, 221
Rib cage, 63
Ribs, 63, 220f
Rickets, 70
Right atrioventricular valve, 174
Right atrium, 172f, 174, 175f, 176f
Right bronchus, 219, 219f
Right primary bronchus, 220f
Right pulmonary arteries, 175f
Right pulmonary veins, 175f
Right ventricle, 172f, 174, 175f, 176f
Rilutek (riluzole), 92
Riluzole (Rilutek), 92
Rods, 130
ROM (range of motion), 67
Root words, 10, 10t
    combining suffixes with, 15, 16t, 18t–19t, 21–22
Roots, 2, 4t, 5t
Rotator cuff injury, 90
RV (residual volume), 222t

S

SA (sinoatrial) node, 175, 176f
Sacral vertebrae, 65f
Sacrum, 34, 34f, 35t, 63, 65f, 66f
Sagittal plane, 32, 32f
Saliva, 243
Salivary glands, 240f, 243
Salpingitis, 286
Salpingo-oophorectomy, 288
Scabicides, 46
Scabies, 44, 44f
Scaphoid, 66f

Scapula, 64, 66f
Schizophrenia, 110
Sclera, 129, 129f, 132f
Scleral buckle, 132, 132f
Scleroderma, 43
Scoliosis, 70, 70f
Scrotum, 281, 281f
Sebaceous (oil) glands, 39, 41, 41f
Sebum, 41
Secondary hypertension, 180
Secretory phase, of menstrual cycle, 284
Seizure, 110
Seizure disorders, 110
Semen, 281
Semicircular canals, 133, 134f
Semilunar valve, 175
Seminal glands, 281, 281f, 282f
Seminal vesicles, 281
Seminiferous tubules, 281f, 282, 282f
Sense. See Hearing; See Sight
Sensorineural hearing loss, 133
Septum, 173, 174f
Sexually transmitted diseases (STDs), 286
Sexually transmitted infections (STIs), 286
Shin splints, 91
Shingles (herpes zoster), 44, 45f
Shoulder blade, 64
Shoulder girdle, 64
    bones of, 66f
Sight, 127–144
    abbreviations, 135, 135t
    case study, 127, 144
    diagnostic tests, 132
    disorders, 131–132
        eyelid disorder, 131
        infection, 131
        other disorders, 131–132
        refractive errors, 131, 131f
    exercises, 145–150
    overview of, 127–128
    practice and practitioners, 132
    structure and function of eye, 128–130, 129f, 130f
    study table, 135t–144t
    surgical procedures, 132
    treatments, 132
    word elements related to, 128, 128t
Sigmoid colon, 243, 243f, 244f
Simple fracture, 67, 69, 69f
Sinoatrial (SA) node, 175, 176f
Sinus rhythm, 179
Sinusitis, 221
Skeletal muscle, 88, 89f, 90f
Skeletal system, 59–85
    abbreviations, 71t
    case study, 59, 79
    diagnostic tests, 70
    disorders related to, 67–70, 70f
    exercises, 79–85
    overview of
    practice and practitioners, 70–71

structure and function of, 61–69
  appendicular skeleton, 61, 61*f*, 63–67, 66*f*, 67*f*
  axial skeleton, 61, 61*f*, 62–63, 63*f*, 64*f*, 65*f*
  joints, 62, 67, 68*f*, 68*t*–69*t*
  study table, 71*t*–78*t*
surgical procedures, 70
treatments, 70
word elements related to, 59–60, 60*t*–61*t*
Skin, 39, 41*f*. *See also* Integumentary system
  with accessory structures, 40, 41*f*
  biopsy of, 45
  cancer, 43, 44*f*
  glands within, 39, 41
  infections, 44, 44*f*, 45*f*
  inflammatory disorders of, 43, 43*f*
  lesions, 42–43, 42*f*
    depressed, 42*f*, 43
    elevated, 42*f*, 43
    flat, 42*f*, 43
SLE (systemic lupus erythematosus), 203
Small intestine, 239, 240*f*, 242, 243*f*, 244*f*
Smooth muscle, 88–90, 90*f*
Somatic nervous system, 103, 104*f*, 107
Special senses. *See* Hearing; *See* Sight
Speed, prefixes of, 10, 11*t*
Sperm, 279, 282*f*
Spermatogenesis, 281, 282
Sphenoidal sinus, 218*f*, 219*f*
Sphincters
  cardiac, 242
  ileocecal, 242
  internal and external urethral, 264
  pyloric, 242
Sphygmomanometer, 178
Spinal cavity, 32, 32*f*
Spinal column, 34–35, 34*f*, 35*t*
Spinal cord, 103, 104*f*, 106*f*, 107, 107*f*, 108*f*
Spinal nerves, 104*f*
Spine, abnormal curvatures of, 70, 70*f*
Spiral fracture, 69, 69*f*
Spirometer, 222
Spleen, 201, 240*f*
Splenectomy, 203
Splenomegaly, 203
Spongy bone, 62, 62*f*
Sports injuries, 90–91, 91*f*, 92, 92*f*
Sprain, 67
Sputum, 221
Squamous cell carcinoma, 43, 44*f*
Squamous suture, 63, 63*f*
Stapedectomy, 134
Stapes, 133, 134*f*
STDs (sexually transmitted diseases), 286
Sternum, 63, 64*f*
STIs (sexually transmitted infections), 286
Stoma, 245
Stomach, 239, 240*f*, 242, 242*f*, 245*f*
Stomatitis, 244
Striated muscle. *See* Skeletal muscle

Stridor, 221
Stroke. *See* Cerebrovascular accident
Structural abnormalities, of reproductive system, 287, 287*f*
Structure and function
  cardiovascular system, 173–178
    blood, 178, 178*t*
    blood vessels, 177–178, 178*f*
    heart, 173–175, 174*f*, 175*f*
    heartbeat, 175–176, 176*f*, 177*f*
  digestive system, 240*f*, 241–244
  ear, 133, 134*f*
  endocrine system, 152–156, 153*f*, 153*t*–154*t*
    adrenal glands, 155, 155*f*
    gonads, 156
    pancreas, 156
    parathyroid glands, 155, 155*f*
    pituitary gland, 152–155
    thyroid gland, 155, 155*f*
  eye, 128–130, 129*f*, 130*f*
  hearing, 133, 134*f*
  integumentary system, 40–42, 41*f*, 42*f*
  lymphatic system, 201–202, 202*f*
  muscular system, 88–90
    cardiac muscle, 90
    muscle movement, 91
    skeletal muscle, 88, 89*f*, 90*f*
    smooth muscle, 88–90, 90*f*
    types of muscle tissue, 88, 89*f*, 90*f*
  nervous system, 105–108
    central nervous system, 104*f*, 106–107, 106*f*, 107*f*
    peripheral nervous system, 104*f*, 107–108, 108*f*
  reproductive system, 280–286
    female reproductive system, 283–284, 283*f*, 284*f*
    male reproductive system, 281–282, 281*f*, 282*f*
  respiratory system, 216–221, 216*f*
    bronchi, bronchioles, and alveoli, 219, 219*f*
    diaphragm, 220, 220*f*
    larynx, 219, 219*f*
    lungs, 219–220, 220*f*
    nasal cavity, 216–218, 218*f*
    nose, 216–218
    paranasal sinuses, 216–218, 218*f*
    pharynx, 218–219, 219*f*
    tonsils, 218–219, 219*f*
    trachea, 219, 219*f*
  sight, 128–130, 129*f*, 130*f*
  skeletal system, 61–69
    appendicular skeleton, 61, 61*f*, 63–67, 66*f*, 67*f*
    axial skeleton, 61, 61*f*, 62–63, 63*f*, 64*f*, 65*f*
    joints, 62, 67, 68*f*, 68*t*–69*t*
  urinary system, 263–264, 263*f*, 264*f*
Study table
  body organization, 35*t*–36*t*
  cardiovascular system, 182*t*–191*t*

digestive system, 246*t*–249*t*
endocrine system, 159*t*–165*t*
hearing, 135*t*–144*t*
immunity, 204*t*–209*t*
integumentary system, 46*t*–51*t*
lymphatic system, 204*t*–209*t*
muscular system, 93*t*–97*t*
nervous system, 112*t*–119*t*
prefixes, 16*t*–17*t*
reproductive system, 289*t*–299*t*
respiratory system, 224*t*–231*t*
sight, 135*t*–144*t*
skeletal system, 71*t*–78*t*
suffixes, 18*t*–19*t*
urinary system, 265*t*–270*t*
Sty. *See* Hordeolum
Subcutaneous layer, 40, 41*f*
Subdural hematoma, 109
Sudoriferous (sweat) glands, 39, 41, 41*f*
Suffixes, 2, 3, 4, 4*t*, 5, 5*t*
  case study of, 9, 19
  categories of, 13–16, 13*t*–16*t*
  exercises for, 21–25
  study table, 18*t*–19*t*
  that denote adjectives, 15–16, 16*t*
  that signify diagnostic terms, test information or surgical procedures, 14, 15*t*
  that signify medical conditions, 13, 13*t*–14*t*
Superior lobe, of lungs, 220, 220*f*
Superior parathyroid glands, 155*f*
Superior position, 30, 31*f*
Superior vena cava, 172*f*, 174, 175*f*, 176*f*
Supine position, 30, 31*f*
Suprarenal glands. *See* Adrenal glands
Surgical procedures
  cardiovascular system, 180
  digestive system, 245–246
  endocrine system, 158
  hearing, 134
  integumentary system, 45–46
  lymphatic system, 203
  muscular system, 91–92
  nervous system, 110
  reproductive system, 288–289
  respiratory system, 222–223
  sight, 132
  skeletal system, 70
  suffixes that signify, 15, 16*t*
  urinary system, 264–265
Sweat glands. *See* Sudoriferous glands
Sympathetic nervous system, 103, 104*f*, 107
Synapses, 106
Synarthrosis, 67
Synovial fluid, 67
Synovial joints, 67
  movements, 68*f*, 68*t*–69*t*
Syphilis, 286
Systemic circuit, 171, 172*f*
Systemic degenerative diseases, 109–110
Systemic lupus erythematosus (SLE), 203

Systems, 28
Systole, 176, 177*f*
Systolic pressure, 178

T

T lymphocytes, 199
Tachycardia, 179
Tachypnea, 221
Talus, 64, 67*f*
Tarsals, 65, 66*f*
Tarsus, 65
TB (tuberculosis), 221
Tear ducts. *See* Lacrimal apparatus
Tear sac. *See* Lacrimal Sac
Temporal bones, 62, 63*f*
Temporal lobe, 106, 107*f*
Tendons, 62, 88
Tennis elbow. *See* Epicondylitis
Test information, suffixes that signify
Testes, 152, 153*f*, 153*t*–154*t*, 156, 279,
    281, 281*f*, 282*f*
Testicle, 280
Testosterone, 156, 282
Thalamus, 107, 107*f*
Thoracentesis, 222
Thoracic cage, 63, 64*f*
Thoracic cavity, 32, 32*f*
Thoracic duct, 199
Thoracic vertebrae, 65*f*
Thorax, 34–35, 34*f*, 35*t*, 63
THR (total hip replacement), 71
Throat. *See* Pharynx
Thrombocytes. *See* Platelets
Thrombocytopenia, 180
Thrombosis, 179
Thrombus, 179
Thymectomy, 203
Thymus gland, 152, 153*f*, 153*t*–154*t*,
    200*f*, 201
Thyroid cartilage, 155*f*
Thyroid gland, 152, 153*f*, 153*t*–154*t*,
    155, 155*f*, 156–157, 157*f*
Thyromegaly. *See* Goiter
Thyroxine, 153*t*–154*t*, 155
TIA (transient ischemic attack), 109
Tibia, 64, 66*f*, 67*f*
Tidal volume (TV), 222*t*
Time, prefixes of, 10, 11*t*
Tinea, 44, 44*f*
Tinnitus, 134
Tissues, 28
TKA (total knee arthroplasty), 71
TLC (total lung capacity), 222*t*
Toes
    bones of, 65
    nail, 42, 42*f*
Tongue, 218*f*
Tonsillectomy, 203
Tonsils, 201, 218–219, 218*f*, 219*f*
Topical medications, integumentary
    system, 46

Total hip replacement (THR), 71
Total knee arthroplasty (TKA), 71
Total lung capacity (TLC), 222*t*
Total parenteral nutrition (TPN), 242
Toxic goiter. *See* Graves' disease
TPN (total parenteral nutrition), 242
Trachea, 155*f*, 215, 216*f*, 217*f*, 219,
    219*f*, 220*f*
Traction, 70
Tradition, 3
Transdermal, 46
Transient ischemic attack (TIA), 109
Transurethral resection of the prostate
    (TURP), 289
Transverse colon, 243, 243*f*, 244*f*
Transverse fracture, 69, 69*f*
Transverse plane, 32, 32*f*
Trapezium, 66*f*
Trapezoid, 66*f*
Trauma, 108–109, 109*f*
Treatments. *See also* Disorders
    cardiovascular system, 180
    digestive system, 245–246
    endocrine system, 158
    hearing, 134
    integumentary system, 45–46
    lung, 222
    lymphatic system, 203
    muscular system, 91–92
    nail, 46
    nervous system, 110
    reproductive system, 288–289
    respiratory system, 222–223
    sight, 132
    skeletal system, 70
    urinary system, 264–265
Treponema pallidum, 286
Tricuspid valve, 174
Triiodothyronine, 153*t*–154*t*, 155
Triquetrum, 66*f*
Troponin, 179
True ribs, 63, 64*f*
Tubal ligation, 288
Tuberculosis (TB), 221
Tumors, 70
    of nervous system, 109
    of reproductive system, 287–288
TURP (transurethral resection of the
    prostate), 289
TV (tidal volume), 222*t*
Tympanectomy, 134
Tympanic cavity, 133
Tympanic membrane, 133, 134*f*
Tympanoplasty, 134
Type 1 diabetes, 158
Type 2 diabetes, 158

U

UC (ulcerative colitis), 245
UGI (upper gastrointestinal) tract,
    239–240, 244

UGIS (upper gastrointestinal series), 245
Ulcerative colitis (UC), 245
Ulcers, 42*f*, 43, 44
Ulna, 64, 66*f*
Ultrasound transducer, 288*f*
Umbilical cord, 284, 285*f*
Umbilical regions, 33, 33*f*, 34*t*
Upper extremity, 64
Upper gastrointestinal series (UGIS), 245
Upper gastrointestinal (UGI) tract,
    239–240, 244
Upper limb bones, 66*f*
Upper respiratory tract, 215, 216*f*
Urea, 263
Ureter, 261, 262*f*, 263*f*, 281*f*
Urethra, 261, 262*f*, 282*f*, 283*f*, 285*f*
Urethritis, 264
Uric acid, 263
Urinary bladder, 261, 262*f*, 281*f*, 283*f*,
    285*f*
Urinary system, 261–277
    abbreviations, 265*t*
    case study, 261, 271
    diagnostic tests, 264–265
    disorders related to, 264
    exercises, 272–277
    organs of, 261, 262*f*
    overview of, 261, 262*f*
    practice and practitioners, 265
    structure and function of, 263–264,
        263*f*, 264*f*
    study table, 265*t*–270*t*
    surgical procedures of, 264–265
    treatments of, 264–265
    word elements related to, 262,
        262*f*–263*f*
Urinary tract infection (UTI), 264
Urination reflex, 263
Urine, 261, 262*f*, 263
Urologists, 265, 289
Urology, 265
Uterine cycle, 284
Uterine tubes, 283, 283*f*
Uterus, 283, 283*f*, 287, 287*f*
    benign tumors of, 287
    with fetus, 285*f*
    prolapsed, 287
    wall of, 285*f*
UTI (urinary tract infection), 264

V

Vaccinations, 203
Vaccines, 200
Vagina, 280, 283, 283*f*, 285*f*, 287
Vaginitis, 286
Varicocele, 288
Varicocelectomy, 289
Vas deferens, 281, 289
Vascular insults, 109, 109*f*
Vascular layer, eye, 129
Vasoconstriction, 177

Vasodilation, 177
Vasopressin, 155
Vasovasostomy, 289
VC (vital capacity), 222*t*
Vein graft, 182*f*
Veins, 41*f*, 171, 177, 178*f*
Ventral cavity, 30, 31*f*
Ventral position, 30, 31*f*
Ventricles, 107, 172*f*, 175*f*, 176*f*
Ventricular fibrillation, 180
Ventricular systole, of cardiac cycle, 177*f*
Venules, 177, 178*f*
Vermiform appendix. *See* Appendix
Vertebrae, 34, 34*f*, 63, 65*f*, 70
Vertebral column, 62, 63, 65*f*
Vertebrochondral ribs, 63, 64*f*
Vertebrosternal ribs, 63, 64*f*
Vertigo, 134
Vesicle, 42*f*, 43
Vessel, 179*f*
Vestibule, 133, 134*f*
Visceral pleura, 220, 220*f*
Vital capacity (VC), 222*t*
Vitiligo, 44, 45*f*
Vitreous humor, 130

Vocal cords, 219, 219*f*
Voice box. *See* Larynx
Volvulus, 245
Vulva, 281, 283

W

Wall of coronary artery, 181*f*
Wall of uterus, 285*f*
Wheal, 42*f*, 43
Wheezing, 221
White blood cells, 178
White of the eye. *See* Sclera
Whooping cough. *See* Pertussis
Windpipe. *See* Trachea
Word elements, 1–8, 5*t*
    body organization, 28, 28*t*
    cardiovascular system, 172, 172*t*–173*t*
    digestive system, 240, 240*t*–241*t*
    endocrine system, 151–152, 152*t*
    hearing, 132–133, 133*t*
    immunity, 200–201, 201*t*
    integumentary system, 40, 40*t*
    lymphatic system, 200–201, 201*t*

    muscular system, 88, 88*t*
    nervous system, 105, 105*t*
    reproductive system, 279–280, 280*t*
    respiratory system, 216, 217*t*
    sight, 128, 128*t*
    skeletal system, 59–60, 60*t*–61*t*
    urinary system, 262, 262*f*–263*f*
Word roots. *See* Root words
Words
    accurate use of, 2, 3, 4*t*, 5
    analysis of, 4*t*
Wrist bones, 66*f*

X

Xerophthalmia, 131
Xiphoid process, 63, 64*f*

Z

Zygomatic bones, 62, 63*f*
Zygote, 279